# WORK AND HEALTH IN INDIA

Edited by Martin Hyde, Holendro Singh Chungkham
and Laishram Ladusingh

First published in Great Britain in 2018 by

Policy Press
University of Bristol
1-9 Old Park Hill
Bristol
BS2 8BB
UK
t: +44 (0)117 954 5940
pp-info@bristol.ac.uk
www.policypress.co.uk

North America office:
Policy Press
c/o The University of Chicago Press
1427 East 60th Street
Chicago, IL 60637, USA
t: +1 773 702 7700
f: +1 773-702-9756
sales@press.uchicago.edu
www.press.uchicago.edu



British Library Cataloguing in Publication Data
A catalogue record for this book is available from the British Library

Library of Congress Cataloging-in-Publication Data
A catalog record for this book has been requested

ISBN 978-1-4473-2736-3 hardback
ISBN 978-1-4473-2738-7 ePdf
ISBN 978-1-4473-3543-6 ePub
ISBN 978-1-4473-3544-3 Mobi



Cover design by Policy Press
Front cover image: www.getty.com
Printed and bound in Great Britain by CPI Group (UK) Ltd, Croydon, CR0 4YY
Policy Press uses environmentally responsible print partners

FSC www.fsc.org MIX Paper from responsible sources FSC® C013604

# Contents


| | | |
|---|---|---|
| List of tables and figures | | v |
| Notes on contributors | | ix |
| Foreword by Johannes Siegrist | | xiv |
| one | Introduction: Work, stress and health in India<br>*Martin Hyde, Holendro Singh Chungkham and Laishram Ladusingh* | 1 |
| two | Work, stress and health: Theories and models<br>*Linda L. Magnusson Hanson, Martin Hyde, Holendro Singh Chungkham and Hugo Westerlund* | 25 |
| three | Work environment, health and the international development agenda<br>*Martin Hyde and Töres Theorell* | 45 |
| four | Employment trends in India: Some issues for investigation<br>*A.V. Jose* | 67 |
| five | Rural-urban and gender differences in time spent in unpaid household work in India<br>*Laishram Ladusingh* | 87 |
| six | Activity status, morbidity patterns and hospitalisation in India<br>*Harihar Sahoo* | 107 |
| seven | Occupational class and chronic diseases in India<br>*Sanjay K. Mohanty and Anshul Kastor* | 133 |
| eight | Stress and health among the Indian police<br>*Vaijayanthee Kumar and T.J. Kamalanabhan* | 153 |
| nine | Health status and lifestyle of the Oraon tea garden labourers of Jalpaiguri district, West Bengal<br>*Subrata K. Roy and Tanaya Kundu Chowdhury* | 177 |
| ten | The role of work-family support factors in helping individuals achieve work-family balance in India<br>*Sarlaksha Ganesh and M.P. Ganesh* | 191 |

| | | |
|---|---|---|
| eleven | Working conditions, health and well-being among the scavenger community<br>*Vimal Kumar* | 213 |
| twelve | Lessons and future research directions from work environment research in India<br>*Martin Hyde, Holendro Singh Chungkham and Laishram Ladusingh* | 237 |
| Index | | 255 |

# List of tables and figures

## Tables


| | | |
|---|---|---|
| 1.1 | Stressful characteristics of work | 4 |
| 4.1 | Indicators of employment in western Europe | 68 |
| 4.2 | Distribution of labour force among three major sectors in selected countries at the start and end of long periods of change as % share of the total labour force | 69 |
| 4.3 | Employment population ratios (age 15–64 years) in selected European countries | 71 |
| 4.4 | Employment and unemployment rates among men and women aged 25–64 by educational attainment, 2011 | 72 |
| 4.5 | Part-time employment as a percentage of total employment | 73 |
| 4.6 | Worker participation rates according to usual status in different NSS rounds | 76 |
| 4.7 | Distribution (per 1,000) of usually employed people by industry divisions, by area of residence and gender | 77 |
| 4.8 | Distribution (per 1,000) of usually employed by status in different NSSO rounds: rural areas | 79 |
| 4.9 | Distribution (per 1,000) of usually employed people by status in different NSSO rounds: urban areas | 79 |
| 5.1 | Average hours spent on daily activities by age and residence in India | 94 |
| 5.2 | Average hours spent on daily activities by sex and age in India | 97 |
| 5.3 | Average hours spent on daily activities by age and residence in India | 98 |
| 5.4 | Tobit regression coefficients and standard errors for time spent on household management and maintenance and time spent on care for children, sick and older people | 100 |
| 5.5 | Monetary value of labour inputs for cooking and childcare by age and sex in Indian Rupees | 101 |
| 6.1 | Prevalence of ailments per 1,000 people by states of India, 2004 | 114 |
| 6.2 | Reported rates of different diseases (per 1,000) during last 15 days by regions of India, 2004 | 115 |
| 6.3 | Prevalence of ailments per 1,000 people on the day before the date of survey by activity status and by age group of India, 2004 | 118 |
| 6.4 | Prevalence of ailments per 1,000 people during last 15 days by activity status and by age group of India, 2004 | 120 |

| | | |
|---|---|---|
| 6.5 | Top five diseases during last 15 days by economic activity groups (total) | 122 |
| 6.6 | Hospitalisation rate per 1,000 people during last year by activity status and by age group of India, 2004 | 125 |
| 6.7 | Average duration of stay in the hospital during last year prior to the survey by nature of ailment and by regions of India, 2004 | 126 |
| 6.8 | Odds ratio showing the effect of usual activity status on any morbidity during the last 15 days and hospitalisation during the year before the survey, India, 2004: results from logistic regression analysis | 128 |
| 7.1 | Sample characteristics of occupation group in 20–65 age group in India, 2011–12 | 142 |
| 7.2 | Differences in selected morbidity among working population in 20–65 age group in India, 2011–12 | 143 |
| 7.3 | Results of the logistic regression analyses for the likelihood of being diagnosed with a chronic illness for different occupational groups in India, 2011–12 | 145 |
| 8.1 | Correlation table for study constructs | 163 |
| 8.2 | Results of regression analysis predicting perceived psychological stress | 164 |
| 8.3 | Summary of hierarchical regression analysis for variables predicting perceived psychological stress | 165 |
| 9.1 | Selected health practices of Oraon tea garden labourers | 181 |
| 9.2 | Selected health traits of Oraon tea garden labourers | 182 |
| 9.3 | Classification based on standard cut off on selected health status of the Oraon tea garden labourers | 183 |
| 11.1 | Educational status of scheduled castes of Haryana | 227 |

## Figures

| | | |
|---|---|---|
| i | Map of the states of India | xvi |
| 1.1 | Proportion of male and female employees who are in vulnerable employment in developing countries | 7 |
| 1.2 | Sectoral composition of the workforce in India: 1994–2013 | 8 |
| 1.3 | Life expectancy at birth by sex and for the population as a whole: 1960–2013 | 12 |
| 1.4 | Percentage of deaths attributable to communicable disease, non-communicable disease and injuries in India 2000–15 | 12 |
| 2.1 | The demand-control model | 30 |
| 2.2 | The effort-reward imbalance model | 31 |

| | | |
|---|---|---|
| 3.1 | Proportion of men and women in vulnerable employment as a % of total employment in 2013: selected countries | 48 |
| 3.2 | Relationship between proportion in vulnerable employment and healthy life expectancy in 2013: women | 49 |
| 3.3 | Relationship between proportion in vulnerable employment and healthy life expectancy in 2013: men | 49 |
| 3.4 | The degree to which work is manual or intellectual: selected countries, 2013 | 55 |
| 3.5 | The degree to which work is routine or creative: selected countries, 2013 | 56 |
| 3.6 | The degree of independence at work: selected countries, 2013 | 57 |
| 3.7 | Proportion of people in manual and intellectual jobs who report poor health in the BRIC countries | 59 |
| 3.8 | Proportion of people in routine and creative jobs who report poor health in the BRIC countries | 59 |
| 3.9 | Proportion of people with more or less independence at work who report poor health in the BRIC countries | 60 |
| 5.1 | The proportion of time spent on average on daily activities in India | 93 |
| 5.2 | Time spent in unpaid household work by activities by women in India | 95 |
| 6.1 | Trends in birth and death rates in India, 1901–2008 | 108 |
| 6.2 | Prevalence of ailments per 1,000 people by regions of India, 2004 | 112 |
| 6.3 | Prevalence of ailments per 1,000 people on the day before the date of survey and for the previous 15 days by activity status, 2004 | 117 |
| 6.4 | Hospitalisation rate per 1,000 population during year before the survey by regions of India, 2004 | 124 |
| 6.5 | Average duration of stay (in days) in the hospital by type of hospital and regions of India, 2004 | 125 |
| 7.1 | Schematic presentation of working adults by type of occupation in India, 2011–12 | 141 |
| 7.2 | Age pattern of cause of death in India, 2001–03 | 141 |
| 8.1 | Two-way interaction effect of lack of interpersonal trust and emotional intelligence on perceived stress | 166 |
| 8.2 | Two-way interaction effect of lack of career growth opportunities and emotional intelligence on perceived stress | 166 |
| 11.1 | The location of Ladwa, Haryana province | 220 |
| 11.2 | The prevalence of health problems among scavengers in Ladwa | 221 |

| | | |
|---|---|---|
| 11.3 | Prevalence of work environment complaints among scavengers in Ladwa | 223 |
| 11.4 | A scavenger cleaning gutters without any protective clothing | 225 |
| 11.5 | Prevalence of alcohol and tobacco use among scavengers in Ladwa | 228 |
| 11.6 | Proportion of scavengers who report discrimination and abuse during work | 231 |

# Notes on contributors

**Tanaya Kundu Chowdhury** is a Senior Research Fellow at the Biological Anthropology Unit, Indian Statistical Institute, Kolkata. She did her Master's degree in Anthropology at the University of Calcutta. Her main area of research is the health and lifestyles of Oraons living in India and she has published several research papers on different health and lifestyle-related issues of Oraons.

**Holendro Singh Chungkham** is working as an Assistant Professor at the Indian Statistical Institute, North-East Centre, Tezpur, India. Before joining the ISI, Dr Chungkham was at the Stress Research Institute (SRI), Stockholm University, as a Researcher from 2011 to 2014. During this time he was mainly involved in statistical modelling to uncover the relationship between psychosocial work characteristics and several health outcomes using the in-house longitudinal survey, the Swedish Longitudinal Occupational Study of Health (SLOSH). Apart from using the SLOSH he has published papers using the RN4CAST data on nurses' practice environment across several EU states including Sweden. Dr Chungkham's research interest is in the application of advanced statistical techniques (such as multilevel, structural equation, mixed-effects and generalised estimating Equations) to look at psychosocial work characteristics and health outcomes. He is still collaborating with some of the researchers at the SRI and is involved in an EU-funded project, Integrated Datasets in Europe for Ageing Research (IDEAR) network.

**M.P. Ganesh** is an Assistant Professor at Department of Liberal Arts, Indian Institute of Technology, Hyderabad. He is an organisational behaviourist by training and has specialised in cross-cultural virtual teams. His other teaching and research interests include ethical decision making, self-leadership, teacher leadership and corporate social responsibility.

**Sarlaksha Ganesh** completed her PhD in organisational behaviour from the Indian Institute of Technology, Madras. Her work was in understanding the role of personal attributes and social support factors in the areas of work-family balance and quality of work life. She is passionate about the area of work-family balance and providing a good working environment to professionals. Apart from this, she has a keen interest in emotional intelligence, employee engagement and employee experience, diversity and inclusion in the workplace and total worker health. She has been a part of conferences at national and international levels. She is a passionate researcher and enjoys writing research articles as well as contributing to book chapters.

**Linda Magnusson Hanson** is an Associate Professor of Public Health as well as the study manager of the Swedish Longitudinal Occupational Survey of Health (SLOSH). She investigates how various psychosocial working conditions are associated with health, mortality and quality of life, with emphasis on mental health, cardiometabolic disease and pain. Linda works mainly with large, longitudinal cohort studies from several different countries, including the Swedish SLOSH, the French GAZEL and British Whitehall II. She has a special interest in modelling data based on repeated measures to provide better evidence about causal relationships between working conditions and health outcomes, and to increase the understanding of pathways explaining the relationships as well as factors modifying the effect of work stressors.

**Martin Hyde** is an Associate Professor at Swansea University. Before this he was Deputy Director of the Epidemiology Unit at the Stress Research Institute at Stockholm University. He has a long-standing interest in the impact of the psychosocial work environment on health and has published articles and book chapters on this issue. He has been involved in large-scale studies including the English Longitudinal Study of Ageing (ELSA), the Survey for Health, Retirement and Ageing in Europe (SHARE) and the Swedish Longitudinal Occupational Study of Health (SLOSH). He also a Deputy Editor for Ageing and Society and an Associate Editor for *BMC Geriatrics*.

**A.V. Jose** is a Development Economist with specialising in labour markets, employment, wages and income distribution. A retired official of the International Labour Office in Geneva, he last worked as the Head of Education Program in the International Institute for Labour Studies. Currently based in Thiruvananthapuram, Kerala, Dr Jose is an Honorary Visiting Professor at the Centre for Development Studies, and associated with the Gulati Institute of Finance and Taxation, Thiruvananthapuram. He is a member of the Standing Committee on Labour Force Statistics, Central Statistical Organization, Government of India.

**T.J. Kamalanabhan** received a PhD in Psychology from the University of Madras, India. He is a Professor at the Department of Management Studies, Indian Institute of Technology, Madras. His research interests include industrial psychology, human resource management and organisational behaviour. He has been a recipient of several prestigious academic awards such as DAAD Fellowship, Fulbright Fellowship and Erasmus Mundus Scholarship.

**Anshul Kastor** is a Doctoral Fellow at the International Institute for Population, Mumbai (India) and is pursuing a PhD on the topic 'health financing transition and its linkages with health outcomes in India'. He has done his M Phil. Dissertation on 'economic well-being and health of older adults in India'. His areas of research interest are: health economics; population ageing and health; maternal and child health; occupational health; family planning; migration and poverty. He possesses a good analytical approach and can easily handle the large-scale data. He has published some research articles in reputed peer-reviewed journals. He has also presented his research papers in many international and national conferences.

**Vaijayanthee Kumar** holds a PhD degree in Management from Indian Institute of Technology, Madras. She has been working in the area of police stress and work-related well-being in India. With a post-graduate and graduate degree in Psychology from University of Delhi, she has contributed in introducing and teaching criminal psychology for law students. She has been part of several research projects such as police suicide in India and mitigation of road rage. Her research interest lies in experimental and longitudinal approach in stress management among police personnel.

**Vimal Kumar** is the founder of the Movement for Scavenger Community (MSC), an organisation committed to the eradication of manual scavenging in India and bringing education and awareness to the existing scavenger community. Under MSC he also operates the Dr B.R. Ambedkar Youth Study Center which provides career counselling and a small library to disadvantaged students in Haryana. As a PhD scholar in social work with a focus on 'caste violence' at the Tata Institute of Social Sciences in Mumbai, he was awarded the Young Professional Fellowship from the Dalit Foundation in 2008. Vimal holds a Bachelor of Arts and Master of Social Work from the University of Kurukshetra in Haryana. He was awarded a DAAD research fellowship in 2016 under the Student Exchange Program with Westfalische Wilhelms, Universitat Münster, Germany. He is also Acumen Fellow at Acumen Funds.

**Laishram Ladusingh** is Head of Department of Mathematical Demography and Statistics at the International Institute for Population Sciences, India. He has written extensively on demographic issues. He is a member of the International Advisory Board of Population, Space and Place, the Indian Society on Probability and Statistics and the Indian Statistical Association.

**Sanjay Kumar Mohanty** is a trained economist and demographer working in the field of population, health and development. Currently, Dr Mohanty is working as Professor at the International Institute for Population Sciences, Mumbai, India. He has 16 years of teaching and research experience. Dr Mohanty was C.R. Parekh Fellow at Asia Research Centre, London School of Economics from January to April 2010 and Visiting Scientist at Harvard School of Public Health from September 2014 to August 2015. He has authored more than 60 research papers in international and national peer-reviewed journals. His research interests include economics of health and healthcare, maternal and child health, multidimensional poverty and exploring the complex relationship of poverty, inequality and health in India.

**Subrata K. Roy** is a Professor in Anthropology at the Biological Anthropology Unit, Indian Statistical Institute, Kolkata. He has a long-standing interest in health-related issues especially occupational health of several indigenous populations of east and north-eastern India and has published several research articles on these issues.

**Harihar Sahoo** is working as Assistant Professor, Department of Development Studies, International Institute for Population Sciences, Mumbai, India. He obtained his doctoral degree in Population Studies from Jawaharlal Nehru University, New Delhi. He has been engaged in teaching and research in India since 2008. His research interests include fertility, family planning, reproductive and child health, population and development. His research papers have been published in *Population Review*, *Marriage and Family Review*, *Journal of Biosocial Science*, *Journal of Comparative Family Studies*, *Social Change*, and *Journal of Family Welfare* among others.

**Töres Theorell** is a retired Professor of Psychosocial Medicine at the Karolinska Institute, Sweden. Between 1995 and 2006 he was also the director of the National Institute for Psychosocial Factors and Health in Stockholm, Sweden. He became a licensed physician in 1967 and wrote his PhD dissertation at the Karolinska Institute in 1971. His research has been on several aspects of stress at work and outside work. Several of the studies of his group have focused on physiological stress mechanisms, epidemiological associations between work environment factors and health, controlled evaluations of interventions both at and outside work and longitudinal studies. During recent years he has participated in the European IPD-Work Consortium and he has also been chairman of two committees working for the Swedish Government with the aim of reviewing international research publications on the association between working conditions and health. Many of his recent research publications have been on the relationship between cultural activities and health. Theorell has collaborated extensively with colleagues in Europe, North America, Asia and Australia.

**Hugo Westerlund** is Professor of Epidemiology as well as Director and Head of the Stress Research Institute at Stockholm University. He investigates how social and psychological exposures across the life course impact on health, mortality and quality of life. A recurrent theme has been labour market participation, and lately a focus has been on ageing workers and retirement, as well as the prerequisites and consequences of extended working lives. Hugo works mainly with large, longitudinal cohort studies from several different countries, including the French GAZEL Cohort Study, British Whitehall II, Swedish Longitudinal Occupational Study of Health (SLOSH) and Work, Lipids and Fibrinogen (WOLF) Study. He leads a multinational project on determinants of healthy life expectancy as well as a Forte-financed research programme on healthy and productive work in later life. He is also engaged in projects about open plan office environments, mental health development in early life, risk factors for sickness absence and presenteeism, and validation of questionnaires to assess the psychosocial work environment.

# Foreword

Good quality of work and employment exerts beneficial effects on working people's health and wellbeing. This is not only due to favourable material and social consequences, but equally so to the opportunities of meeting important psychological needs, such as the experience of autonomy and personal control, of self-esteem and recognition, and of purpose in life. Conversely, exclusion from work, precarious and poor work act as powerful threats to human health and wellbeing. These opportunities and threats are unequally distributed across the globe, and in particular between economically advanced and less developed countries. Among the latter, large parts of the adult population are working in the informal sector, with poor earnings and low security, and often exposed to occupational hazards and discrimination. Despite international proscription, child labour and forced labour still exist, and a tremendous burden of disease due to adverse working and employment conditions calls for preventive activities at local, national, and international levels.

India, a rapidly developing country, shares some of the benefits of economically advanced countries, but is also faced with serious challenges of social inequalities in life chances and health, and with far-reaching socioeconomic and socio-cultural disruptions. As the labour market underwent a substantial transformation more recently, industrial and service sectors have expanded quite extensively, and while some traditional occupational hazards disappeared, chronic psychosocial stress at work is now becoming an important threat to the health of employees. At the same time, different from most western countries, the agricultural sector continues to grow, exposing its workforce often to physical adversity and noxious environments.

Against this background the book *Work and health in India* offers a timely, most welcome and important contribution to a growing public awareness that this country, too, needs major investments into improved working and employment conditions as a main pathway towards sustainable human development. The three aims of the book support this goal – first, to draw attention to this matter by describing and explaining the broader Indian context, second, to demonstrate the topicality of the problem by presenting selective empirical evidence, and third, to offer recommendations to policy makers on how to improve working life in this country.

The editors are to be congratulated for their balanced synthesis of chapters that deal with theoretical, methodological and socio-cultural or historical aspects with chapters that present findings from recent population surveys, from administrative data analysis, or from small-scale quantitative and qualitative medical-sociological studies. For instance, one learns about the amount of gender segregation of unpaid work, leaving young women with the highest burden. Other chapters deal with the unequal distribution of illnesses across occupations, where some higher status occupational groups still suffer from a higher prevalence. Occupational stressors vary considerably between hotel workers, policemen, tea garden labourers, and the low status group of scavengers, but each occupational group is exposed to distinct adversities which call for targeted interventions.

The book is one of the first to address the topic of work environment, stress and health in a rapidly developing country by offering impressive scientific quality and substance. For these reasons, this book is highly recommended to those involved in occupational life in India as professionals, students, employers, managers, trade union representatives, or policy makers. It is equally recommended to a wider national and international public interested in this topic.

*Johannes Siegrist*
*Senior Professor 'Work Stress Research',*
*Faculty of Medicine, Heinrich-Heine, University of Düsseldorf*
*July 2017*

**Figure i: Map of the states of India**

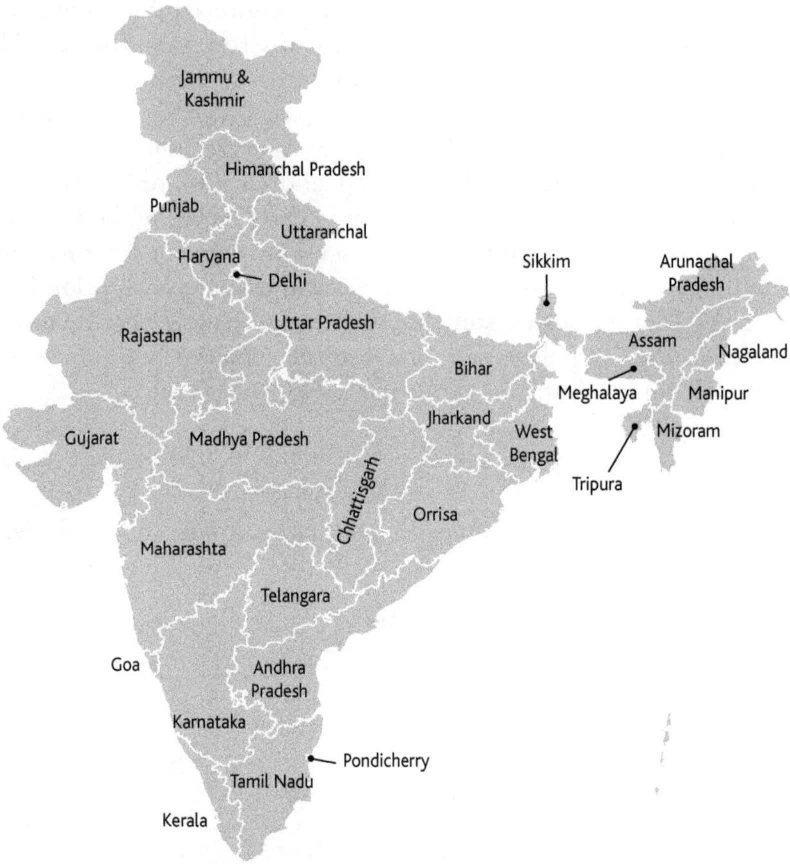

ONE

# Introduction: Work, stress and health in India

*Martin Hyde, Holendro Singh Chungkham and Laishram Ladusingh*

## Introduction

India is one of the fastest growing economies in the world (Gupta et al., 2014). Although growth in gross domestic product (GDP) has been quite volatile at times, India has still maintained an average annual growth rate of more than 7% since 2000, even reaching double-digit growth in 2010. This compares with just over 2% in the UK over the same period (World Bank, 2016a). The growth of the Indian economy has been matched by the steady increase in its labour force, which has risen from 330 million in 1990 to nearly half a billion people in 2014. This is roughly double the size of the labour force of the entire European Union. Not only has the workforce grown but it has also changed from one dominated by agriculture to one with vibrant and growing service and manufacturing sectors (World Bank, 2016b). Yet, despite drawing hundreds of millions of people into work and reducing levels of absolute poverty it is estimated that there are still 600 million Indians who lack access to necessities such as clean drinking water (Gupta et al., 2014). These privations are most keenly felt by those who are already in the most disadvantaged positions in society, such as poor people, wage labourers, agricultural labourers in rural areas, Scheduled Tribes and Scheduled Castes (Kumar, 2015). As Dreze and Sen (2014) critically note the benefits of India's tremendous economic growth have been unevenly distributed across society.

The same is true of developments in the health of the Indian population. On the one hand, there have been great improvements across a wide range of health indicators. Life expectancy has risen steadily for both sexes, largely owing to falling infant and maternal mortality rates. Life expectancy in India today (about 66 years) is more than twice what it was in 1951 (32 years) and infant mortality is about a quarter of what it used to be – 44 per thousand live births today as opposed to 180 or so in 1951 (Dreze and Sen, 2014). Infectious diseases have declined over the past few decades with some key diseases, such as maternal and neonatal tetanus and polio, being eliminated or even eradicated (Centers for Disease Control and Prevention, 2015; Narain et al., 2015; WHO, 2015). However, this fall in infectious diseases has been accompanied by a rise in non-communicable diseases (NCD), which now account for the top three causes of death in India (Centers for Disease Control and Prevention, 2015). As Popkin and colleagues (2001) note India is also going through a nutritional transition in which undernutrition is being rapidly reduced but the proportion of those who are overweight and the prevalence of early onset diabetes are increasing, most notably among urban residents and high-income rural residents. So not only is the Indian economy and workforce beginning to more closely resemble those of the advanced industrial economies so too are its disease and mortality profiles. Hence, given the wealth of evidence on the link between stressful work and many NCD outcomes (see CSDH, 2008) this underlines the importance of looking at the impact of work and working conditions on health in India.

## Work, stress and health

Stress seems to have become part of our daily vocabulary. Everyday people talk about getting stressed out about everything from getting stuck in traffic jams or taking exams to not being able to get a mobile signal or find the outfit they want when shopping. Countless newspaper columns, magazines articles and books offer ways to de-stress your lives and cope with the many demands that the increasingly fast-pace of modern living places on us. However, the concept of stress has a much longer history. The term was first coined by Hans Selye in 1936 to define 'a non-specific response of the body to any demand of change'. Alongside this he was also interested in identifying those factors that triggered a physiological and psychological stress response, which he called 'stressors'. This research laid the foundations for numerous research areas on stress. Among them was the development of research on the causes and consequences of work-related stress from the 1950s onwards (Sauter et al., 1989). Research in this area gained further impetus with the emergence of psychosocial work environment research and occupational psychology in the 1960s (Johnson and Hall, 1996) with a shift in focus from an individual perspective to the impact of certain aspects of the work environment on health (Cox et al., 2000). The International Labour Organization (ILO, 2016:2) defines work-related stress as:

> 'the harmful physical and emotional response caused by an imbalance between the perceived demands and the perceived resources and abilities of individuals to cope with those demands. Work-related stress is determined by work organisation, work design and labour relations and occurs when the demands of the job do not match or exceed the capabilities, resources, or needs of the worker, or when the knowledge or abilities of an individual worker or group to cope are not matched with the expectations of the organisational culture of an enterprise.'

Research in this area really exploded the 1990s and today there are many academic papers, conferences, books and even entire journals dedicated to the topic. This reflects the fact that workers today are facing increasingly intense working conditions. Employees around the world are finding it harder and harder to meet the demands of modern working life. High speed, 24/7 internet and communications technology means that many workers are always 'on' and the boundaries which used to separate work life from leisure time are becoming increasingly blurred. Increased global competition means that workers in all parts of the world feel their jobs are less secure and their wages buy them less than in the past. Many observers are worried that these factors and others like them are leading to a global rise in work-related stress which might have dramatic consequences for the health of the workforce. (EU 2007; NIOSH, 2002). Even the World Health Organization (WHO, 2010) has warned that work-related stress is a significant emerging risk to public health.

Work-related stress represents a major and costly health problem for individuals, companies and nations (EC, 2002, 2007). The EU has identified four particularly important areas of work-related stress: intensification of work (increased demands), emotional demands, new forms of employment contracts (short term, lack of security), and work-life balance (work hours). These areas build on earlier work by Cox and colleagues (2000) in which they identified a number of areas that might contribute to work-related stress (Table 1.1)

As Magnusson-Hansson and colleagues discuss in Chapter 2 the psychological and social experiences people have in the workplace, often referred to as the psychosocial work environment, have become an important component in studies related to stress and occupational health. The consequences of chronic work-related stress are extensive and include cardiovascular disease (Kivimaki et al., 2008), obesity (Nyberg et al., 2011) type II diabetes (Agardh et al., 2003), depression

**Table 1.1: Stressful characteristics of work**

| Category | Conditions defining hazard |
|---|---|
| **Content of work** | |
| Work environment and work equipment | Problems around the reliability, availability, suitability and maintenance or repair of both equipment and facilities |
| Task design | Lack of variety or short work cycles, fragmented or meaningless work, underuse of skills, high uncertainty |
| Workload/work pace | Work overload or underload, lack of control over pacing, high levels of time pressure |
| Work schedule | Shift working, inflexible work schedules, unpredictable hours, long or unsocial hours |
| **Context of work** | |
| Organisational culture and function | Poor communication, low levels of support for problem-solving and personal development, lack of definition of organisational objectives |
| Role in organisation | Role ambiguity and role conflict, responsibility for people |
| Career development | Career stagnation and uncertainty, under-promotion or over-promotion, poor pay, job insecurity, low social value of work |
| Decision latitude/control | Low participation in decision-making, lack of control over work (control, particularly in the form of participation, is also a contextual and wider organisational issue) |
| Interpersonal relationships at work | Social or physical isolation, poor relationships with superiors, interpersonal conflict, lack of social support |
| Home-work interface | Conflicting demands of work and home, low support at home, dual career problems |

*Source:* Adapted from ILO (2016)

(Stansfeld and Candy, 2006; Hanson et al., 2008), extreme fatigue/cognitive impairment (McEwen, 2008) and musculoskeletal disorders (Theorell, 2008). There is even some evidence that it is associated with an increased risk of cancer (Achat et al., 2000; Kuper et al., 2007). In addition, a growing body of evidence indicates both a direct and indirect role of the psychosocial working environment on organisational health indices (such as absenteeism, sickness absence, productivity, job satisfaction and intention to quit) (Spurgeon et al., 1997; Michie, 2002; Kivimaki et al. 2003a,b; Vahtera, 2004; van den Berg et al., 2009). Among the broader family of stress theories there are a set of models that focus on the effects of psychosocial work environment factors on mental strain and physical illness. The two most commonly used models to study the relationships between the psychosocial work environment and health are the 'demand-control model' and the 'effort-reward imbalance model'. In a broad sense the demand-control model holds that the demands workers experience at the point of production interact with the opportunities they have to influence work tasks and procedures to create different levels of stress. High job demands, in the form of high workloads and intense time pressure coupled with lack of control, are likely to lead to mental strain and cardiovascular disease, particularly when social support is low (Karasek, 1979; Theorell and Karasek, 1996). The demand-control model is one of the most widespread theoretical models used in psychosocial work environment research during the past decades. The effort-reward imbalance model on the other hand identifies the imbalance employees experience between high work effort and low rewards, lack of promotional opportunities and job insecurity as important sources of stress, and other negative health effects. Studies have shown that effort-reward imbalance is associated with an increased risk for cardiovascular disease (Siegrist, 1996). To date these two quite similar models have been used most in studies in Europe and North America. However, alongside these models, research in the field has grown to encompass a wide range of other potential workplace stressors, such as managerial leadership (Bernin and Theorell, 2001; Nyberg, 2008), organisational justice (Kivimaki et al., 2003; Ferrie et al., 2006; Ferrie et al., 2007; Elovainio et al., 2010; Elovainio et al., 2012) organisational instability (Westerlund et al., 2001; Westerlund et al., 2004), job insecurity (Sverke, 2002; Hellgren and Sverke, 2003) and the use of information and communication technology (ICT) (Sanchez, 2008). Hence this is a vibrant and growing field of research that incorporates a wide range of disciplinary perspectives from sociology, organisational psychology, occupational health and epidemiology.

However, although the effects of poor psychosocial working conditions on health are well known in Europe and North America, there is growing awareness of the need for similar studies in developing countries.

This is important given the rapid rate of economic growth in low and middle income countries alongside increased globalisation and technological progress. These have transformed the world of work, introducing new forms of work organisation, working relations and employment patterns which could contribute to the increase of work-related stress and its associated disorders. Economic globalisation in particular has been associated with changes in employment patterns such as greater flexibility in the work process, more part-time and temporary employment and independent contracting of staff. In turn these can result in higher job demands and job insecurity, lower control and an increased likelihood of layoff of workers (ILO, 2016). This makes combatting work-related stress a key priority for governments and international organisations. The WHO Commission on Social Determinants of Health (CSDH) identified fair employment and decent work as a key factor for decreasing the inequalities in health both between and within nations. Prof Sir Michael Marmot, the Chair of the Commission, has repeatedly pointed out that poor working conditions, especially in the informal sector, is a major driver behind the high levels of poor health in the developing world (CSDH, 2008). A small but growing number of studies from middle income countries lend support to this argument. Studies in China (Cheng et al., 2003; Li et al., 2004; Li et al., 2007; Xu et al., 2010; Chien et al., 2011; Xu et al., 2011), Brazil (Alves et al., 2009; Lopes et al., 2010) and Eastern Europe (Salavecz et al., 2010) have all shown that poor work environments are detrimental to health and well-being. Building on this research Hyde and Theorell (Chapter 3) discuss these issues in the wider international context. The Millennium Development Goal (MDG) 1.b committed the international community to 'achieve full and productive employment and decent work for all, including women and young people'. The MDGs have now been replaced with the new Sustainable Development Goals but fair and equitable work remains at the heart of the UN's vision for a 'human race [free] from the tyranny of poverty and want' (Maurice, 2015). These goals highlight work and the workplace as key sites for improving health and well-being in developing countries. As Figure 1.1 shows the World Bank estimates that around 80% of those in work in developing countries are in vulnerable employment, defined as unpaid family workers and own-account workers. Hence in this chapter Hyde and Theorell aim to move beyond the workplace and situate the research on the work environment and health within the broader debates on international development. However, rather than try to present a comprehensive picture covering all the low and middle income countries, they focus on the other BRIC[1] nations as their current conditions and recent histories of rapid social and industrial change are comparable to those in India. Like India, Brazil and China have experienced a declining agricultural sector, rapid industrialisation and the emergence of a service sector over the past few decades. Russia has undergone a different, although no less radical transformation, with the shift from a state-planned economy to neo-liberal capitalist forms of organisation and production which, although more extreme,

[1] Brazil, Russia, India and China.

**Figure 1.1: Proportion of male and female employees who are in vulnerable employment in developing countries**

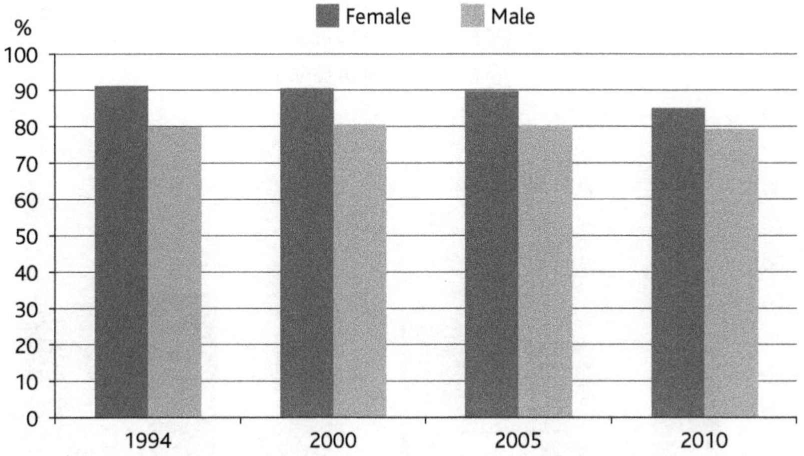


*Source:* World Bank (http://data.worldbank.org/indicator)

mirrors the successive liberalisation and deregulation of the Indian economy. To date, however, despite these radical transformations in the organisation and nature of work in these countries there is relatively little research that has looked at either the state of working conditions or their relationship with stress of health in Russia, Brazil or China. Yet, as previously noted, the research there is indicates that notions and measures of the work environment that were developed in Western Europe and North America several decades ago are meaningful and relevant for describing the situation of these emerging industrial and service classes in the BRIC countries. Moreover, they show that, in line with research in the more advanced industrial economies, a poor work environment can be detrimental to health and well-being. Chapter 3 begins with a review of the current debates on the role of work and working conditions in the discourse on international development before moving on to explore the impact of vulnerable work and poor psychosocial working conditions on health in the developing world in general and the BRIC countries in particular.

## Work in India

As already noted, over the past few decades India has undergone a period of rapid economic development and is now the 11th largest economy in the world. Alongside this economic growth the nature and composition of the Indian economy has changed. As Figure 1.2

**Figure 1.2: Sectoral composition of the workforce in India: 1994–2013**

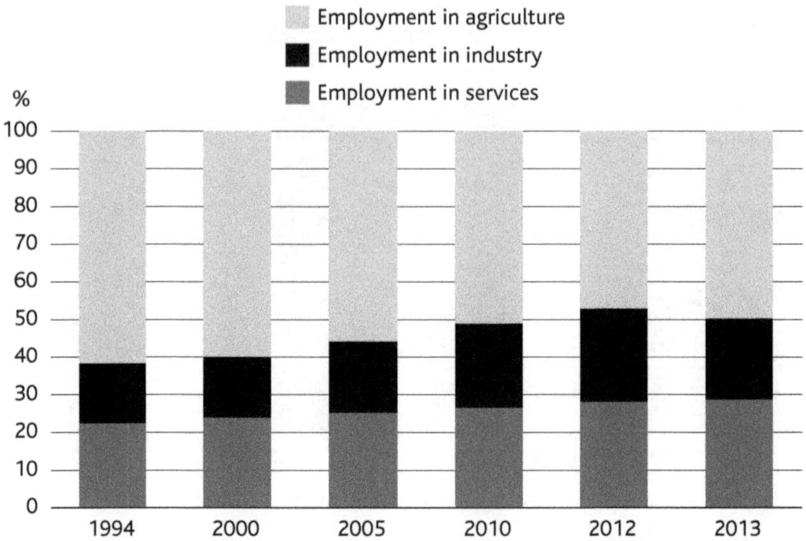


*Source:* World Bank (http://data.worldbank.org/indicator)

shows India has gone from being a largely agricultural economy to a much more industrialised economy with a growing service sector. Employment in agriculture has declined from around 60% of the workforce in 1994 to just under 50% in 2014. Conversely those employed in manufacturing have risen dramatically over the same period, from around 15% to 21% of the workforce over the same period. This shift in the sectoral composition of the workforce has been accompanied by rapid expansion of the middle classes in India (Murphy, 2011). This is expected to grow from 5% of the population to 40% over the next 10 to 15 years (Ablett et al., 2007). Thus, as more and more workers are pulled into the growing manufacturing and service sectors, it is likely that they will be subject to the same sorts of workplace stressors as their European and American counterparts, such as 'flexiwork', ICT use and organisational change. At the same time, India remains a country dominated by small and medium-sized enterprises. Enterprises with fewer than 49 workers accounted for 84% of India's manufacturing employment in 2009, compared with 70% in the Philippines, 46% in Thailand, and a mere 25% in China. This is likely to have an impact on future economic growth as smaller companies in India tend to be less productive and their employees less protected than larger companies (Gupta et al., 2014).

In Chapter 4 A.V. Jose critically discusses the direction and magnitude of changes in key domains such as the labour force, employment and productivity in India in relation to some historical antecedents of Western industrial economies. The 19th century was a key historical period during which major changes affecting the size and composition of the labour force took place throughout Europe and North America. Together with urbanisation, the shift from agriculture to more productive sectors, improvements in living standards and reductions in the drudgery of work all occurred during this period. To assess whether we are seeing a similar transformation in India, Prof Jose reviews the work of eminent economic historians, notably Kuznets, on the chain of causation and synergy leading to the maturing of labour markets under the aegis of modern economic growth. Following this he looks at recent evidence from major industrial economies on the evolution of markets that culminated in the establishment of a European social model. The structural changes that unfolded in industrial economies are used as a template for assessing similar changes, if any, in the Indian context. To do this, he critically examines the emerging employment situation based on data from the National Sample Survey. The findings suggest that India is at the early stages of a qualitative transformation leading to improvement in worker participation rates along with structural changes in the distribution of workforce into sectors, status groups, gender divisions and skill categories. There have also been some impressive gains in managing the labour market from the supply side by way of improving the age-structure and skill-content of the workforce. On the downside, the post-war construct of employment and industrial relations adapted from the toolkit of Western economies, based on which the transformation of labour market was planned and nurtured in the Indian context, is literally falling apart under the onslaught of globalisation. In conclusion, Prof Jose finds that there is a long way to go for markets to mature and appropriate institutions to develop that can safeguard the legitimate rights and interests of all in the world of work. At best one can accelerate the pace of progress towards this goal with the right mix of policy interventions.

Following on from this in Chapter 5 Prof Ladusingh addresses the crucial issues of gender and rural-urban differences in the time spent on unpaid household work in India. These are particularly pressing issues given the wide disparities between these groups. Women are particularly under-represented in the workforce in India. According to a McKinsey Global Institute report on gender parity:

> '[w]omen in India only represent 24% of the labour force that is engaged in any form of work in the market economy, compared with an average of 40% globally. India's position on share of women in workforce is on a par with countries in the Middle East and North Africa, where, unlike India, legal provisions can restrict many forms of female employment in many countries.' (Woetzel, et al., 2015, 1)

The report goes on to note that women in India are almost 10 times more likely to be engaged in unpaid work such as cooking, cleaning and taking care of children and older members of the family than are men. This compares with a global average of roughly three times the amount of time spent by men. Indeed, they calculate that if this unpaid work were to be valued and compensated in the same way as paid work, it would contribute $0.3 trillion to India's economic output. As Prof Ladusingh (Chapter 5) notes in a developing country like India where the participation of women in market-based production activities is low and the division of labour between men and women is governed by cultural norms, women spend considerably more time than men in non-market household production. To explore this in more depth this chapter draws on a unique source of time-use survey data in India carried out by the National Sample Survey Organisation. Analysis of these data shows that people aged 6 years and older spent an average of 2.20 hours a day doing unpaid household work, such as preparing, cooking and serving food and drinks; cleaning, washing clothes and sewing; maintaining the household, shopping for food and non-personal goods; and caring for pets. There was marginal variation between rural and urban residents. Men, regardless of residential background, spent on average 0.30 hours a day on household work compared with women who spent 4.15 and 4.45 hours per day on average in unpaid household activities. Furthermore the time spent by women in unpaid household work varied significantly by age. Those aged 20 to 30 years spent as much as 5.69 hours per day doing unpaid household work while women aged 50 to 64 spent 3.96 hours. Care for children, sick, older and disabled people of one's own household is another form of unpaid household work considered traditionally as women's work. Those aged 6 years and older spent 0.39 hours per day caring for others in the household. The rural-urban figures are 0.38 and 0.41 hours respectively. Women in rural and urban areas spent 0.64 and 0.72 hours per day respectively caring for people who need help in the household. Moreover, women aged between 20 and 34 years had the double burden of caring for their own children and other sick, older and disabled people and spent on an average 1.16 hours per day doing so. The findings that women spend more time than men in unpaid household activities related to management and maintenance and care of children, sick, elderly and disabled household members provide clear evidence that there is gender division of unproductive and productive activities which is induced by prevailing sociocultural norms and practices.

## Health in India

Alongside its tremendous economic growth India has experienced a series of dramatic demographic changes. There has been a dramatic decline in most demographic indicators between 2000 to 2011 (World Bank, 2012). These are reflected in changes in the crude birth rate, crude death rate, total fertility rate and growth rate. The crude birth rate has dropped from 24.79 to 20.97, which means that fewer children are being born per 1,000 people in the population. Another way of looking at this is the total fertility rate: the number of children born to each woman in the country. This too has fallen from 3.11 to 2.62. These two trends have led to a fall in the population growth rate from 1.58% per year to 1.34% per year. So although the size of the population continues to grow it is doing so at a slower rate. While at the other end of the lifecycle the crude death rate has fallen from 8.88 to 7.48, which means that fewer people are dying per 1,000 people. As Figure 1.3 shows life expectancy has risen dramatically from just over 40 years in 1960 to almost 70 years in 2014. Alongside this demographic transition India has also passed through an epidemiological transition (Omran, 1971). This transition is characterised by a shift in the burden of disease away from communicable diseases, such as TB and cholera, to NCD and lifestyle-related diseases, such as cardiovascular diseases (see Figure 1.4). NCDs now account for 53% of total deaths from all causes in India (WHO, 2011) and have been projected to increase to over 57% by 2020 (Rajagopalan, 2000). According to the 2016 WHO ischemic heart disease was the leading cause of death in 2012, followed by chronic obstructive pulmonary disease and stroke. However, as evidence from Europe, North America and Japan shows, the risk of suffering from a NCD are highly associated with socioeconomic position, with those in the most disadvantaged groups having the highest risks. Yet, to date there is little research that has looked at socioeconomic differences in rates of NCD in India.

To redress this Dr Harihar Sahoo (Chapter 7) looks at patterns of health across different economic activity groups, such as those in work,

**Figure 1.3: Life expectancy at birth by sex and for the population as a whole: 1960–2013**

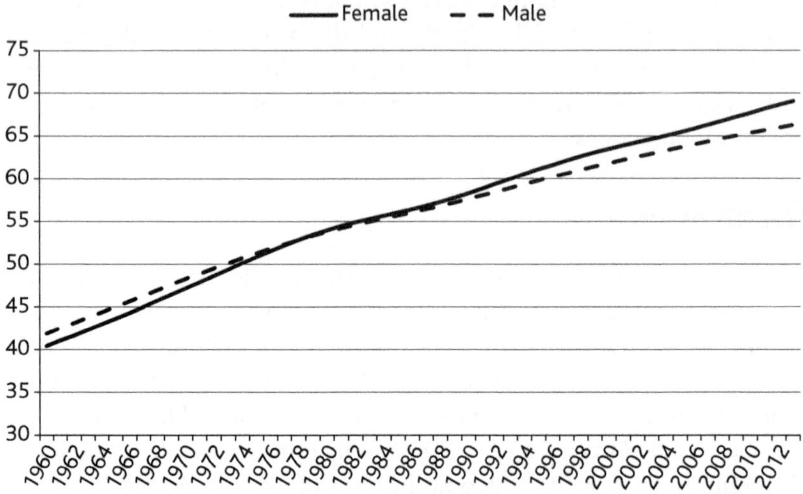


*Source:* World Bank (http://data.worldbank.org/indicator)

**Figure 1.4: Percentage of deaths attributable to communicable disease, non-communicable disease and injuries in India 2000–15**

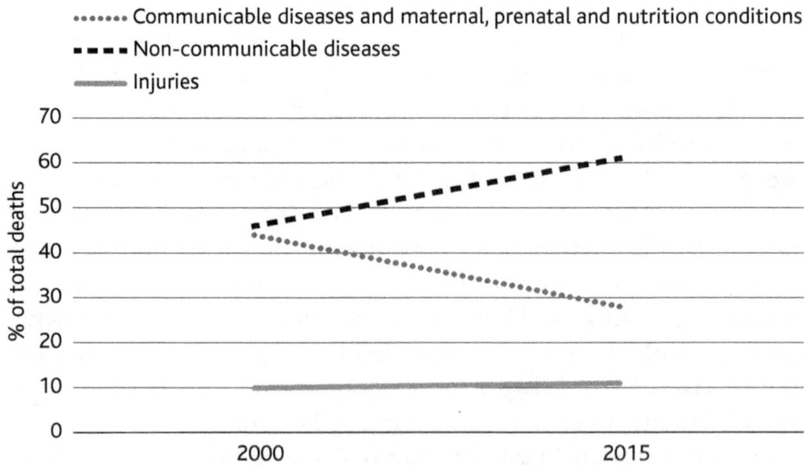


*Source:* World Bank (http://data.worldbank.org/indicator/SH.DTH.INJR.ZS)

studying full time or unemployed. Research from Europe and North America has long since shown that a person's main economic activity, notably if one is unemployed, is an important social determinant of health (Chirikos, 1993; Ferrie, 1997; Kerkhofs and Lindeboom, 1997). This is hardly surprising as much everyday life is spent in work. Not only do people work for many years over their lifetime but they also work for many hours per day. Therefore, a person's activity status has the potential to impact on health. However, activity status has received relatively little attention in the literature on the determinants of health in India. Hence this chapter will examine the impact of economic activity status on the health of its population. The data come from the 60th round of National Sample Survey conducted from January to June 2004. Different indicators of health are used to give as comprehensive picture as possible. The survey asked whether the respondent has suffered from a range of illnesses in the 15 days preceding the date of interview. For hospitalisation, however, information was collected for the 365 days before the date of enquiry. The results show that those who are engaged as own-account workers in a household enterprise have the highest rate of reported disorders in joints and bones, respiratory illnesses including ear/nose/throat ailments, and bronchial asthma during the last 15 days of the survey. The leading diseases among employers are diabetes, cardiovascular disease, disorders of the joints and bones, hypertension and gastritis. The average duration of hospital stays is greater for those who suffered from tuberculosis (16.7 days), followed by skin diseases (16.2 days). Surprisingly, it is found that the burden of the ailments is reported to be higher among the better-off sections of society than among poorer groups. This could be largely due to under-reporting of morbidity by poor people. Furthermore, the higher reported prevalence of NCDs resulting from higher prevalence of lifestyle-related diseases among richer groups could also have contributed to the greater burden of illness among them. It is imperative that health budgets target these populations with very different pattern of disease profile and health care access.

Building on this work, Dr Sanjay Mohanty (Chapter 6) focuses on those in paid employment to explore patterns of chronic illness across different occupational classes in India. Along with economic development, India's economy has become increasingly monetarised and diversified. On the other hand, the demographic and epidemiological transition is leading to an increase in NCDs and largely affecting the prime working age group (Gupte et al., 2001; Joshi et al., 2006). In this context, this chapter examines the differentials of major morbidities among waged and salaried workers in India using data from the India Human Development Survey-II (2011–12) that covered 42,152 households and 204,569 people. Waged and salaried workers account for about two thirds of India's workforce and the analyses are confined to those in the working-age population (20–65 years). Individual occupations are classified into seven broad groups based on National Classification of Occupation 1968: professional, technical and related; administrative, executive and managerial; clerical and related; sales; service; agriculture and allied; and production and related workers. The chronic diseases include diabetes, heart diseases, high blood pressure, diabetes, cancer, Asthma which were diagnosed at some point of time. Descriptive and multivariate analyses were used to understand the differentials of major morbidities among occupational groups in India. Results indicate that economic status and educational level varies significantly by type of occupation. While the mean household annual income was lowest among agricultural and allied workers (US$1,454) it was highest among managerial and administrative workers (US$7,972). The prevalence of any chronic diseases varies from a low of 4.1% among production and transport workers, 4.5% among farming-related workers, 4.7% among sales workers, 7.5% among professional and technical workers, 8.7% among each of service and clerical workers and 12.0% among managerial and administrative workers. Controlling for sociodemographic and economic characteristics, the odds of chronic disease was about twice as high among managerial/administrative workers and 1.4 times higher among clerical worker compared with agricultural and allied worker. These are interesting findings as they appear contrary to the patterns found throughout the more advanced industrial economies. This suggests that India is still passing through the epidemiological transition and it is likely that the relatively low rates of NCD among those in lower social classes might be because of the higher rates of premature mortality due to infectious diseases that still afflict these groups.

## Work, stress and health in India

Globalisation and rapid industrial growth in India in the last few years has led to occupational health-related issues emerging. Gupte and colleagues (2001) have argued that the major factors that contribute to the high prevalence of cardiovascular diseases and neuropsychiatric disorders in India include the increase in life expectancy, changes in lifestyles, stressful living and working conditions and general lack of support systems that enable better coping mechanisms. As noted earlier research in the advanced industrial economies that focused on the relationship between working environment and health, particularly cardiovascular diseases, has already established the severe effects of unfavourable working environments on health (Theorell and Karasek, 1996; Kivimäki, 2012; Heikkilä et al., 2013; Nyberg et al. 2013). Most of the research in this area used the well-known demand-control model (Karasek, 1979). This model measures the balance between psychological work demand, control over work and their impact on health, particularly cardiovascular diseases. Yet to date there is relatively little research on the impact of the work environment on health in India. Where this does exist, it tends to fall under the rubric of occupational health research (for example Saiyed et al., 2004). However, the focus of this research tends to be on the impact of physical work on health hazards rather than measuring the psychological perceptions about working environment on health. Yet as already noted, although physically demanding jobs such as labouring and construction still clearly make up a considerable portion of the Indian workforce, the numbers of workers in service, technical and 'white-collar' jobs has increased considerably. Taken together with the findings that those in these types of occupations have higher rates of chronic illness and hospitalisation and the evidence from psychosocial work environment studies in the advanced industrial economies this strongly suggests that increasing number of workers in these new jobs are being exposed to work-related stress, which is impacting on their health. This calls for greater research into these issues to ensure that India's economic development does not come at the cost of increased levels of chronic illness and poor health. The next four chapters seek to answer this call by looking at various aspects of work, stress and health across a wide range of occupations from the police to tea pickers.

In Chapter 8, Dr Vaijayanthee Kumar and Dr T.J. Kamalanabhan examine the predictors of psychological stress among police personnel and the role that emotional intelligence might play in moderating the relationship between the determinants of psychological stress and the subjective experience of stress itself. They draw on a unique sample of sub-inspectors and inspectors (N=493) from the capital city, Delhi. Standardised scales were employed to measure stress. However, to measure the potential police stressors, new scales were developed by the authors based on their previous qualitative work with this group. Given that previous research in India has shown that different police ranks experience different stressors (Singh and Kar, 2015), these scales provide a better assessment of the specific stressors that this group of police officers face. The results of multiple hierarchical regression revealed that factors such as inflexible work schedules, work-family conflict, political interference and lack of fairness significantly influenced stress. Emotional intelligence was found to buffer the relationship between a number of stressors and the experience of stress.

In Chapter 9 Prof Subrata K. Roy and Dr Tanaya Kundu Chowdhury examine the health and lifestyle factors among tea garden labourers in West Bengal. Tea picking remains a major industry in India. Yet little is known about the health and health behaviours of those employed in the industry. Tea garden labourers enjoy access to some free facilities like education for children, medical facilities, piped drinking water, housing and subsidised food. Yet they still suffer from several health problems. This might be due to insufficient or inadequately maintained facilities, poor lifestyles or a mixture thereof. The present study aims to investigate the work environment, lifestyles and physical health status of Oraon tea garden labourers of Jalpaiguri district, West Bengal. A total of 286 male and 214 female labourers were surveyed. Health was assessed using a range of anthropometric and haematological measures, including body mass index, packed cell volume, haemoglobin level, systolic and diastolic blood pressure. The results reveal that around 60% of the labourers are underweight, despite reporting that they were getting sufficient food to eat. Poor hygienic practices may explain these results. Moreover, around 52% of males fell below the normal range for packed cell volume, although women show a reverse trend. Anaemia was high for both sexes. The overall health condition of the labourers may be explained by the poor health lifestyles that they have adopted in response to their work environment.

In Chapter 10 Dr Sarlaksha Ganesh and Dr M.P. Ganesh review the research and policies on work-family balance in India. Research has shown that balancing work and family demands has become an important topic of research for organisations, researchers and practitioners alike (Guest, 2002; Crompton and Lyonette, 2006). The positive consequences of achieving such a balance are immense, not only for the individual employee, but also for the organisation and their family. Many Western countries have realised the importance of striking this balance, and have addressed the issue not only from a research or theoretical perspective, but have managed to implement work-family balance programmes in their organisations. Yet in India, research on work-family issues is still at a nascent stage. Specifically, issues such as designing work-family balance policies, customising and implementing these and evaluating employee's work-family balance experiences are not frequently addressed in organisations. Aside from the organisation itself, the support given by individuals within the organisation (supervisors and co-workers) as well as the employee's family members (parents, siblings, spouse and children) are also key factors that would help the employees to achieve a good work-family balance. Hence the chapter critically explores the current state of policies and practices in India that aim to promote a good work-family balance, as well as the obstacles to their realisation.

Finally, in Chapter 11 Dr Vimal Kumar examines the working conditions, health and well-being among the scavenger community. Scavenging is one of the occupations performed by particular castes in Indian society. They play a crucial role in maintaining cleanliness, hygiene and sanitation in the towns and cities across India. Scavengers are socially ascribed and made responsible for cleaning roads, streets, sewage, animal dung, toilets and even human excreta. Due to the practice of these activities, scavengers are ignored and excluded from community life in society. The debates around the lives of scavengers are both a human rights issue and an issue of dignity and survival. In his chapter Vimal Kumar draws on the findings from qualitative research, using a mix of participant observation and in-depth interviews conducted in Ladwa, Haryana, Northern India. Through these methods the study exposes the realities of mental stress that members of scavenger community are experiencing. These stress factors include low wages, irregular salaries, debt, fear of job loss, low status in society, shame attached to work, occupational related diseases, injuries, unpleasant work environment and caste-based discrimination during work. Perhaps unsurprisingly exposure to these factors results in high levels of poor health among scavengers. This is an incredibly important study that looks at a highly marginalised group in India which faces a unique set of challenges in work and in society at large.

## Conclusion

At the global and regional level, we now have a growing body of evidence about the burden of disease attributable to a number of environmental and occupational risk factors (WHO, 2010; ILO, 2016). However, due to the dearth of reliable global data, we still lack information about the health impacts of some risk factors, such as the including negative aspects of work organisation. More importantly, in a 2004 WHO report, the authors acknowledged that:

> 'While evidence for a causal relationship is strong, lack of data on accumulated exposure, especially in developing countries, restricted the ability to provide a detailed

> assessment of attributable mortality and disease burden for these outcomes.' (Concha-Barrientos et al., 2004: 1,655)

We hope that this book goes some way to redress this knowledge gap by looking at the impact of work and health across different groups and regions of India. The chapters collected represent some of the state-of-the-art research in the fast-growing field of work environment studies and health in India. As such they make a valuable contribution to our understanding of these issues in one of the world's fastest growing economies.

## References

Ablett, J., Baijal, A., Beinhocker, E., et al. (2007). *The 'bird of gold': The rise of India's consumer market.* McKinsey Global Institute: London.

Achat, H., Kawachi, I., Byrne, C., et al. (2000). A prospective study of job strain and risk of breast cancer. *International Journal of Epidemiology*, 29(4), 622–628.

Agardh, E.E., Ahlbom, A., Andersson, T., et al. (2003). Work stress and low sense of coherence is associated with type 2 diabetes in middle-aged Swedish women. *Diabetes Care*, 26(3), 719–724.

Alves, M.G., Chor, D., Faerstein, E., et al. (2009). Job strain and hypertension in women: Estudo Pro-Saude (Pro-Health Study). *Revista de Saúde Pública*, 43(5), 893–896.

Bernin, P., and Theorell, T. (2001). Demand-control-support among female and male managers in eight Swedish companies. *Stress and Health*, 17(4), 231–243.

Centers for Disease Control and Prevention. (2015). India at a glance. http://www.cdc.gov/globalhealth/countries/india/pdf/india_factsheet.pdf. Accessed 20/3/2016.

Cheng, Y., Luh, W.M., and Guo, Y.L. (2003). Reliability and validity of the Chinese version of the Job Content Questionnaire in Taiwanese workers. *International Journal of Behavioral Medicine*, 10(1), 15–30.

Chien, T.W., Lai, W.P., Wang, H.Y., et al. (2011). Applying the revised Chinese Job Content Questionnaire to assess psychosocial work conditions among Taiwan's hospital workers. *BMC Public Health*, 11, 478.

Chirikos, T.N. (1993). The relationship between health and labor market status. *Annual Review of Public Health*, 14(1), 293–312.

Concha-Barrientos, M., Imel, N.D., Driscoll, T., et al. (2004). Selected occupational risk factors. In M. Ezzati, A.D. Lopez, A. Rodgers and C.J.L. Murray (Eds.), *Comparative Quantification of Health Risks.* Geneva: WHO.

Cox, T., Griffiths, A., and Rial-Gonzalez, E. (2000). *Research on work-related stress*. European Agency for Safety and Health at Work. Luxembourg: Office for Official Publications of the European Communities.

Crompton, R., and Lyonette, C. (2006). Work-life 'balance' in Europe. *Acta Sociologica*, 49(4), 379–393.

CSDH. (2008). *Closing the Gap in a Generation: Health Equity Through Action on the Social Determinants of Health*. Commission on Social Determinants of Health Final Report. Geneva: WHO.

Dreze J., and Sen A. (2014). *An Uncertain Glory: India and its Contradictions*. London: Penguin.

EC. (2002). *Communication from the Commission. Adapting to change in work and society: a new community strategy on health and safety at work 2002–2006*. Commission of the European Communities.

EC. (2007). European Agency for Safety and Health at Work. *Expert forecast on emerging psychosocial risks related to occupational safety and health*. Luxembourg: Office for Official Publications of the European Communities.

Elovainio, M., Ferrie, J.E., Singh-Manoux, A., et al. (2010). Organisational justice and markers of inflammation: the Whitehall II study. *Occupational and Environmental Medicine*, 67(2), 78–83.

Elovainio, M., Singh-Manoux, A., Ferrie, J.E., et al. (2012). Organisational justice and cognitive function in middle-aged employees: the Whitehall II study. *Journal of Epidemiology and Community Health*, 66(6), 552–556.

Ferrie, J.E. (1997). Labour market status, insecurity and health. *Journal of Health Psychology*, 2(3), 373–397.

Ferrie, J.E., Head, J.A., Shipley, M.J., and Vahtera, J. (2007). Injustice at work and health: causation, correlation or cause for action? *Occupational and Environmental Medicine*, 64(6), 428–428.

Ferrie, J.E., Head, J., Shipley, M.J., et al. (2006). Injustice at work and incidence of psychiatric morbidity: the Whitehall II study. *Occupational and Environmental Medicine*, 63(7), 443–450.

Guest, D.E. (2002). Perspectives on the study of work-life balance. *Social Science Information*, 41(2), 255–279.

Gupta, R., Sankhe, S., Dobbs, R., et al. (2014). *From poverty to empowerment: India's imperative for jobs, growth, and effective basic services*. London: McKinsey Global Institute.

Gupte, M.D., Ramachandran, V., Mutatkar, R.K. (2001). Epidemiological profile of India: historical and contemporary perspectives, *Journal of Biosciences*, 26(4): 437–464.

Hanson, L.L.M., Theorell, T., Oxenstierna, G., et al. (2008). Demand, control and social climate as predictors of emotional exhaustion symptoms in working Swedish men and women. *Scandinavian Journal of Public Health*, 36(7), 737–743.

Heikkilä, K., Fransson, E.I., Nyberg, S.T., et al. (2013). Job strain and health-related lifestyle: findings from an individual-participant meta-analysis of 118,000 working adults. *American Journal of Public Health*, 103(11), 2090–2097.

Hellgren, J., and Sverke, M. (2003). Does job insecurity lead to impaired well-being or vice versa? Estimation of cross-lagged effects using latent variable modelling, *Journal of Organizational Behavior*, 24(2), 215–236.

ILO. (2016). *Workplace stress: A collective challenge*. ILO: Geneva.

Johnson, J.V., and Hall, E.M. (1996). Dialectic between conceptual and causal enquiry in psychosocial work-environment research, *Journal of Occupational Health Psychology*, 1(4), 362–374.

Joshi, R., Cardona, M., Iyengar, S., et al. (2006). Chronic diseases now a leading cause of death in rural India – mortality data from the Andhra Pradesh Rural Health Initiative. *International Journal of Epidemiology*, 35(6), 1522–1529.

Karasek, R.A. (1979). Job demands, job decision latitude, and mental strain. implications for job redesign, *Administrative Science Quarterly*, 24(2), 285–308.

Kerkhofs, M., and Lindeboom, M. (1997). Age related health dynamics and changes in labour market status, *Health Economics*, 6(4), 407–423.

Kivimaki, M., Elovainio, M., Vahtera, J., and Ferrie, J.E. (2003b). Organisational justice and health of employees: prospective cohort study, *Occupational and Environmental Medicine*, 60(1), 27–33.

Kivimaki, M., Vahtera, J., Elovainio, M., et al. (2008). What are the next steps for research on work stress and coronary heart disease? *Scandinavian Journal of Work Environment and Health*, Suppl 2008(6), 33–40.

Kivimäki, M., Head, J., Ferrie, J.E., et al. (2003a). Sickness absence as a global measure of health: Evidence from mortality in the Whitehall II prospective cohort study, *British Medical Journal*, 327(7411), 364–368.

Kivimäki, M., Nyberg, S.T., Batty, G.D., et al. (2012). Job strain as a risk factor for coronary heart disease: a collaborative meta-analysis of individual participant data, *The Lancet*, 380(9852), 1491–1497.

Kumar A. (2015). Rural Households' Access to Basic Amenities in India: Deprivation and Socio-economic Exclusions, *Social Change*, 45(4); 561–586.

Kuper, H., Yang, L., Theorell, T., et al. (2007). Job strain and risk of breast cancer, *Epidemiology*, 18(6), 764–768.

Li, J., Yang, W., Liu, P., et al. (2004). Psychometric evaluation of the Chinese (mainland) version of Job Content Questionnaire: a study in university hospitals, *Industrial Health*, 42(2), 260–267.

Li, W., Zhang, J.Q., Sun, J., et al. (2007). Reliability and validity of Job Content Questionnaire in Chinese petrochemical employees, *Psychological Reports*, 100(1), 35–46.

Lopes, C.S., Araya, R., Werneck, G.L., et al. (2010). Job strain and other work conditions: relationships with psychological distress among civil servants in Rio de Janeiro, Brazil, *Social Psychiatry and Psychiatric Epidemiology*, 45(3), 345–354.

Maurice, J. (2015) UN set to change the world with new development goals, *The Lancet*, 386(9999), 1121–1124.

McEwen, B.S. (2008). Central effects of stress hormones in health and disease: Understanding the protective and damaging effects of stress and stress mediators, *European Journal of Pharmacology*, 583(2–3), 174–185.

Michie, S. (2002). Causes and management of stress at work, *Occupational and Environmental Medicine*, 59, 67–72.

Murphy, J. (2011). Indian call centre workers: vanguard of a global middle class? *Work Employment and Society*, 25(3), 417–433.

Narain, J.P., Jain, S.K., Bora, D. and Venkatesh, S. (2015). Eradicating successfully yaws from India: The strategy and global lessons, *Indian Journal of Medical Research*, 141(5), 608–13.

NIOSH (2002). The changing organization of work and the safety and health of working people: Knowledge gaps and research directions, *National Institute for Occupational Safety and Health*, 2002 (116): Department of Health and Human Services.

Nyberg, A., Westerlund, H., Hanson, L.L.M., and Theorell, T. (2008). Managerial leadership is associated with self-reported sickness absence and sickness presenteeism among Swedish men and women, *Scandinavian Journal of Public Health*, 36(8), 803–811.

Nyberg, S.T., Heikkilä, K., Fransson, E.I., et al. for the IPD Work Consortium. (2011). Job strain in relation to body mass index: pooled analysis of 160,000 adults from 13 cohort studies, *Journal of Internal Medicine*, 272(1), 65–73.

Nyberg, S.T., Fransson, E.I., Heikkilä, K., et al., (2013). Job strain and cardiovascular disease risk factors: meta-analysis of individual-participant data from 47,000 men and women. *PloS one*, 8(6).

Omran, A. (1971). The epidemiologic transition: A theory of the epidemiology of population change. *The Milbank Memorial Fund Quarterly*, 49(4): 509–538.

Popkin, B.M., Horton, S., Kim, S., et al. (2001). Trends in Diet, Nutritional Status, and Diet-related Noncommunicable Diseases in China and India: The Economic Costs of the Nutrition Transition. *Nutrition Reviews*, 59(12), 379–390.

Rajagopalan, M. (2000). Health and nutrition profile of India. *Health education in South East Asia*, 1, 15–26.

Saiyed, H.N., Tiwari, R.R., 2004. Occupational health research in India. *Industrial Health*, 42: 141–148.

Salavecz, G., Chandola, T., Pikhart, H., et al. (2010). Work stress and health in Western European and post-communist countries: An East-West comparison study. *Journal of Epidemiology and Community Health*, 64(1), 57–62.

Sanchez, A.M.R., Gallego, E.C., Scoria, M.S., and Aborg, C. (2008). Technoflow among Spanish and Swedish students: A confirmatory factor multigroup analysis. *Anales De Psicologia*, 24(1), 42–48.

Sauter, S.L., Hurrell, J.J., and Cooper, C.L. (1989). *Job Control and Worker Health*. Chichester: Wiley & Sons.

Siegrist, J. (1996). Adverse health effects of high-effort/low-reward conditions. *Journal of Occupational Health Psychology*, 1(1), 27–41.

Singh, S. and Kar, S.K. (2015). Sources of occupational stress in the police personnel of North India: An exploratory study. *Indian Journal of Occupational and Environmental Medicine*; 19, 56–60.

Spurgeon, A., Harrington, J.M., and Cooper, C.L. (1997). Health and safety problems associated with long working hours: A review of the current position. *Occupational and Environmental Medicine*, 54(6), 367–375.

Stansfeld, S., and Candy, B. (2006). Psychosocial work environment and mental health – a meta-analytic review. *Scandinavian Journal of Work, Environment & Health*, 32(6), 443–462.

Sverke, M., Hellgren, J., and Naswall, K. (2002). No security: a meta-analysis and review of job insecurity and its consequences. *Journal of Occupational Health Psychology*, 7(3), 242–264.

The World Bank. 2011. *World Development Indicators*, World Bank, http://data.worldbank.org/data-catalog/world-development-indicators

Theorell, T. (2008). After 30 years with the demand-control-support model – how is it used today? Introduction. *Scandinavian Journal of Work Environment and Health*, 3–5.

Theorell, T., and Karasek, R.A. (1996). Current issues relating to psychosocial job strain and cardiovascular disease research. *Journal of Occupational Health Psychology*, 1(1), 9–26.

Vahtera, J., Pentti, J. and Kivimäki, M. (2004). Sickness absence as a predictor of mortality among male and female employees. *Journal of Epidemiology and Community Health*, 58(4), 321–326.

van den Berg, T.I.J., Elders, L.A.M., de Zwart, B.C.H., and Burdorf, A. (2009). The effects of work-related and individual factors on the Work Ability Index: A systematic review. *Occupational and Environmental Medicine*, 66, 211–220.

Westerlund, H., Ferrie, J., Hagberg, J., Jeding, K., et al. (2004). Workplace expansion, long-term sickness absence, and hospital admission. *The Lancet*, 363(9416), 1193–1197.

Westerlund, H., Theorell, T., and Bergstrom, A. (2001). Psychophysiological effects of temporary alternative employment. *Social Science & Medicine*, 52(3), 405–415.

Woetzel, J., Madgavkar, A., Gupta, R., et al. (2015). *The power of parity: Advancing women's equality in India*. McKinsey Global Institute: London.

World Bank. (2016a). GDP growth (annual %). http://data.worldbank.org/indicator/NY.GDP.MKTP.KD.ZG Accessed 18/03/2016.

World Bank. (2016b). India. World Development Indicators. http://data.worldbank.org/country/india Accessed 17/02/2016.

WHO. (2010). *Health Impact of Psychosocial Hazards at Work: An Overview*. Geneva: WHO.

WHO. (2011). Non-communicable diseases, Country Profiles. http://www.who.int/nmh/countries/ind_en.pdf

WHO. (2015). Maternal and Neonatal Tetanus (MNT) elimination. http://www.who.int/immunization/diseases/MNTE_initiative/en/index1.html Accessed 20/3/1016.

WHO. (2016). India: WHO statistical profile. http://www.who.int/gho/countries/ind.pdf?ua=1

Xu, W.X., Yu, H.Y., Gao, W., et al. (2011). When Job Stress Threatens Chinese Workers Combination of Job Stress Models Can Improve the Risk Estimation for Coronary Heart Disease-the BADCAR Study. *Journal of Occupational and Environmental Medicine*, 53(7), 771–775.

Xu, W.X., Zhao, Y.M., Guo, L.J., et al. (2010). The Association Between Effort-Reward Imbalance and Coronary Atherosclerosis in a Chinese Sample. *American Journal of Industrial Medicine*, 53(7), 655–661.

TWO

# Work, stress and health: Theories and models

*Linda L. Magnusson Hanson, Martin Hyde, Holendro Singh Chungkham and Hugo Westerlund*

## Introduction

Work is necessary to provide people with the means to live healthily, but since time immemorial, it has also been obvious that work can harm people's health through occupational accidents and the wear and tear of heavy and repetitive physical labour. It is far less obvious, but not necessarily less important, that work can also harm through chemical, social and psychological exposures. In this chapter, we will discuss how psychosocial factors at work can impact on people's health, and how such factors have been conceptualised and measured by researchers in this field. For decades, technological development has meant that fewer people work in agriculture, that factories acquire more modern machinery, and that increasing numbers of people work in office and service occupations – for example as salespersons, computer programmers, call centre operators and nurses. As described in Chapter 4, this is also increasingly true in India. Related to this is a decrease in physical work injuries. At the same time, the development of vaccines, antibiotics and good hygiene practices have helped to reduce the relative burden of infectious diseases. In contrast, cardiovascular disease, diabetes and cancer have become more salient as causes of death (Lonzano et al., 2012) and disability more globally (Murray et al., 2012). These are diseases which are known to be affected by health behaviours and are also believed to be stress related. Mental and substance use disorders, while contributing relatively little to premature mortality, are now the leading cause of years lived with disability worldwide, with depressive disorders contributing about 40% of this burden of ill health (Whiteford et al., 2013). These disorders are also commonly held to be stress related, and thus likely to be affected by the psychosocial work environment. A 2006 study, part of the World Health Organization (WHO) Global Burden of Disease studies, reported that 8% of depression globally can be attributed to environmental factors, in particular occupational stress (Prüss-Üstün and Corvalán, 2006).

It can therefore be argued that psychosocial factors are likely to have gained in relative importance for public health, at least in industrialised welfare states. The situation is less clear in developing countries, where a large proportion of the population still works in agriculture and physically demanding factory work, and where issues such as malnutrition, lack of clean water and poor access to healthcare are still salient for substantial parts of the population. It has, however, been argued that psychosocial issues are also of major importance in such environments (Marmot, 2004), and it should not be forgotten that in countries like India and China, there is a large middle class whose working conditions may be very like those in the industrialised countries. Moreover, as the relative material and social inequalities are larger in low and middle income countries, it can be argued that they contribute even more to health there than they do in high income countries (Marmot et al., 2008).

Interest in the effects of the psychosocial work environment emerged during the 1960s when studies looked at the effects of long working hours or shift work (Hinkle et al., 1968). The scope of the research has since grown to include, for example, job insecurity, job demands, control and resources, perceived fairness and organisational justice, coping, leadership practices, threats of violence, and bullying and discrimination. Most research to date, however, has focused on the balance between demands on the one hand, and control, resources or rewards on the other, and this will also be the focus of this chapter. After a brief introduction to stress theory and an overview of the major models of occupational stress used to date, we will return to the empirical evidence for health effects of work.

## Stress

To survive, all living organisms have to cope with various changes and challenges in their environment, ranging from heat and cold, to hunger and thirst, and being hunted by predators. This must be done while maintaining a relatively steady internal state – homeostasis – in, for instance, temperature, salinity and levels of oxygen and carbon dioxide. The concept of stress is not well defined in the research literature (Monroe, 2008), but encompasses adapting to time-limited challenges to survival or homeostasis that typically require energy mobilisation, such as finding food or fighting off or fleeing from a predator. Stress in this sense is not intrinsically good or bad, but a natural feature of life for all living organisms. There are, however, conditions where stress can be harmful to health. One is if the environmental challenge – or stressor – is so large that the organism cannot cope successfully (Selye, 1980; Brunner and Marmot, 2001). Another is if sustained stress activation over the long term leads to a cumulative burden ('wear and tear') on physiological systems eventually resulting in dysregulation and failure (McEwen, 2003). Examples of the former are a worker doing hard physical labour in a hot environment who dies from overheating, and an antelope that runs itself exhausted and is eaten by a lion. An example of the latter is the accumulation of risk factors for coronary heart disease in people with stressful jobs (Nyberg et al., 2013).

The basic human stress responses are similar to those of other mammals and have evolved over the course of evolution. In fact, all living organisms have some kind of adaptive responses to environmental changes. The most common physiological stress responses, involving activation of the autonomic nervous and neuroendocrine systems, have evolved to mobilise energy for fight or flight in the face of immediate danger or need, with a possible third alternative being to 'play dead' to avoid the attention of predators. These responses were highly useful for our forebears, and continue to be useful in situations needing short-term energy mobilisation. Yet they are arguably less well suited to handle modern life stressors, such as high job demands or fear of unemployment, that can be long lasting and impossible to fight or flee from in a physical sense. The standard stress responses, while adaptive in the short run, could thus instead be maladaptive in the longer-time perspective. One example is that the increased levels of circulating blood lipids are part of energy mobilisation may over the long term lead to atherosclerosis and cardiovascular disease. Another is the high availability of relatively cheap calories in high-income countries means that too much energy intake, rather than too little, tends to be a major problem, leading to obesity, atherosclerosis and related diseases.

In humans, however, the psychological assessment of the situation plays a larger role in forming the stress response than in other life forms. How a person experiences and interprets the potentially stressful situation may thus determine if it is associated with positive or negative consequences (Katz and Kahn, 1978; Monroe, 2008). While some people interpret a situation as threatening and overwhelming, others may view it as stimulating and rewarding (Frankenhaeuser and Johansson, 1981). A person's experience may be influenced by factors such as personality, preferences and previous experiences, expectations on the situation and what coping resources are available. It is also assumed that recovery is important in avoiding the strain associated with sustained energy mobilisation (Geurts and Sonnentag, 2006).

## Work and health

Although work can be harmful, extensive studies and theoretical analyses of work and of unemployment, and comparisons between work and unemployment, support the basic concept that work in general is beneficial for health and well-being. In most societies paid employment is the most important means of getting adequate economic resources, which are essential for material well-being and the ability to participate in social and civic activities (Jahoda, 1982; Brenner and Mooney, 1983; Nordenmark and Strandh, 1999; Saunders, 2002; Saunders and Taylor, 2002; Shah and Marks, 2004; Layard, 2004; Coats and Max, 2005). Moreover, work meets important psychosocial needs in societies where employment is the norm and is central to individual identity, social roles and social status (Jahoda, 1982; Warr, 1987; Brenner and Mooney, 1983; Ezzy, 1993; Nordenmark and Strandh, 1999; Dodu, 2005). However, studies note that not all forms of work are equally beneficial for health and in fact some can have a detrimental impact. Cross-national research in Europe has shown that people with precarious forms of employment, such as temporary jobs or fixed-term contracts, consistently reported greater levels of stress, fatigue, backache and muscular pains as compared with full-time permanent workers. (Benavides et al., 2000).

There is a substantial literature showing a strong association between unemployment and mortality (Brenner and Mooney, 1983; Platt, 1984; Jin et al., 1995; Lynge and Andersen, 1997; Mathers and Schofield, 1998; Brenner, 2005), poorer physical health (Jin et al., 1995; Mathers and Schofield, 1998; Cohen, 1999), poorer general health, somatic complaints, long-standing illness, limiting long-standing illness, disability (Jin et al., 1995; Shortt, 1996; Mathers and Schofield, 1998; Lakey, 2001), poorer mental health and psychological well-being (Platt, 1984; Murphy and Athanasou, 1999; Fryers et al., 2003). There are a number of possible mechanisms by which unemployment might have adverse effects on health. Bartley (1994) notes that there are four possible mechanisms by which job loss might impact on health: poverty, stress, health-related behaviour and the effect of unemployment on the rest of the work career. Unemployment can often lead to material deprivation through the loss of income. However, it can also lead to other forms of deprivation. Employment provides non-economic, latent, functions, such as structure and regular activity, identity and status that are lost when a person is forced out of work (Jahoda, 1982; Nordenmark and Strandh, 1999). Losing one's job can also be an extremely stressful life event (Bartley, 1994; Henkens et al., 2008) and therefore may affect physical health via a stress pathway involving physiological changes such as hypertension and lowered immunity. Hence, although these studies show that work has a generally positive effect on health, certainly relative to being unemployed, many researchers have argued that work alone is not enough for health but that it needs to be good quality work. This sentiment lies at the heart of work environment research which attempts to measure the quality of psychosocial conditions at work and their impact on health. In the next section, we will present the three main, separate but conceptually related, theoretical models used in psychosocial work environment and health research.

## The demand-control-support model

In the late 1970s, against a backdrop of changes in workplace organisation in some Scandinavian countries, Robert Karasek formulated a two-dimensional model that has become known as the 'demand-control model' (Karasek, 1979; Karasek and Theorell, 1990). This model has since dominated the research on psychosocial working conditions. It postulates that stress and health may be affected by psychological job demands that are not matched by enough control, also called decision latitude (Karasek and Theorell, 1990). *Psychological demands* relate to how hard a person has to work, for example how much a factory labourer is expected to produce in a certain time period or how many patients a nurse has to care for. How fast or intensively employees have to work, how much effort the work requires, and if there is enough time to complete work tasks may all contribute to the experience of psychological demands. In contrast, control (decision latitude) relates to the possibilities that workers are provided with to exert control and make decisions about their work. Control can also be divided into two sub-components. One of these is *decision authority* or authority over decisions, that is the possibilities to influence what to do at work and how the work tasks are performed. The other, *skill discretion*, measures how the knowledge and skills of workers are used and developed. It is hypothesised that competence, for example learning new things, increases the possibilities that workers have to control their work situation, thus reducing stress. In many research studies, however, control is studied as decision latitude rather the specific sub-components (cf. de Lange et al., 2003).

The relationship between demands and control is often visualised by a two-by-two table (see Figure 2.1). The combination of high demands and low control is predicted to be the most stressful, with possible consequences for health. This 'high-strain' combination is referred to as *job strain*. The anticipated most favourable combination, on the other hand, is called *low strain* and represents a work situation with low psychological demands and high control. The combination of low demands and low control is labelled *passive* work, and the combination of high demands and high control *active work*. In the long run, job strain is hypothesised to lead to accumulated strain that inhibits learning, thus lowering control, while an active job provides experiences that promote a feeling of mastery which inhibits strain perception (Karasek and Theorell, 1990). At a later stage, social support was added to the demand-control model as an additional ameliorating factor (Johnson and Hall, 1988). A work environment with high demands, low control as well as low support, referred to as *iso-strain*, may according to this hypothesis increase the risk of disease even more than job strain alone (Johnson and Hall, 1988).

**Figure 2.1: The demand-control model**

| Decision latitude (control) | Psychological demands: Low | Psychological demands: High |
| --- | --- | --- |
| High | Low-strain | Active |
| Low | Passive | High-strain |

## The effort-reward imbalance model

The other main model commonly employed in work environment studies is the effort-reward imbalance model (Siegrist, 2008), based on contract or role theory (see Figure 2.2). It is argued that social reciprocity lies at the heart of the employment contract which defines tasks to be performed and the associated rewards, wages or promotion. Any substantial breach of the perceived equity or fairness of a social exchange at work is hypothesised to result in stress reactions that can have adverse health effects for the disfavoured party. A situation of effort-reward imbalance (failed reciprocity) can arise if efforts, originating in the demands or obligations at the workplace, are perceived as exceeding the rewards received, which can be material (such as salary), social (such as prospects for promotions and job security) and psychological (such as appreciation and positive feedback). Such an effort-reward imbalance can constitute a threat to self-regulatory needs such as acquiring self-efficacy (such as, successful performance), self-esteem (such as, recognition) and self-integration (such as, belonging to a significant group) and may be unfavourable for health and well-being. An unreasonably strong motivation, and the related unrealistic expectations of rewards, referred to as 'overcommitment', is usually associated with an experience of imbalance between efforts and rewards and reduced health.

**Figure 2.2: The effort-reward imbalance model**

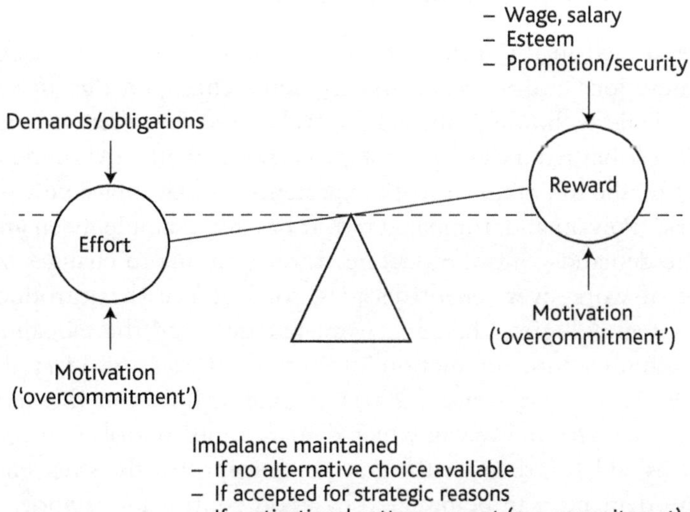


*Source:* Universitätsklinikum Düsseldorf (www.uniklinik-duesseldorf.de/unternehmen/institute/institut-fuer-medizinische-soziologie/forschung/the-eri-model-stress-and-health/theoretical-background-of-the-effort-reward-imbalance-model/)

## Organisational justice

The organisational justice model also builds on equity theory and refers to the employee's perception of fairness in the workplace/organisation (Greenberg et al., 1978). A perception of equity is usually formed by an employee through comparing his/her inputs to that of others in a similar situation; these could include effort, time, skill, loyalty, tolerance, flexibility and integrity and outputs, such as salary and bonuses, job security, recognition, reputation and responsibilities/promotions (Adams, 1965). Several types of organisational justice have, however, been suggested. One is *distributive justice*, which concerns perceptions about fairness in how resources and benefits are distributed, for example. Another is *interactional justice*, which relates to perceptions about treatment at work and interpersonal relationships. A third is *informational justice*, which concerns the perception of the way in which outcomes were distributed and why (Bies and Moag, 1986). Finally, *procedural justice* refers to perceptions of fairness of the decision processes concerning the distribution of resources and benefits in the organisation (Greenberg et al. 1987). It has been hypothesised that a lack of organisational justice could have negative consequences for both organisational citizenship behaviour (Moorman, 1991) and health (Elovainio et al., 2002).

## Criticisms of the dominant models

As mentioned in the introduction, the nature of work is changing, with new jobs and working arrangements emerging due to social, financial and technological changes. Related to this, there is concern that the established measures of the psychosocial work environment fail to capture the full range of work experiences in this 'brave new world of work' (Polyani and Tompa, 2004). It has, for example, been argued that the demand-control model needs revising due to changes in the nature of work over recent decades, for instance the introduction of new technologies, changing work practices and the globalisation of communication, production and services (Lash and Urry, 1987; Castells, 1996; Sparks et al., 2001). Arguably, however, this may be more accurate for the way in which demands and control are measured (as discussed later) than for the general concept that the stress elicited by high demands can be buffered by good control and support. The development in many Western countries of a more flexible labour force also means that organisational changes and job insecurity are potentially prominent modern work-related stressors which are not explicitly addressed in the main models. Moreover, the combination of Internet and mobile computer technology has, for instance, enabled many white-collar workers to work flexibly, including working from home and telecommuting. While potentially helping people to better combine work and private life, there are also worries that being online – and theoretically available to work 24 hours a day, 7 days a week – might lead to increased stress. At the same time, there are also people, especially in agriculture, who work in the pre-modern manner, without clear distinctions between work and leisure time. In contrast, most models of work stress developed so far have implicitly assumed that people work as employees in the manner typical of the industrial society, with distinct working hours and clear boundaries between paid work and private life. Working schedules with long working hours are common to date and may also be important for health and well-being. Especially, working schedules involving night work or other forms of shift work may be associated with changes in biological circadian rhythms, reduced length and poor quality of sleep, and conflicting work-home demands which contribute to increasing levels of stress and fatigue.

Related to this is the criticism that job stress should not be seen as distinct from stress in private life, but rather as part of a complex interaction of life spheres (Bellavia and Frone, 2005). Work-home interference has been shown to predict major depression/antidepressant treatment after adjustment for work characteristics too (Magnusson Hanson et al., 2014). Stressors in private life may, conversely, impact on people's ability to cope with work demands, and possibly also to earn their living. Within the working situation itself, there may be stressors that are not fully captured by the dominating work stress theories – or at least not by the instruments most often used to measure them. Emotional demands, for example, which are usually not measured well in the existing scales for measuring overall demands, have been shown to predict mental health problems (Madsen et al., 2014).

## Other commonly used models

In work psychology, in contrast to the health sciences, the job demands-resources (JD-R) model is today the by far most commonly used, especially in relation to occupational burnout. It proposes that burnout develops due to two processes: the demanding aspects of work may ultimately lead to exhaustion, and the lack of resources makes it difficult to meet job demands, potentially leading to withdrawal behaviour (Demerouti et al., 2001). Compared with the demand-control model of Karasek, the job demands-resources model considers a wider range of resources, and does not postulate any interaction between demands and resources. It also allows for a positive path from resources to motivation.

The cognitive activation theory of stress (CATS; Ursin and Eriksen, 2004) focuses on how past experiences of attempts to cope with environmental challenges will form expectancies around future coping. A lack of a positive outcome expectancy, derived from earlier failures, is in the presence of stressors predicted to lead to sustained physiological activation that can eventually lead to illness and disease. While not specifically concerned with work, the CATS framework may be helpful in explaining both how individual differences in reactions to a certain environment arise, and how experiences from one environment can have long-term consequences by impacting on the coping outcome expectancies of those exposed.

## Measurement of psychosocial work characteristics

The psychosocial environment is inherently difficult to measure objectively since it is largely determined by interpersonal relationships. Self-reports are therefore by far the most common source of information, and arguably the most valid since only the person can have the full picture of his or her working situation. Self-reports are, however, also likely to be biased by a range of factors, such as individual differences, including health status, recall bias and social desirability (Monroe, 2008). This makes them vulnerable to reverse causality (that poorer health leads to changes in perception of psychosocial work environment rather than the other way around) and confounding (that the association is explained by third factors). In these situations, structured interviews may be preferable, but tend to be costly and hence difficult to use in large-scale quantitative studies. Some researchers have therefore attempted to assess psychosocial working conditions by expert ratings or by applying so-called job exposure matrices which assign a certain score on various working conditions to people based on their occupations or job titles. However, observations require quite extensive resources to carry out and may miss important aspects of the social and psychological environment. Job exposure matrices, while largely circumventing subjective biases, are even more crude, since they completely ignore differences between workplaces and individuals in workplaces, potentially leading to gross misclassification of people's work situation. Subjective measures, in contrast, are less expensive and more practical. However, widely accepted standard instruments are still lacking. Many different instruments have been developed over the years, some of which are translated into several different languages (Tabanelli et al., 2008).

The demand-control-support model is usually measured with the extensive Job Content Questionnaire (JCQ; www.jcqcenter.org) developed by Karasek and colleagues, or the shorter, originally Swedish Demand-Control Questionnaire (DCQ) developed by Karasek's colleague and collaborator Töres Theorell (Karasek and Theorell, 1992; Chungkham et al., 2013). In practice, variants and abbreviated versions of these questionnaires are often used, but an international comparative study found that certain partial scales may be acceptable proxies of the respective dimensions of demand-control model (Fransson et al., 2012).

The effort-reward imbalance components are usually measured with variants of the questionnaire developed by Johannes Siegrist, the originator of the effort-reward imbalance model. Several versions are available (Siegrist et al., 2009; Leineweber et al., 2010), and validation studies have shown that short proxy measures and partial versions of the original scales can be used to assess effort-reward imbalance (Siegrist et al., 2014). An example of a more generic questionnaire, which has been translated into more than 20 languages, is the Copenhagen Psychosocial Questionnaire (COPSOQ; Kristensen, 2010; Pejtersen, 2010). It was originally constructed both for scientific studies and workplace risk assessment, and is currently available in three versions. COPSOQ draws from several different models of job stress rather than being based on a specific theory. For instance, it differentiates between six different types of demands: quantitative demands, work pace, cognitive demands, emotional demands, demands for hiding emotions and sensory demands. COPSOQ may therefore be more suited to support workplace interventions since it may help identify the precise targets of interventions. In epidemiological research, on the other hand, a more generic model of job stress, such as the demand-control model, may be more successful at predicting disease risk.

## Conclusions

In this chapter, we have aimed to show that works plays an important role in health. Many studies have shown being in work can confer health benefits compared with being unemployed. However, it is not as simple as this. As many researchers have shown not all work is equal. Moreover, poor working conditions can lead to stress which, if unchecked, can lead to poor health. There is now a large body of work, albeit largely from the advanced industrialised countries, showing the association between these psychosocial working factors and the health of the workforce. Although research in this field can be complicated by the use of different measures of the work environment, the evidence that poor working conditions are bad for your health are pretty consistent regardless of the measure being used.

Research on the demand-control-support model has indicated that there may be risks associated with iso-strain, that is the combination of job strain (high demands, low control) and low social support (Amick et al., 1998; van der Doef et al., 2000, Chandola et al., 2006; Lindeberg et al., 2011; Mather et al., 2015). However, most studies on the connection between the psychosocial work environment and health have focused on jobs strain or on the individual components of the demand-control model. A large body of research shows that job strain, or at least one of the demand and control or support components, is associated with increased risk of many different health problems (de Lange et al., 2003). Job strain has for example been shown to predict mental health problems in terms of symptoms of depression (Swedish Council on Health Technology Assessment, 2014; Theorell et al., 2015; Madsen et al., 2017), coronary heart disease (Kivimaki et al., 2014), stroke (Fransson et al., 2015), metabolic syndrome (Bergmann et al., 2014), diabetes (Nyberg et al., 2014), musculoskeletal problems in terms of back/neck pain (Lang et al., 2012, Swedish Council on Health Technology Assessment, 2014), but not the most common forms of cancer (Heikkilä et al., 2013). Job demands and low job control have also been associated with emotional exhaustion (Aronsson et al., 2017) among other issues. Social support at work has also been linked to mental and physical health outcomes including depressive symptoms (Nieuwenhuijsen et al., 2010, Theorell et al., 2015), emotional exhaustion (Aronsson et al., 2017), musculoskeletal problems such as low back pain (Lang et al., 2012, Swedish Council on Health Technology Assessment, 2014), and cardiovascular disease (Theorell et al. 2016). Most of the evidence is, however, based on studies in Europe, North America and Japan. It is uncertain if associations are similar in developed countries with less developed welfare systems (see Chapter 3 in this volume).

Furthermore, an imbalance between efforts and rewards has been shown to predict some health outcomes, such as mental health problems (Nieuwenhuijsen et al., 2010; Swedish Council on Health Technology Assessment, 2014; Rugulies et al., 2017) and coronary heart disease (Theorell et al., 2016; Dragano et al., 2017). Most of the evidence is, however, based on studies in Europe. A growing literature also focuses on the possible health consequences of organisational injustice. Although the different types of organisational justice may predict various health-related outcomes, the potential influence of procedural justice on health and well-being is the most documented empirically. Mental health (Elovainio et al., 2010; Nieuwenhuijsen et al., 2010; Ndjaboué et al., 2012; Robbins et al., 2012, Swedish Council on Health Technology Assessment, 2014), the metabolic syndrome (Bergmann et al., 2014), and coronary heart disease (Theorell et al., 2016) have all been shown to be related to lack of procedural justice. However, research on organisational justice and health has yet mainly been performed in Europe particularly in the Scandinavian countries.

Beyond the main models, relatively consistent support is also emerging for associations between work stressors, such as long working hours and job insecurity, and health outcomes. Recently a large-scale study has related long working hours to coronary heart disease and stroke (Virtanen et al., 2015). Some evidence also links long working hours to poorer mental health such as depressive symptoms (Bannai and Tamakoshi, 2014; Theorell et al., 2015). Similarly, job insecurity has been associated with coronary heart disease (Virtanen et al., 2013), diabetes (Ferrie et al., 2016) and musculoskeletal problems (Lang et al. 2012). The relationship with coronary heart disease was, however, partly attributed to poorer socioeconomic circumstances and less favourable profile of risk factors among those with job insecurity (Virtanen et al., 2013).

Overall, there is scientific evidence that indicates associations between various psychosocial working conditions and several physical and mental health conditions although the estimated risks are often small or modest. However, the evidence can still be seen as insufficient to determine whether there are associations on a range of factors beyond the main theoretical models presented in this chapter. More research is needed on the relationship between, for example, organisational justice, long working hours, job insecurity, emotional demands, violence, threats and conflicts, and a range of health outcomes.

## References

Adams, J.S. (1965) Inequity in social exchange. *Advances in Experimental Social Psychology*, 2:267e99.

Amick, B.C., Kawachi, I., Coakley, E.H. et al. (1998) Relationship of job strain and iso-strain to health status in a cohort of women in the United States. *Scandinavian Journal of Work Environment and Health*, 24(1), 54–61.

Aronsson, G., Theorell, T., Grape, T., Hammarström, A., Hogstedt, C., Marteinsdottir, I., Skoog, I., Träskman-Bendz, L. and Hall, C. (2017) A systematic review including meta-analysis of work environment and burnout symptoms. *BMC Public Health*, 17, 264.

Bannai, A. and Tamakoshi, A. (2014) The association between long working hours and health: A systematic review of epidemiological evidence. *Scandinavian Journal of Work Environment and Health*, 40(1), 5–18. doi:10.5271/sjweh.3388.

Bartley, M. (1994). Unemployment and ill health: understanding the relationship. *Journal of epidemiology and community health*, 48(4), 333–337.

Bellavia, G., Frone, M. (2005) Work–family conflict. In: Barling, J., Kelloway, E.K., Frone, M. (Eds), *Handbook of work stress*. Sage Publications, Thousand Oaks, 113–147.

Benavides, F.G., Benach, J., Diez-Roux, A.V. and Roman, C. (2000). How do types of employment relate to health indicators? Findings from the Second European Survey on Working Conditions. *Journal of Epidemiology and Community Health*, 54(7), 494–501.

Bergmann, N., Gyntelberg, F., Faber, J. (2014). The appraisal of chronic stress and the development of the metabolic syndrome: a systematic review of prospective cohort studies. *Endocrinology Connect*, 3(2), R55–80. doi: 10.1530/EC-14-0031. Epub 17/4/2017.

Bies, R.J. and Moag, J.F. (1986). Interactional justice: Communication criteria of fairness. In Lewicki, R.J., Sheppard, B.H., and Bazerman, M.H. (Eds.), *Research on negotiations in organizations* (Vol. 1, 43–55). Greenwich, CT: JAI Press.

Brenner, M.H. (2005). Commentary: Economic growth is the basis of mortality rate decline in the 20th century – experience of the United States 1901–2000. *International Journal of Epidemiology*, 34(6), 1214-1221.

Brenner, M.H. and Mooney, A. (1983). Unemployment and health in the context of economic change. *Social Science & Medicine*, 17, 1125–1138.

Brunner, E. and Marmot, M. (2001). Social organisation, stress and health. In Marmot, M. and Wilkinson, R.G. (Eds). *Social determinants of health*. Oxford University Press: Oxford: 17–43.

Castells, M. (1996). *The rise of the network society*. Oxford: Blackwells.

Chandola, T., Brunner, E., Marmot, M. (2006). Chronic stress at work and the metabolic syndrome: prospective study. *BMJ*, 332(7540), 521–5.

Chungkham, H.S, Ingre, M., Karasek, R. et al. (2013) Factor structure and longitudinal measurement invariance of the demand control support model: an evidence from the Swedish Longitudinal Occupational Survey of Health (SLOSH). *PLoS ONE*, 8(8), e70541.

Coats, D. and Max, C. (2005). *Healthy work: productive workplaces. Why the UK needs more "good jobs"*. London: The Work Foundation. www.theworkfoundation.com/research/healthy_work.jsp

Cohen, S. (1999). Social status and susceptibility to respiratory infections. *Annals New York Academy of Sciences*, 896, 246–253.

de Lange, A.H., Taris T.W., Kompier, M.A.J. et al. (2003). "The very best of the millennium": Longitudinal research and the demand-control-(support) model. *Journal of Occupational Health Psychology*, 8(4), 282–305.

Demerouti, E., Bakker, A., Nachreiner, F., and Schaufeli, W. (2001). The Job demands resources model of burnout. *Journal of Applied Psychology*, 86(3), 499–512.

Dodu, N. (2005). Is employment good for well-being? A literature review. *Journal of Occupational Psychology, Employment and Disability*, 7, 17–33.

Dragano, N., Nyberg, S.T. (2014). Validating abbreviated measures of effort-reward imbalance at work in European cohort studies: the IPD-Work Consortium. *Int Arch Occup Environ Health*, 87(3), 249–56.

Dragano, N., Siegrist, J., Nyberg, S.T. et al. for IPD-Work Consortium. (2017). Effort-reward imbalance at work and incident coronary heart disease: a multi-cohort study of 90,164 individuals. *Epidemiology*. doi: 10.1097/EDE.0000000000000666. [Epub ahead of print]

Elovainio, M., Kivimäki, M., and Vahtera, J. (2002). Organizational justice: evidence of a new psychosocial predictor of health. *American Journal of Public Health*, 92(1), 105–108.

Elovainio, M., Heponiemi, T., Sinervo, T., and Magnavita, N. (2010). Organizational justice and health: Review of evidence. *Giornale Italiano di Medicina del Lavoro ed Ergonomia*, Supplemento B, Psicologia, 32(3), 5–9.

Ezzy, D. (1993).Unemployment and mental health: a critical review. *Social Science & Medicine*, 37, 41–52.

Ferrie, J.E., Virtanen, M., Jokela, M., Madsen, I.E., Heikkilä, K., Alfredsson, L., Batty, G.D., Bjorner, J.B., Borritz, M., Burr, H. and Dragano, N. (2016). Job insecurity and risk of diabetes: a meta-analysis of individual participant data. *Canadian Medical Association Journal*, 188(17-18), pp E447–E455.

Frankenhaeuser, M. and Johansson, G. (1981). Stress at work: psychobiological and psychosocial aspects. *Journal of Applied Psychology*, 35(3), 287–299.

Fransson, E., Nyberg, S.T., Heikkilä, K., et al. (2012). Comparison of alternative versions of the job demand-control scales in 17 European cohort studies: the IPD-Work Consortium. *BMC Public Health*, 20(12), 62. doi: 10.1186/1471-2458-12-62.

Fransson, E.I., Nyberg, S.T., Heikkila, K. (2015). Job strain and the risk of stroke: an individual-participant data meta-analysis. *Stroke*, 46(2), 557–9.

Fryers, T., Melzer, D. and Jenkins, R. (2003). Social inequalities and the common mental disorders. *Social psychiatry and psychiatric epidemiology*, 38(5), 229–237.

Geurts, S.A. and Sonnentag, S. (2006). Recovery as an explanatory mechanism in the relation between acute stress reactions and chronic health impairment. *Scandinavian Journal of Work Environment and Health*, 2(6), 482–92.

Greenberg, J. (1987). A taxonomy of organizational justice theories. *Academy of Management Review*, 12, 9–22.

Heikkila, K., Nyberg, S.T., Theorell, T. et al. for IPD-Work Consortium. (2013). Work stress and risk of cancer: meta-analysis of 5700 incident cancer events in 116,000 European men and women. *BMJ*, 346:f165.

Henkens, K., van Solinge, H. and Gallo, W.T. (2008). Effects of retirement voluntariness on changes in smoking, drinking and physical activity among Dutch older workers. *The European Journal of Public Health*, 18(6), 644–649.

Hinkle, L.E., Whitney, L.H., Lehman, E.W. et al. (1968). Occupation, education and coronary heart disease. *Science*, 161, 238–46.

Jahoda, M. (1982). *Employment and unemployment*. Cambridge: Cambridge University Press.

Jin, R.L., Shah, C.P., Svoboda, T.J. (1995). The impact of unemployment on health: a review of the evidence. *Canadian Medical Association Journal*, 153, 529–540.

Johnson, J. and Hall, E.M. (1988). Job strain, workplace social support and cardiovascular disease: A cross-sectional study of a random sample of the Swedish working population. *American Journal of Public Health*, 78, 1336–42.

Karasek, R.A. (1979). Job demands, job decision latitude and mental strain: implications for job redesign. *Administrative Science Quartely*, 24, 285–307.

Karasek, R. and Theorell, T. (1990). *Healthy work*. New York: Basic Books.

Karasek, R. and Theorell, T. (1992). *Healthy work: stress, productivity, and the reconstruction of working life*. New York: Basic Books.

Katz, D. and Kahn, R.L. (1978). *The social psychology of organizations*. Wiley: New York.

Kivimäki, M., Batty, G.D., Ferrie, J.E., Kawachi, I. (2014). Cumulative meta-analysis of job strain and CHD. *Epidemiology*. 25(3), 464–5. doi: 10.1097/EDE.0000000000000087.

Kristensen, T.S. (2010). A questionnaire is more than a questionnaire. *Scandinavian Journal of Public Health*, 38(3 suppl), 149–55.

Lakey, J. (2001). *Youth unemployment, labour market programmes and health*. London: Policy Studies Institute.

Lang, J., Ochsmann, E., Kraus, T., and Lang, J.W.B. (2012). Psychosocial work stressors as antecedents of musculoskeletal problems: A systematic review and meta-analysis of stability-adjusted longitudinal studies. *Social Science & Medicine*, 75(7), 1163–1174.

Lash, S., and Urry, J. (1987). *The end of organised captialism*. Oxford: Polity Press.

Layard, R. 2004. CEP Occasional Paper No 19 April 2004. *Good jobs and bad jobs*. London: Centre for Economic Performance.

Leineweber, C., Wege, N., Westerlund, H., et al. (2010). How valid is a short measure of effort-reward imbalance at work? A replication study from Sweden. *Occupational and Environmental Medicine*, 67(8), 526–31.

Lindeberg, S.I., Rosvall, M., Choi, B. et al. (2011). Psychosocial working conditions and exhaustion in a working population sample of Swedish middle-aged men and women. *European Journal of Public Health*, 21(2), 190–6.

Lozano, R., Naghavi, M., Foreman, K. et al. (2012). Global and regional mortality from 235 causes of death for 20 age groups in 1990 and 2010: a systematic analysis for the Global Burden of Disease Study 2010. *The Lancet*, 380(9859), 2095–128.

Lynge, E. and Andersen, O. (1997). II: Unemployment and cancer in Denmark, 1970-1975 and 1986-1990, in: M. Kogevinas, N. Pearce, M. Susser and P. Boffetta (eds), *Social inequalities and cancer*. ARC Scientific Publications No. 138. Lyon: International Agency for Research on Cancer.

Madsen, I.E., Hanson, L.L., Rugulies, R. et al. (2014). Does good leadership buffer effects of high emotional demands at work on risk of antidepressant treatment? A prospective study from two Nordic countries. *Social Psychiatry and Psychiatric Epidemiology*.

Madsen, I.E., Nyberg, S.T., Magnusson Hanson, L.L. for IPD-Work Consortium. (2017). Job strain as a risk factor for clinical depression: systematic review and meta-analysis with additional individual participant data. *Psychol Med.* doi: 10.1017/S003329171600355X. [Epub ahead of print].

Magnusson Hanson, L.L., Leineweber, C., Chungkham, H.S. and Westerlund, H. (2014). Work-home interference and its prospective relation to major depression and treatment with antidepressants. *Scandinavian Journal of Work, Environment & Health*, 40, 66–73.

Marmot, M.G. (2004). *The status syndrome: how social standing affects our health and longevity*. 1st American ed. New York: Times Books

Marmot, M., Friel, S., Bell, R., et al. 2008. Closing the gap in a generation: health equity through action on the social determinants of health. *The Lancet*, 372, 1661–9.

Mather, L., Bergström, G., Blom, V., Svedberg, P. (2015). High Job Demands, Job Strain, and Iso-Strain are Risk Factors for Sick Leave due to Mental Disorders: A Prospective Swedish Twin Study With a 5-Year Follow-Up. *Journal of Occupational and Environmental Medicine*, 57(8), 858–65. doi: 10.1097/JOM.0000000000000504.

Mathers, C.D., Schofield, D.J. (1998). The health consequences of unemployment: the evidence. *Medical Journal of Australia*, 168, 178–182.

McEwen, B.S. and Wingfield, J.C. (2003). The concept of allostasis in biology and biomedicine. *Hormones and Behavior*, 43(1), 2–15.

Monroe, S.M. (2008). Modern approaches to conceptualizing and measuring human life stress. *Annual Review of Clinical Psychology*, 4, 33–52.

Moorman, R.H. (1991). Relationship between organizational justice and organizational citizenship behaviors: Do fairness perceptions influence employee citizenship? *Journal of Applied Psychology*, 76(6), 845.

Murphy, G.C, Athanasou, J.A. (1999). The effect of unemployment on mental health. *Journal of Occupational and Organizational Psychology*, 72: 83–99.

Murray, C.J., Vos, T., Lozano, R. et al. (2012). Disability-adjusted life years (DALYs) for 291 diseases and injuries in 21 regions, 1990–2010: a systematic analysis for the Global Burden of Disease Study 2010. *The Lancet*, 380, 2197–2223.

Ndjaboué, R., Brisson, C., and Vézina, M. (2012). 'Organisational justice and mental health: a systematic review of prospective studies', *Occupational and Environmental Medicine*, 69, 694–700.

Nieuwenhuijsen, K., Bruinvels, D., and Frings-Dresen, M. (2010). Psychosocial work environment and stress-related disorders, a systematic review. *Occupational Medicine*, 60, 277–286.

Nordenmark, M. and Strandh, M. (1999). Towards a sociological understanding of mental well-being among the unemployed: the role of economic and psychosocial factors. *Sociology*, 33, 577–597.

Nyberg, S.T., Fransson, E.I., Heikkila, K. et al. for IPD-Work Consortium. (2013). Job strain and cardiovascular disease risk factors: meta-analysis of individual-participant data from 47,000 men and women. *PLoS ONE*, 8(6), e67323.

Nyberg, S.T., Fransson, E.I., Heikkila, K. et al. for IPD-Work Consortium. (2014). Job strain as a risk factor for type 2 diabetes: a pooled analysis of 124,808 men and women. *Diabetes Care*, 37(8), 2268–2275.

Pejtersen, J.H., Kristensen, T.S., Borg, V., Bjorner, J.B. (2010). The second version of the Copenhagen Psychosocial Questionnaire. *Scandinavian Journal of Public Health*, 38(3 Suppl), 8–24.

Platt, S. (1984). Unemployment and suicidal behaviour: a review of the literature. *Social Science & Medicine*, 19, 93–115.

Polanyi, M., and Tompa, E. (2004). Rethinking work-health models for the new global economy: A qualitative analysis of emerging dimensions of work. *Work*, 23, 3–18.

Prüss-Üstün, A. and Corvalán, C. (2006). *Preventing disease through healthy environments: Towards an estimate of the environmental burden of disease*. Geneva: World Health Organization.

Robbins, J.M., Ford, M.T., and Tetrick, L.E. (2012). Perceived unfairness and employee health: A meta-analytic integration. *Journal of Applied Psychology*, 97(2), 235–272.

Rugulies, R., Aust, B., Madsen, I.E. (2017). Effort-reward imbalance at work and risk of depressive disorders. A systematic review and meta-analysis of prospective cohort studies. *Scandinavian Journal of Work, Environment & Health*. doi: 10.5271/sjweh.3632. [Epub ahead of print]

Saunders, P. and Taylor, P. 2002. *The price of prosperity. The economic and social costs of unemployment*. University of New South Wales Press, Sydney.

Saunders, P. 2002. *The direct and indirect effects of unemployment on poverty and inequality* (SPRC discussion paper 118). Sydney: Social Policy Research Centre. www.sprc.unsw.edu.au/dp/DP118.pdf

Selye, H. (Ed). (1980). *Selyes guide to stress research*. New York: Van Nostrand Reinhold Company.

Shah, H., Marks, N. (2004). *A well-being manifesto for a flourishing society*. London: New Economic Foundation.

Shortt, S.E.D. (1996). Is unemployment pathogenic? A review of current concepts with lessons for policy planners. *International Journal of Health Services*, 26, 569–589.

Siegrist, J. (1996). Adverse health effects of high effort-low reward conditions at work. *Journal of Occupational Health Psychology*, 1, 27–43.

Siegrist, J., Wege, N., Puhlhofer, F., Wahrendorf, M. (2009). A short generic measure of work stress in the era of globalization: effort-reward imbalance. *International Archives of Occupational and Environmental Health*, 82(8), 1005–13.

Sparks, K., Faragher, B. and Cooper, C.L. (2001). Well-being and occupational health in the 21st century workplace. *Journal of Occupational and Organizational Psychology*, 74, 489–509.

Swedish Council on Health Technology Assessment. (2014). *Occupational Exposures and Back Disorders*. Stockholm: Swedish Council on Health Technology Assessment (SBU), 2014 Oct. SBU Yellow Report No. 227. SBU Systematic Review Summaries.

Tabanelli, M.C., Depolo, M., Cooke, R.M., Sarchielli, G., Bonfiglioli, R., Mattioli, S. and Violante, F.S. (2008). Available instruments for measurement of psychosocial factors in the work environment. *International Archives of Occupational and Environmental Health*, 82(1), 1–12.

Theorell, T., Hammarström, A., Aronsson, G. (2015). A systematic review including meta-analysis of work environment and depressive symptoms. *BMC Public Health*, 1(15), 738. doi: 10.1186/s12889-015-1954-4.

Theorell, T., Perski, A., Åkerstedt, T. (1988). Changes in job strain in relation to changes in physiological state. A longitudinal study. *Scandinavian Journal of Work Environment and Health*, 14, 189–196.

Ursin, H. and Eriksen, H.R. (2004). The cognitive activation theory of stress. *Psychoneuroendocrinology*, 29(5), 567–592.

Van der Doef, M., Maes, S. and Diekstra, R. (2000). An examination of the job demand-control-support model with various occupational strain indicators. *Anxiety, Stress, and Coping*, 13, 165–185.

Virtanen, M., Nyberg, S.T., Batty, G.D. et al. for IPD-Work Consortium. (2013). Perceived job insecurity as a risk factor for incident coronary heart disease: systematic review and meta-analysis. *BMJ*, 347, 4746. doi: 10.1136/bmj.f4746.

Warr, P. (1987). *Work, unemployment, and mental health*. Oxford: Oxford University Press.

Whiteford, H.A, Degenhardt, L., Rehm, J. (2013). Global burden of disease attributable to mental and substance use disorders: findings from the Global Burden of Disease Study 2010. *The Lancet*, 382(9904), 1575–86.

THREE

# Work environment, health and the international development agenda

*Martin Hyde and Töres Theorell*

## Introduction

Global sociopolitical developments including increased economic globalisation, the spread of neo-liberal ideas, the changing nature of work, the development of information and communication technology, and significant demographic changes have had a major impact on the nature of today's working conditions (Hyde et al., 2006; Kompier, 2006; EU-OSHA, 2007). As a result, psychosocial conditions in the workplace have been identified as significant emerging risks in the global public health agenda (NIOSH, 2002; EU-OSHA 2007). Towards the end of 2015 the UN launched the Sustainable Development Goals which it hopes will 'free the human race from the tyranny of poverty and want and [will] heal and secure our planet for present and future generations' (Maurice, 2015). Among the list of 17 goals it has identified the need to 'Promote sustained, inclusive and sustainable economic growth, full and productive employment, and decent work for all' (Goal 8) as a key issue. This builds on the previous Millennium Development Goal that committed the international community to 'achieve full and productive employment and decent work for all, including women and young people'. It is reassuring to see the UN continues to recognise the centrality of decent work for ensuring good health and well-being among the population. This is even more pressing when considered alongside the latest results from the Global Burden of Disease project which show that non-communicable diseases, such as cardiovascular disease, are on the increase in developing countries. These diseases have long been associated with poor working conditions in Europe and North America (Wilkinson et al., 2003; Marmot and Wilkinson, 2005). Hence combatting these conditions and promoting decent work in developing countries will be key to ensuring a healthy workforce in these countries. Encouragingly there is evidence that occupational health and safety priorities in developing countries have changed during the last decade and there is greater awareness about psychosocial risks and addressing work-related stress, violence, harassment and unhealthy behaviours (Kortum and Leka, 2014).

## Vulnerable and insecure employment

A first step to meeting the goal to create decent jobs for all must be ensuring that all workers have secure employment. Job insecurity has been shown to have a deleterious effect on the health of employees and their families in a wide range of studies (Ferrie, 2001; Wilkinson et al., 2003). A study of 16 European countries, covering all parts of the continent, found that workers with insecure jobs were at an increased risk of poor health in most of these countries (László et al., 2010). This is supported by longitudinal data from the Whitehall II study in the UK, one of the longest running occupational health studies, which showed that prolonged job insecurity was associated with higher self-reported morbidity and increased blood pressure (Ferrie et al., 2002). Similarly, a US study found that persistent perceived job insecurity is a significant predictor of poorer self-rated health among American workers (Burgard et al., 2009). These findings are particularly concerning as the rates of job insecurity and (new forms of) precarious working, such as zero-hours contracts, are on the rise throughout Europe and North America (Standing, 1997; Standing, 2011).

However, to date there is little work that has looked at the impact of job insecurity on the health and well-being of workers in developing countries. Yet it is assumed that economic globalisation and market liberalisation have led to increasing job insecurity in these countries (Loewenson, 2001; Huynen et al., 2005; Swende et al., 2008). Although the evidence base is relatively low, two Taiwanese studies have shown that job insecurity was strongly associated with poor health (Cheng et al., 2005) and psychological distress (Yiengprugsawan et al., 2015). Moreover, the prevalence of job insecurity was high with half of all employees reporting it. However, rates were even higher among employees with lower education attainment, in blue-collar and construction workers, those employed in smaller companies, and in older women (Cheng et al., 2005). These figures are extremely disturbing as they suggest that almost half of those in work in developing countries could be at risk of poor physical and psychological health due to working in unsecure or precarious jobs. Meanwhile, it must be acknowledged that there has been an increased intensification of work among those in employment in middle income countries. As Gómez Ortiz and Juárez-García (2016) observe Mexico, Costa Rica and Chile have the longest working hours in the Organisation for Economic Co-operation and Development (OECD), while over 50% of Peruvian workers report doing 48 hours of overtime a week.

Hence, if the UN, other international agencies and national governments are to create decent jobs for all and promote health and well-being in all developing countries, it is important that we get an idea of the extent of insecure employment in these countries. To begin to do this we have used data from the International Labour Organization (ILO) on rates of what it calls 'vulnerable employment' and linked these to data on healthy life expectancy from the Global Burden of Disease study (Murray et al., 2015). Figure 3.1 shows the proportions of men and women in various developing countries who are in vulnerable employment according to the ILO. Vulnerable employment is defined as those working as unpaid family workers or own-account workers. Furthermore, the ILO states that those who occupy these labour market positions 'are less likely to have formal work arrangements, and are therefore more likely to lack decent working conditions, adequate social security and "voice" through effective representation by trade unions and similar organisations. Vulnerable employment is often characterised by inadequate earnings, low productivity and difficult conditions of work that undermine workers' fundamental rights' (2010). The data clearly show that although there are wide variations among these countries there are still significant proportions of workers in precarious positions. Over half of both male and female workers in some countries, such as Vietnam and Azerbaijan, are in vulnerable employment. These figures are highest in Tanzania where almost 80% of women workers and 69% of male workers are trapped in this type of work. Even in countries with relatively low rates of vulnerable employment, such as Malaysia and Venezuela, around a quarter of workers experience these conditions. These figures show that there are significant challenges for governments and international non-governmental organisations to realise the goal of creating decent working conditions in all countries.

Figures 3.2 and 3.3 show the relation between the proportion of male and female employees in vulnerable employment and healthy life expectancy at the national level. To explore this relationship more widely, developed countries have been included. The results for both women and men show that as the proportion of those in

**Figure 3.1: Proportion of men and women in vulnerable employment as a % of total employment in 2013: selected countries**

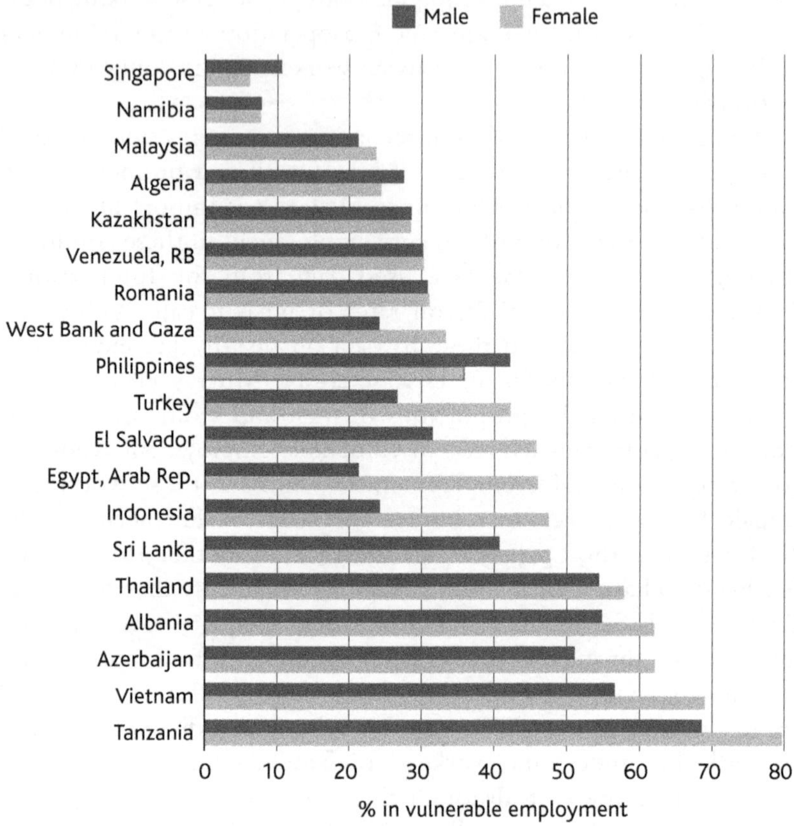


*Source:* World Bank (http://data.worldbank.org/indicator)

vulnerable employment increases the average number of years someone can expect to remain in good health decreases. The strength of this negative relationship is stronger for women (r=–0.53) than for men (r=–0.41). However, it is important to remember that these results are based on aggregate cross-sectional data and therefore we need to be cautious when interpreting them as there are doubtless other factors that might contribute to both these measures. Nonetheless, in conjuncture with existing research, these initial findings do suggest that insecure work is prevalent in developing countries and that this might contribute to poor health in these countries. To explore this further it is important to look at how people feel about their work and how it relates to their health.

**Figure 3.2: Relationship between proportion in vulnerable employment and healthy life expectancy in 2013: women**

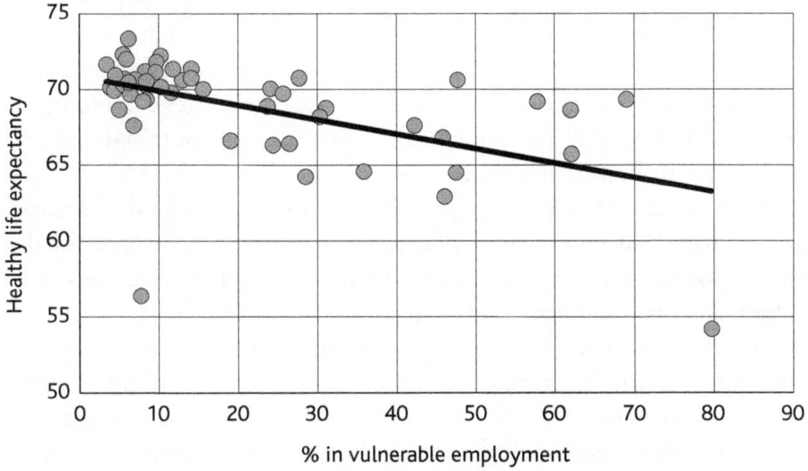


*Source:* World Bank (http://data.worldbank.org/indicator)

**Figure 3.3: Relationship between proportion in vulnerable employment and healthy life expectancy in 2013: men**

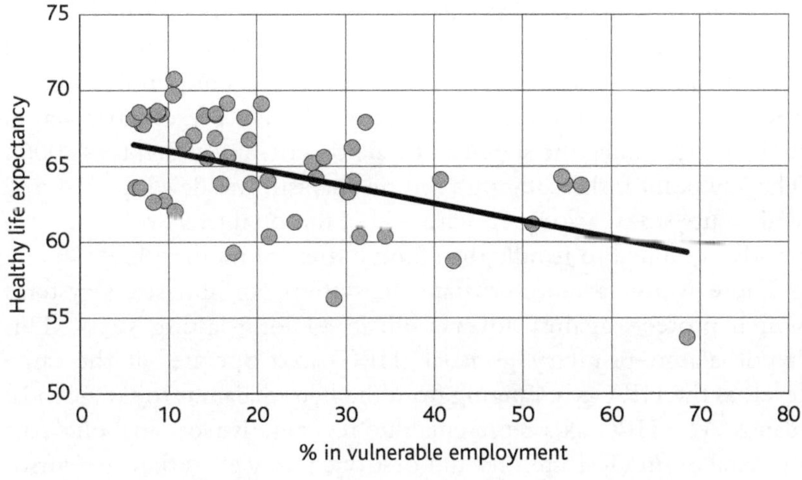


*Source:* World Bank (http://data.worldbank.org/indicator)

## Psychosocial working conditions and health in developing countries

There is a long tradition of psychosocial work environment research in Europe and the USA. This stretches back to the early 1990s and some key developments can be identified in the development of this field of research. Early research in this area developed out of primate studies which looked at the impact of hierarchies on health. Drawing on these studies Professor Sir Michael Marmot argued that those at the bottom of the hierarchy suffered from chronic stress responses which caused them to have poorer health. The notion that stress, in biological terms, is responsible for poor health was not new but Marmot and colleagues placed it in a socio-environmental context (Marmot and Wilkinson, 2005). Crucially, external stressors, such as deprivation, are mediated through a range of intermediate levels or factors. Finally, the exposure is assessed via some forms of psychological processes which in turn stimulate a biological response. The model that they draw on to explain this socio-psychological-biological response is the 'fight-or-flight' mechanism. The mechanism for flight-or-fight response involves two main pathways which coordinate a range of metabolic and physiological actions. These are the sympathy-adrenal pathway and the hypothalamic-pituitary-adrenal (HPA) axis. They are known collectively as the neuroendocrine pathways. The former releases almost instantaneous levels of noradrenaline and adrenaline into the blood. Although this has many functions key among them are to stimulate the heart to pump greater amounts of blood through the body, thus oxygenating the muscles for action, and the brain to increase alertness. Overall the effect is one of increased psychological arousal and energy mobilisation. The HPA axis is responsible for the release of cortisol into the bloodstream. This is a pre-emptive action designed to reduce the shock and scale of any injury (Steptoe, 2006). The key point is that although this mechanism was developed to deal with acute stress, associated with early Homo sapiens evolution, it is poorly equipped to handle the chronic stress of modern life.

There is also a counterbalancing system (an anti-stress system) which protects against adverse effects of long-lasting stress. This hypothalamo–pituitary–gonadal (HPG) axis operates at the same levels as the HPA axis, ranging from the hypothalamus to the gonadal glands. The HPG axis represents the 'regenerative' or 'anabolic' part of metabolism. Testosterone and oestrogen, as well as their precursor dehydroepiandrosterone sulphate (DHEA-S), are examples of corticosteroids with a mainly anabolic/regenerative function. DHEA-S facilitates regeneration. Other hormones also participate in this, such as the pituitary growth hormone. There is a balance between the HPA axis and the HPG axis. This means that the HPG axis tends to lower its activity when the HPA axis has maximal activity (in stressful situations). It also means that damaging effects of long-lasting stress can be dampened by high activity in the HPG axis. Thus, the balance between HPA and HPG activity is an important principle in health promotion. Hence from this position it is not sufficient that the employer simply reduces or eliminates adverse work environment conditions, they also have a responsibility for developing positive factors that can promote good health (EU-OSHA, 2013).

A second major field of psychosocial research that has developed has been around the role of work. The psychobiological pathways that are seen to cause poor health are similar to those already described, but rather than status being viewed as the main risk factor for stress it is working practice. In fact, one of the main criticisms of the Whitehall II findings is that it did not initially control for working conditions which might differ across grades and be responsible for the gradient, thus making the conclusion that status was responsible spurious (Bosma et al., 1997). This approach has been labelled the psychosocial work environment approach. There are two main and distinct models in this approach (Bosma et al., 1998). The first and most longstanding is known as the demand-control model, developed by Karasek and Theorell (Karasek and Theorell, 1992), and the second is known as the effort-reward imbalance model (ERI), developed by Siegrist and colleagues (2004). Despite their differences, they share a similar fundamental approach – if you have a poor working environment, whether it is measured by having too many demands and not enough control or by receiving insufficient rewards for your effort, you will experience stress and if this becomes chronic then your health will suffer.

To date most of the research in this field has come from developed countries. There is now a fairly robust body of research that shows that a poor work environment can have a deleterious effect on a wide range of physical and psychological dimensions of health (Wilkinson et al., 2003; Nyberg et al., 2013; Heikkila et al., 2013a,b; Heikkila et al., 2014a,b,c; Nyberg et al., 2014). However, to date, there is relatively little research on the impact of the psychosocial work environment on health in middle and low income countries. Kortum-Margot (2001) has stressed the need for systematic studies to examine the effects of psychosocial work factors in developing countries where work-related stress and other occupational illnesses remain under-reported and underestimated. This is all the more urgent as a number of these countries, notably the BRIC countries (Brazil, Russia, India and China), are undergoing rapid rates of economic development with continued rates of industrialisation coupled with the emergence of a substantial service sector. In short, we are seeing the growth of the types of jobs which are characterised by these psychosocial working conditions. According to the ILO (2016) there is a significant and growing prevalence of poor psychosocial working conditions among workers in middle and low income countries. For example, in the first Korean Working Conditions Survey carried out in the Republic of Korea (2006), work-related stress affected 18% of male and 15% of female workers, and was significantly related to working hours and job demands. In the second Korean Working Conditions Survey (2010), overall fatigue had increased from 18% in 2006 to 27% in 2010. A similar picture emerges from the Americas. According to the First Central American Survey on Working Conditions and Health (2012) over 10% of respondents reported having felt constantly under stress or strain due to concerns about work. In Argentina, the First National Survey on Employment, Work Conditions, Labour Environment and Health (2009) showed that over a quarter of workers reported that their workload was excessive. In Chile, according to the 7th National Survey of Working Conditions (2011), over a quarter of workers reported that stress and depression were present in their enterprises. In Colombia, according to the first National Survey on Working Conditions and Health on the General System of Occupational Risks (2007), a quarter of male workers and 28% of female workers ranked their level of stress as very high. However, to date there is no information on the prevalence or incidence of psychosocial risks and work-related stress in Africa and the Arab States.

These figures suggest that, alongside more traditional occupational health risks, the emergence of these psychosocial risks could also have an impact on the health of workers in developing countries. Indeed, the research that does exists suggests that this is the case. Studies from China (Yu et al., 2008), Taiwan (Cheng et al., 2005), Thailand (Yiengprugsawan et al., 2015), Iran (Yadegarfar et al., 2013) and Russia (Pikhart et al., 2004) have all shown that workers with a poor psychosocial work environment experience worse physical and psychological health. More recently in a comprehensive review of the state of research in China on work stress and health, using the effort-reward imbalance model, Li (2016) found that an effort-reward imbalance was strongly associated with an increased risk of poor mental health, high blood pressure, coronary heart disease and musculoskeletal disorders. Likewise, in their review of the literature on ERI and health in Latin America Gómez Ortiz and Juárez-García (2016) found that an effort-reward imbalance was associated with poorer mental health, depression, lower quality of life, worse self-rated health and poor health behaviours, including alcohol and drug use.

In India research in this field is rapidly emerging, led by a number of excellent scholars and producing interesting findings (Rajadhyaksha and Smita, 2004; Cowling et al., 2014). Earlier research (Singh and Wherry, 1963; Lahiri and Choudhuri, 1966; Rao and Ganguly, 1971) showed that Indian factory workers tended to be more concerned with material factors, such as job security, than 'psychological' factors, such as learning on the job. However, as Saiyed and Tiwari (2004) observe globalisation and rapid industrial growth have resulted in the emergence of occupational health-related issues in India. This is supported by Mohan and colleagues (2008) who found that lack of control over work, hazardous conditions and employment status led to job strain among Indian steel workers. However, the study was rather limited (N=54) and the authors recommend a large-scale study for the country as a whole to be able to generalise their findings. A more recent study in two Indian provinces found that work environment factors, such as challenging work, were important for job satisfaction for health workers (Peters et al., 2010). Similarly, in their study of rural development workers in India Duraisingam and Dollard (2005) found that high job demands had a significant impact on the risk of exhaustion, while high poor job demands and low rewards contributed to levels of psychological distress. In a study of 129 IT workers in India, Darshan and colleagues (2013) found that over half of the workforce reported work-related stress and that those who had high levels of stress were more likely to be depressed and have a higher prevalence of harmful alcohol use. Roy and Chowdhury (2013) also find that poor working conditions lead to poor health and poor health behaviours. Studies among call centre workers in India show that that employees in this sector suffer from high levels of stress which leads to poorer sleep and a range of physical health complaints (Rameshbabu et al., 2013). Basnet and colleagues (2010) also found significant associations between occupational stress and physical, emotional and social life including limitations of day-to-day activities in their study of people employed as underground construction workers in Sikkim.

These studies strongly suggest not only that poor psychosocial working conditions are a real factor in developing countries but that they are having the same negative impact on health that has been seen in developed countries. To explore these issues in a wider number of countries we can use data from the most recent wave of the World Valiues Survey from 2013. In this study respondents were asked several questions about their work which, although not exactly the same as the more established measures, map on to key dimensions of the work environment. These are 1) whether work is more manual or more intellectual, 2) whether work is more routine or more creative and 3) the degree of independence they have at work. Each of these was measured on a 10-point scale with a high score indicating a more preferable type of work. The mean values for a wide number of countries are presented in Figures 3.4 to 3.6.

The results show some key findings about the nature of work in developing countries. On average work tends to be more manual than intellectual (Figure 3.4). In some countries, such as Brazil, Mexico and Morocco, there appears to be very little intellectual work. Indeed very few countries have scores towards the intellectual end of the scale. Perhaps unsurprisingly the pattern for routine versus creative types of work follows a similar pattern. Hence work is not only overwhelmingly more manual it is also quite routine in these countries. The results for the degree of independence that people can exert at work are more positive. Here workers in some countries, such as the Philippines, Mexico and Thailand, report that they have a good deal of independence at work. However, there are still countries, including India, where workers feel that they have less independence.

The effects of globalisation on work environments have been discussed by other authors (Moutsatsos, 2009). Globalisation is seen to have left workers in developing countries unprotected and therefore at greater risk of having to work in adverse working conditions and accept low wages. A key historical reason for this is that rates of unionisation have been slow and the unions are perceived to be largely ineffective in these countries. In many countries, this is a product of years of either powerful opposition to the unionisation of the workforce and/or the political control and corruption of the major unions. This turbulent history has left its mark and, as a result, old-fashioned leadership styles are still prevalent among managers. For instance, in an ethnographic study of the working conditions in industries in Bangladesh it was shown that supervisors (usually male) in textile factories (with mostly female workers) feel that the most important task for them is to induce fear in the employees (Ashraf and Strümpell, 2011). This authoritarian approach to management has been shown to have serious health consequences for employees (Hyde et al., 2006) and goes against human relations and organisational psychology research on the benefits of transformational styles of leadership.

Structured interview studies of Bangladeshi workers have shown that key work stress components partly differ from those in Western workplace settings (Steinisch et al., 2013). This is not surprising in view of the differences in historical contexts between developing and

**Figure 3.4: The degree to which work is manual or intellectual: selected countries, 2013**

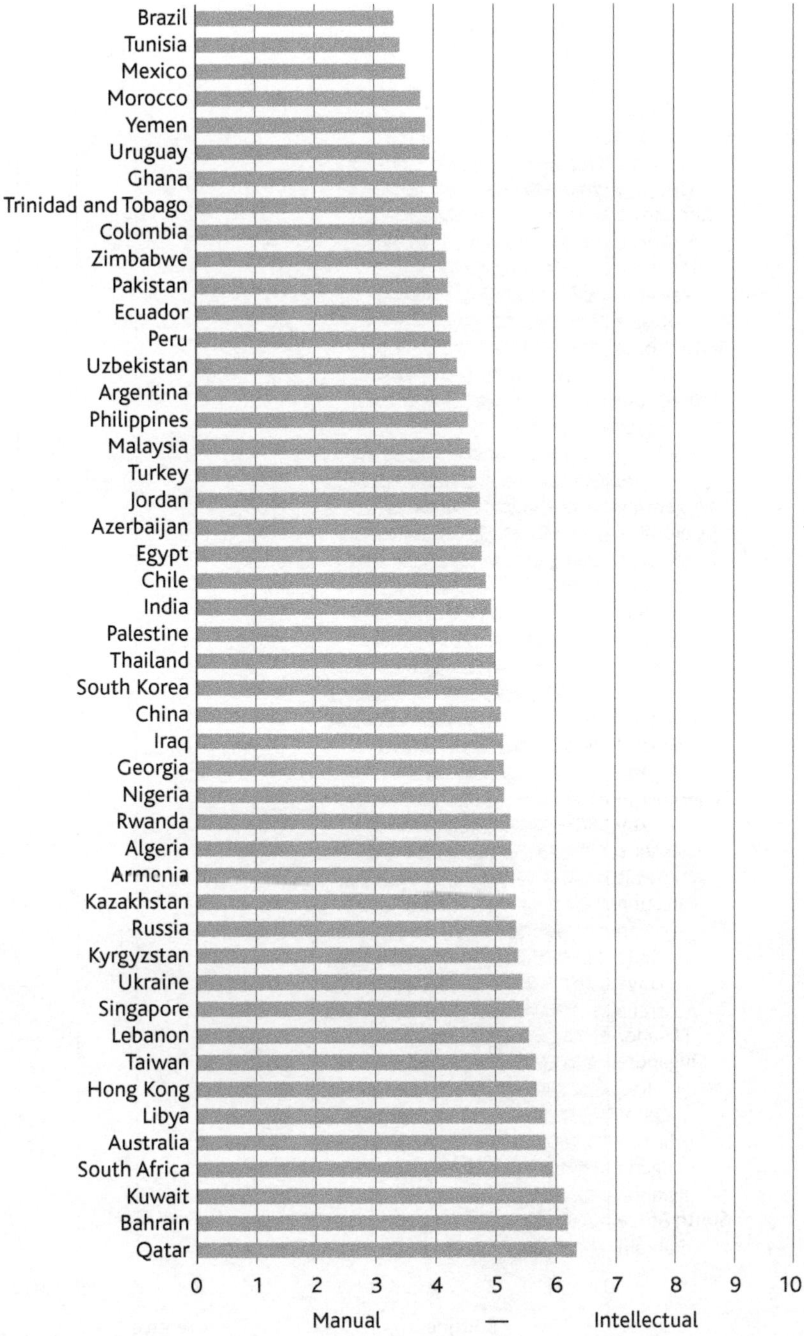


*Source:* International Social Survey Programme (ISSP)

**Figure 3.5: The degree to which work is routine or creative: selected countries, 2013**

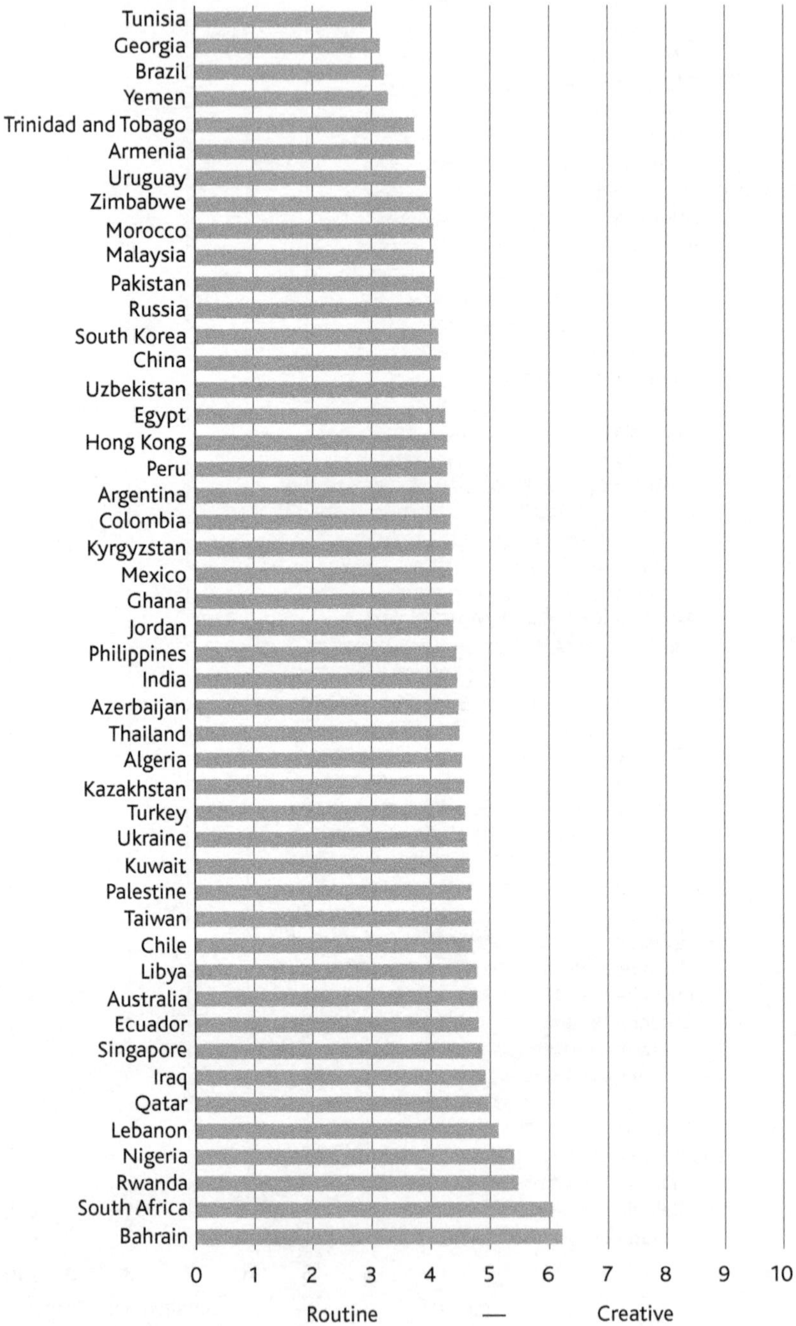


*Source:* ISSP

**Figure 3.6: The degree of independence at work: selected countries, 2013**

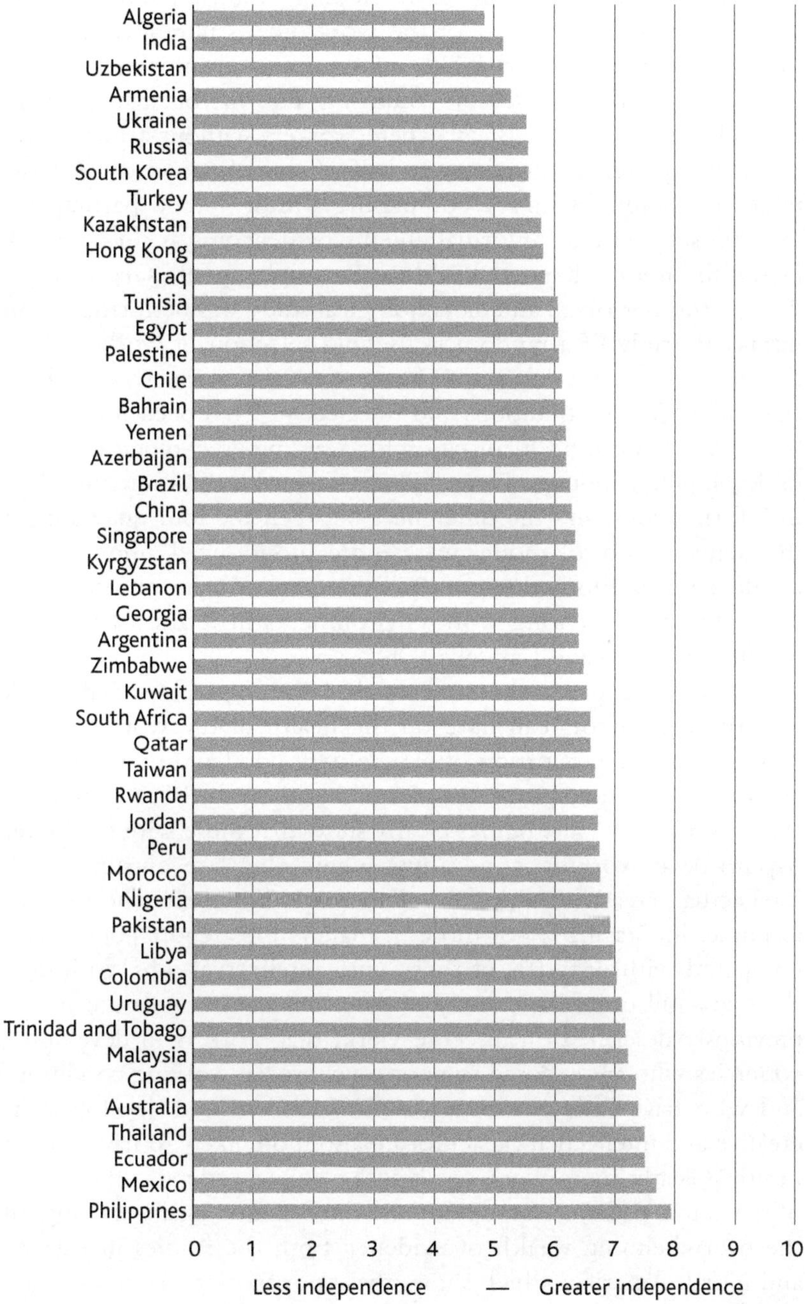


*Source:* ISSP

developed countries. Accordingly, psychosocial work research must be adapted to the conditions in developing countries, and must also take into account that part of the workforce is illiterate. Another important difference is that the informal sector comprises a large part of the workers in several countries. This has been in focus in research for instance in Brazil where workers without a formal job contract represent approximately half of the labour force. A large national household survey comprising almost 90,000 participants in 2003 showed that 'informal' unemployment was as strong a risk factor for poor self-rated health as unemployment (Giatti et al., 2008). Another Brazilian epidemiological study was performed as an interview study of a random household selection of workers. The demand-control model (Job Content Questionnaire) was used for assessing working conditions and the SRQ-20 has been introduced by the World Health Organization for assessing psychological distress in developing countries. Overall ill mental health was more prevalent in informal jobs, and the differences between the four quadrants of the demand-control model were more pronounced among those employed in the formal sector. Still the demand-control model was useful for differentiating work environments in relation to mental health (de Araújo and Karasek 2008).

Finally, to explore the impact that these psychosocial work environment factors can have on the health of the workforce we shall look at the proportion of people with good and poor working environments who report poor general health in the BRIC countries (Figures 3.7–3.9). The figures clearly show that those with the better psychosocial working conditions, where they are engaged with intellectual, creative and independent work, have better health. For example, in Brazil 31% of those in manual jobs report poor health compared with just 19% of those with intellectual jobs. Although these are still quite basic analyses they indicate, as with the results previously described on insecure work, that workers in developing countries who are exposed to poor psychosocial working conditions and who have little chance to be independent and develop their creative and intellectual capacities are also more likely to have poorer health. Clearly more work needs to be done to identify the nature of the causal pathways between these factors. But, again drawing on the overwhelming wealth of evidence from the studies in Europe and North America, which shows that poor working conditions are more likely to cause poor health than vice versa, these results should raise serious concerns for the health of the workforce in developing countries.

**Figure 3.7: Proportion of people in manual and intellectual jobs who report poor health in the BRIC countries**

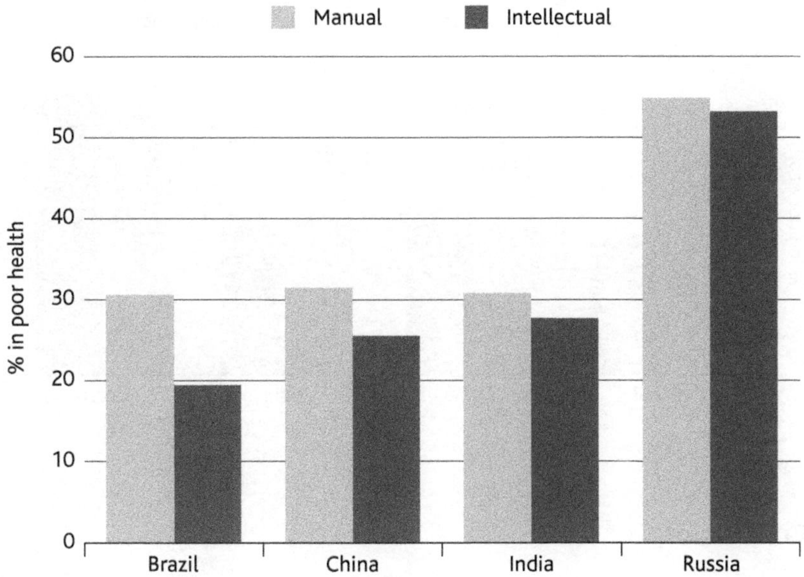


*Source:* ISSP

**Figure 3.8: Proportion of people in routine and creative jobs who report poor health in the BRIC countries**

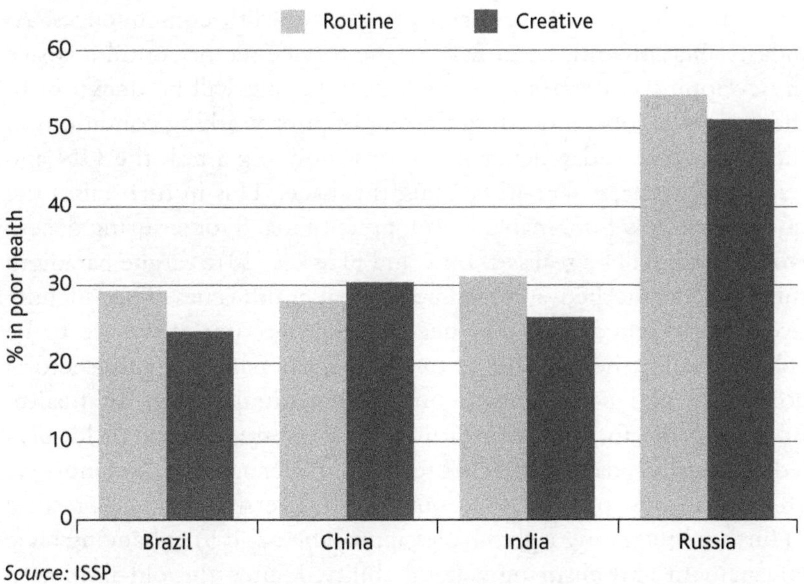


*Source:* ISSP

**Figure 3.9: Proportion of people with more or less independence at work who report poor health in the BRIC countries**

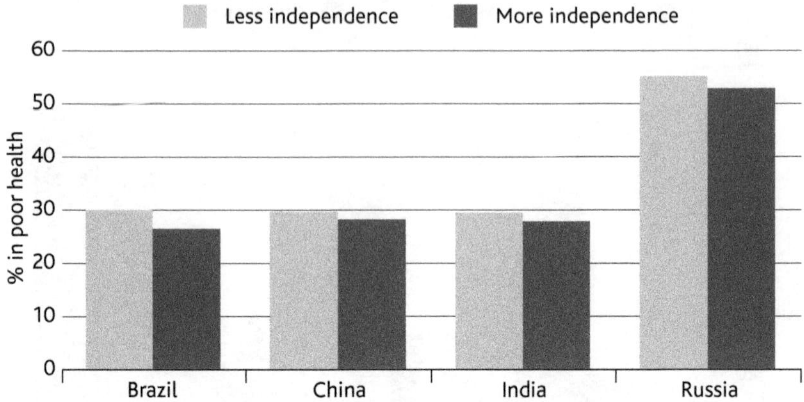


*Source:* ISSP

## Conclusion

The launch of the Sustainable Development Goals in 2015 is a welcome addition in the fight to secure decent work and ensure health and well-being in developing countries. For decades research from Europe and North America has consistently shown that being exposed to poor psychosocial working conditions, such as not having sufficient control to meet the demands at work or being inadequately rewarded for your efforts, can have serious negative health consequences. As industrialisation and the growth of the service sector continue apace in developing countries more and more people will be drawn in to these types of jobs. Indeed, the extent of poor working conditions in these countries today demonstrates just how big a task the UN and associated agencies face in tackling this issue. This in turn raises the question of how Sustainable Development Goal 8, of ensuring decent work for all, will be realised. Buse and Hawkes (2015) argue paradigm shift is needed in the way we address global health issues. They identify five key challenges that will need to be overcome if we are to be able to realise these goals: 1) ensuring leadership for intersectoral coherence and coordination on the structural drivers of health; 2) shifting the focus from treatment to prevention through locally-led, politically-smart approaches to a far broader agenda; 3) identifying effective means to tackle the commercial determinants of ill-health; 4) further integrating rights-based approaches; and 5) enhancing civic engagement and ensuring accountability. Hence the old-fashioned top-down, state-led approach based on the medical model of health is no longer adequate. To achieve these goals, we will need a different, multi-actor, network-based approach that puts public health at the centre and seeks to prevent poor health and promote well-being for all.

## References

Ashraf, H. and Strümpell, C. (2011). Stress and modern work: ethnographic perspectives from industries in Bangladesh. *Viennese Ethnomedicine Newsletter*, 13, 24-33.

Basnet, P., Gurung, S., Pal, R., et al. (2010). Occupational stress among tunnel workers in Sikkim. *Industrial Psychiatry Journal*, 19(1), 13–19. http://doi.org/10.4103/0972-6748.77626.

Bosma, H., Marmot, M.G., Hemingway, H. et al. (1997). Low job control and risk of coronary heart disease in Whitehall II (prospective cohort) study. *BMJ*, 314(7080), 558.

Bosma, H., Peter, R., Siegrist, J., and Marmot, M. (1998). Two alternative job stress models and the risk of coronary heart disease. *American Journal of Public Health*, 88(1), 68–74. doi:10.2105/AJPH.88.1.68

Burgard, S.A., Brand, J.E., and House, J.S. (2009). Perceived job insecurity and worker health in the United States. *Social Science & Medicine*, 69(5), 777–785. doi:http://dx.doi.org/10.1016/j.socscimed.2009.06.029

Buse, K., and Hawkes, S. (2015). Health in the sustainable development goals: ready for a paradigm shift? *Global Health*, 11(1), 13. Retrieved from http://www.globalizationandhealth.com/content/11/1/13

Cheng, Y., Chen, C., Chen, C., and Chiang, T. (2005). Job insecurity and its association with health among employees in the Taiwanese general population. *Social Science & Medicine*, 61, 41–52.

Cowling, K., Dandona, R., and Dandona, L. (2014). Social determinants of health in India: progress and inequities across states. *International Journal for Equity in Health*, 8(13), 1.

de Araújo, T.M. and Karasek, R. (2008). Validity and reliability of the job content questionnaire in formal and informal jobs in Brazil. *SJWEH Supplements*, 6, 52–59.

Duraisingam, V., and Dollard, M.F. (2005). The management of psychosocial risk factors amongst rural development workers in India. *International Journal of Rural Management*, 1(1), 97–123.

Darshan, M.S., Raman, R., Rao, T.S. (2013). A study on professional stress, depression and alcohol use among Indian IT professionals. *Indian Journal of Psychiatry*, 55(1), 63–69.

EU-OSHA. (2007). *Expert forecast on emerging psychosocial risks related to occupational safety and health*. Luxembourg: Office for Official Publications of the European Communities.

EU-OSHA. (2013). *Well-being at work: creating a positive work environment*. Luxembourg: Publications Office of the European Union.

Ferrie, J. E. (2001). Is job insecurity harmful to health? *Journal of the Royal Society of Medicine*, 94(2), 71–76. Retrieved from http://www.ncbi.nlm.nih.gov/pmc/articles/PMC1297910/

Ferrie, J.E., Shipley, M.J., Stansfeld, S.A., and Marmot, M.G. (2002). Effects of chronic job insecurity and change in job security on self reported health, minor psychiatric morbidity, physiological measures, and health related behaviours in British civil servants: the Whitehall II study. *Journal of Epidemiology and Community Health*, 56(6), 450–454. doi:10.1136/jech.56.6.450.

Giatti, L., Barreto, S.M. and César, C.C. (2008). Informal work, unemployment and health in Brazilian metropolitan areas, 1998 and 2003. *Cadernos de Saúde Pública*, 24(10), 2396–2406.

Gómez Ortiz, V. and Juárez-García, A. (2016). Working Conditions and Effort-Reward Imbalance in Latin America. In: Siegrist, J. and Wahrendorf, M. (Eds.), *Work Stress and Health in a Globalized Economy, Aligning Perspectives on Health, Safety and Well-Being*. Springer International Publishing: Switzerland: 235–271.

Heikkila, K., Fransson, E.I., Nyberg, S.T. et al. for IPD-Work Consortium. (2013a). Job Strain and Health-Related Lifestyle: Findings From an Individual-Participant Meta-Analysis of 118 000 Working Adults. *American Journal of Public Health*, 103(11), 2090–2097. doi:10.2105/ajph.2012.301090

Heikkila, K., Nyberg, S.T., Theorell, T., et al. for IPD-Work Consortium. (2013b). Work stress and risk of cancer: meta-analysis of 5700 incident cancer events in 116 000 European men and women. *BMJ*, 346. doi:10.1136/bmj.f165

Heikkila, K., Madsen, I.E.H., Nyberg, S.T. et al. for IPD-Work Consortium. (2014a). Job Strain and the Risk of Inflammatory Bowel Diseases: Individual-Participant Meta-Analysis of 95 000 Men and Women. *Plos One*, 9(2), doi:10.1371/journal.pone.0088711

Heikkila, K., Madsen, I.E.H., Nyberg, S.T. et al. for IPD-Work Consortium. (2014b). Job strain and COPD exacerbations: an individual-participant meta-analysis. *European Respiratory Journal*, 44(1), 247–251. doi:10.1183/09031936.00205113

Heikkila, K., Madsen, I.E.H., Nyberg, S.T. et al. for IPD-Work Consortium. (2014c). Job strain and the risk of severe asthma exacerbations: a meta-analysis of individual-participant data from 100 000 European men and women. *Allergy*, 69(6), 775–783, doi:10.1111/all.12381

Huynen, M.M., Martens, P., and Hilderink, H.B. (2005). The health impacts of globalization: a conceptual framework. *Global Health*, 1, 14. doi:10.1186/1744-8603-1-14.

Hyde, M., Jappinen, P., Theorell, T. and Oxenstierna, G. (2006). Workplace conflict resolution and the health of employees in the Swedish and Finnish units of an industrial company. *Social Science & Medicine*, 63, 2218–2227.

ILO. (2010). Vulnerable employment and poverty on the rise, Interview with ILO chief of Employment Trends Unit. Retrieved from http://www.ilo.org/global/about-the-ilo/newsroom/features/WCMS_120470/lang--en/index.htm.

ILO. (2016). *Workplace stress: A collective challenge*. International Labour Organization: Geneva.

Karasek, R., and Theorell, T. (1992). *Healthy Work: Stress, Productivity, and the Reconstruction of Working Life*. New York: Basic Books.

Kompier, M.A.J. (2006). New systems of work organization and workers' health. *Scandinavian Journal of Work Environment and Health*, 32(6, special issue), 421–430.

Kortum, E., and Leka, S. (2014). Tackling Psychosocial Risks and Work-Related Stress in Developing Countries: The Need for a Multilevel Intervention Framework. *International Journal of Stress Management*, 21(1), 7–26. doi:10.1037/a0035033

Kortum-Margot, E. (2001). Psychosocial Factors in the Workplace. *The Global Occupational Health Network*, 2, 7–10. http://www.who.int/och/OCHWeb/OSHpages/ Gohnet/GOHNET2/ Gohnet2English.pdf

Lahiri, D.K. and Choudhuri, P.K. (1966). Perceived importance of job factors by technical and nontechnical employees. *Personnel Psychology*, 19(3), 287–296.

László, K.D., Pikhart, H., Kopp, M.S. et al. (2010). Job insecurity and health: A study of 16 European countries. *Social Science & Medicine*, 70(6), 867–874. doi:http://dx.doi.org/10.1016/j.socscimed.2009.11.022

Li, J. (2016) Working Conditions and Health in China: Evidence on the ERI Model. In: Siegrist, j and Wahrendorf, M. (Eds.), *Work Stress and Health in a Globalized Economy, Aligning Perspectives on Health, Safety and Well-Being*. Switzerland: Springer International Publishing, 219–234

Loewenson, R. (2001). Globalization and occupational health: a perspective from southern Africa. *Bulletin of the World Health Organization*, 79, 863–868. Retrieved from http://www.scielosp.org/scielo.php?script=sci_arttextandpid=S0042-96862001000900012andnrm=iso

Marmot, M., and Wilkinson, R. (2005). *Social Determinants of Health*, 2nd edition. Oxford: Oxford University Press.

Maurice, J. (2015) UN set to change the world with new development goals. *The Lancet*, 386(9999), 1121–1124. doi:10.1016/S0140-6736(15)00251-2

Mohan, G.M., Elangovan, S., Prasad, P.S.S., et al. (2008). Prevalence of job strain among Indian foundry shop floor workers, *Work*, 30, 353–357.

Moutsatsos, C. (2009). Economic globalization and its effects on labor. In: PL Schnall, M. Dobson and E. Rosskam (eds), *Unhealthy work: Causes, consequences and cures*, Amityville, NY: Baywood Press, pp 21-36.

Murray, C.J.L., Barber, R.M., Foreman, K.J. (2015). Global, regional, and national disability-adjusted life years (DALYs) for 306 diseases and injuries and healthy life expectancy (HALE) for 188 countries, 1990–2013: quantifying the epidemiological transition. *The Lancet*, Online first. doi:10.1016/S0140–6736(15)61340-X

NIOSH. (2002). The changing organization of work and the safety and health of working people: Knowledge gaps and research directions. *NIOSH* (Vol. 2002-116): DHHS (NIOSH).

Nyberg, S.T., Fransson, E.I., Heikkila, K. for IPD-Work Consortium. (2013). Job Strain and Cardiovascular Disease Risk Factors: Meta-Analysis of Individual-Participant Data from 47,000 Men and Women. *Plos One*, 8(6). doi:10.1371/journal.pone.0067323.

Nyberg, S.T., Fransson, E.I., Heikkila, K. for IPD-Work Consortium. (2014). Job Strain as a Risk Factor for Type 2 Diabetes: A Pooled Analysis of 124,808 Men and Women. *Diabetes Care*, 37(8), 2268–2275. doi:10.2337/dc13-2936.

Peters, D.H., Chakraborty, S., Mahapatra, P. and Steinhardt, L. (2010). Job satisfaction and motivation of health workers in public and private sectors: cross-sectional analysis from two Indian states. *Human resources for health*, 8(1), 27.

Pikhart, H., Bobak, M., Pajak, A. (2004). Psychosocial factors at work and depression in three countries of Central and Eastern Europe. *Social Science & Medicine*, 58(8), 1475–1482. doi:http://dx.doi.org/10.1016/S0277-9536(03)00350-2.

Rajadhyaksha, U., and Smita, S. (2004). Tracing a Timeline for Work and Family Research in India. *Economic and Political Weekly*, 39(17), 1674–1680. doi:10.2307/4414926.

Rameshbabu, A., Reddy, D.M., and Fleming, R. (2013). Correlates of negative physical health in call center shift workers. *Applied Ergonomics*, 44(3), 350–354. doi:10.1016/j.apergo.2012.09.002.

Rao, G.S. and Ganguly, T. (1971). Perceived need satisfaction and importance of supervisory and clerical personnel. *Indian Journal of Psychology*, 46, 31–43.

Roy, S.K. and Chowdhury, T.K. (2013). Differences in Selected Health Traits between Occupational Groups among Oraons of Jalpaiguri District, West Bengal. *Journal of Anthropology*. doi:10.1155/2013/582036.

Saiyed, H.N. and Tiwari, R.R. (2004). Occupational health research in India. *Industrial Health*, 42(2), 141–148.

Siegrist, J., Starke, D., Chandola, T. (2004). The measurement of effort–reward imbalance at work: European comparisons. *Social Science & Medicine*, 58(8), 1483–1499. doi:http://dx.doi.org/10.1016/S0277-9536(03)00351-4.

Singh, P.N. and Wherry, R.J. (1963). Ranking of job factors by factory workers in India. *Personnel Psychology*, 16(1), 29–33.

Standing, G. (1997). Globalization, Labour Flexibility and Insecurity: The Era of Market Regulation. *European Journal of Industrial Relations*, 3(1), 7–37. doi:10.1177/095968019731002.

Standing, G. (2011). *The Precariat: The New Dangerous Class*. London: Bloomsbury Academic.

Steinisch, M., Yusuf, R., Li, J., Rahman, O., Ashraf, H.M., Strümpell, C., Fischer, J.E. and Loerbroks, A. (2013). Work stress: Its components and its association with self-reported health outcomes in a garment factory in Bangladesh – findings from a cross-sectional study. *Health & Place*, 24, 123–130.

Swende, T.Z., Sokpo, J., and Tamen, F.I. (2008). Globalization and health: a critical appraisal. *Nigerian Journal of Medicine*, 17(2), 135–138.

Wilkinson, R.G., Marmot, M.G. (2003). *Social Determinants of Health: The Solid Facts*. Geneva: World Health Organization, Regional Office for Europe.

Yadegarfar, G., Alinia, T., Hosseini, R. (2013). Psychometric properties of the Farsi version of effort-reward imbalance questionnaire: a longitudinal study in employees of a synthetic fibre factory in Iran. *International Archives of Occupational and Environmental Health*, 86(2), 147–155. doi:10.1007/s00420-012-0750-z.

Yiengprugsawan, V., Lazzarino, A., Steptoe, A. et al. (2015). Psychosocial job characteristics, wealth, and culture: differential effects on mental health in the UK and Thailand. *Global Health*, 11(1), 31. Retrieved from http://www.globalizationandhealth.com/content/11/1/31

Yu, S., Gu, G., Zhou, W. and Wang, S. (2008). Psychosocial work environment and well-being: a cross-sectional study at a thermal power plant in China. *J Occup Health*, 50(2), 155–162.

FOUR

# Employment trends in India: Some issues for investigation

*A.V. Jose*

## Introduction

During the last 20 years, the Indian economy has grown dramatically, at around 6% per year in real terms in the 1990s, rising to more than 7% at the start of the 21st century. Over this period India became the second fastest-growing large economy, second only to China (Dreze and Sen, 2014). As we try to understand the direction and magnitude of changes taking place in India in relation to key variables such as labour force, employment and income it is important to look at some historical antecedents of the experience of western industrial economies during the 19th century. Labour market analysts have long argued that long-term economic growth sets in motion profound structural changes in the size and composition of the economy and concomitantly that of the labour force. The changes that unfolded in western industrial economies since the onset of the Industrial Revolution, studied at length by scholars in the tradition of Simon Kuznets (1972) and Angus Maddison (2003), provide fascinating insights into the manner in which history might repeat itself in developing countries that are currently at the threshold of experiencing major structural changes. This will help us to place the development of the Indian labour market in a historical perspective and perhaps also equip us to formulate labour market policies appropriate to the time and space in which we find ourselves. To do this, we need to start with a brief review of changes that have impacted on the size and composition of the labour force in the industrial economies during the 19th and 20th centuries. This is crucial as it was also a period of demographic explosion and a pronounced increase in the size of the labour force. These developments occurred along with significant increases in the productivity of labour and a conspicuous shift of population and workforce from agriculture towards more productive sectors of the economy.

The most important consequence of rising productivity levels was that it set the stage for radical improvements in the living standards of people in the industrial economies. Associated with this rise in living standards was yet another unparalleled phenomenon, a reduction in the drudgery of work, which can be seen in the evidence of a consistent decline in the number of hours worked per person per year. The rise in productivity and reduction in working hours signalled the advent of technological changes that reduced the toil of work and facilitated a substantial entry of new workers, in particular women, into the paid labour force. These were indeed tectonic changes in the world of work, set against the background of an emerging industrial society.

Some of these changes, captured in the long-term quantitative data compiled by Angus Maddison (2003) are presented in Table 4.1. The figures are for total employment, gross domestic product (GDP) per person employed, GDP per hour worked and annual hours worked per person. They correspond to averages during a period stretching from 1870 to 1998 among 12 countries of Western Europe.[1] The figures show that during a span of 120 years, when the employed population of these countries doubled itself, GDP per person employed increased 8-fold. More importantly during the same period, productivity per hour worked increased by a factor of 15 and there was a consistent decline in the hours worked per person per annum from 1,293 in 1870 to 657 by 1998.

**Table 4.1: Indicators of employment in western Europe**

| | 1870 | 1913 | 1950 | 1973 | 1990 | 1998 |
|---|---|---|---|---|---|---|
| Total employment in western Europe (000 at mid-year) | 72,030 | 104,152 | 111,383 | 130,215 | 140,806 | 140,213 |
| Labour productivity GDP$/hour worked in 1990* | 1.61 | 3.12 | 5.54 | 16.21 | 24.06 | 28.53 |
| Annual hours worked per head of population | 1,295 | 1,181 | 904 | 750 | 701 | 657 |
| Employment in western Europe, as % of population* | 44.4 | 45.7 | 43.4 | 43.3 | 45 | 43.5 |

*Note:* *Weighted average of 12 western European countries.

*Source:* Maddison (2003), Tables E-1, E-3, E-7, B-10

[1] The countries are: Austria, Belgium, Denmark, Finland, France, Germany, Italy, Netherlands, Norway, Sweden, Switzerland and the United Kingdom.

The long-term changes in employment and productivity could be read together with a more impressive set of data on changes in the sectoral composition of the workforce in the industrialising countries as compiled by another eminent economic historian: Simon Kuznets (1972). His data are somewhat more difficult to compress into a simplified table, for they correspond to different countries at different points of time. Some representative figures from his compilation are summarised in Table 4.2. Countries included in the table are Great Britain (1801–1951), France (1866–1951), Netherlands (1899–1947), Italy (1871–1951), United States (1870–1980) and Japan (1872–1960). In all these countries, starting with Great Britain which pioneered the Industrial Revolution and ending with Japan, an Asian agrarian economy which entered the industrialisation era only in the latter half of the 19th century, there were significant reductions in the relative share of the agricultural workforce along with impressive increases in the share of manufacturing and service industries.

Kuznets' study on the growth experience of nations is a prodigious piece of work full of rich and incisive observations on the chain of causation and synergy underlying various factors of production and factor incomes leading to a rapid increase in income and consumption levels under the aegis of modern economic growth. It is worth summarising some of these observations, since they help us place the empirical evidence on the labour market situation in India at the right historical juncture and to postulate some predictive hypotheses about its likely course of evolution.

During the entire period of structural transformation, the growth rates of productivity per worker in agriculture fell short of corresponding rates in the manufacturing and service industries. This in turn spurred the shift of population towards urban locales

**Table 4.2: Distribution of labour force among three major sectors in selected countries at the start and end of long periods of change as % share of the total labour force**

| | | Agriculture | | Industry | | Services | |
|---|---|---|---|---|---|---|---|
| | | Start | End | Start | End | Start | End |
| Great Britain | 1801–1951 | 35 | 5 | 29 | 57 | 36 | 38 |
| France | 1866–1951 | 43 | 20 | 38 | 47 | 19 | 33 |
| Netherlands | 1899–1947 | 28 | 17 | 36 | 37 | 36 | 46 |
| Italy | 1871–1951 | 51 | 35 | 35 | 40 | 14 | 25 |
| USA | 1870–1950 | 51 | 12 | 30 | 45 | 19 | 43 |
| Japan | 1872–1960 | 85 | 33 | 6 | 35 | 9 | 32 |

*Source:* Kuznets (1972) Table 3.2, 106

and to more productive or remunerative sectors of the economy. Urbanisation in itself was a profoundly important factor that led to huge migratory movements of people all over the industrialising world. For instance, in the UK, which had already attained high levels of urbanisation during the 18th century, the share of the population living in urban areas reached 81% by 1951. In Germany close to 70% of people lived in urban areas by 1939 while in the USA, urbanites accounted for 60% of the population by 1950.[2] A declining share of agriculture in the total labour force also meant a substantial drop in the share of self-employed and own account workers. The obverse of this phenomenon was a trend towards a rising share of employees. For instance, in the USA, which was well on its way to becoming an industrial powerhouse by the early 20th century, the share of employees in the labour force increased to 93% by 1960. A rising share of the category of employees meant that the factor share of employee compensation or wages became the principal source of income for most of the workforce in the industrial economies and a prime determinant of further economic growth. Modern economic growth led to changes in the structure of the employed labour force in terms of age distribution, occupational status and sex composition. As for age distribution, there was a substantial rise in the age of entry into the labour force and a reduction in the age of retirement. As the combined share in the labour force of the very young and the very old declined, workers become concentrated in the prime age groups thus contributing to a higher efficiency and to a narrow spread of age-specific attributes. In terms of occupational status, there has been a general shift of employees from wage earners or blue-collar workers to salaried people or white-collar workers, reflecting a change in industrial structure with a decline in the share of commodity-producing sectors and a rise in the share of service sectors. The causal factors behind this change, such as technological changes and a rising demand for professional, technical, managerial and skilled labour, were conditioned by the stage of economic development attained in the country concerned. The proportion of women among employees increased throughout the period of modern economic growth. In the USA the proportion increased from 23% in 1900 to 34% by 1960. The occupational groups that showed the greatest increase within total body of employees – professional, technical, clerical, sales and service workers – were characterised by large proportions of women workers.

[2] Detailed data on urbanisation are in Table 5.8 of Kuznets (1972).

## Recent labour market developments

Many countries of the industrialised world, notably in Western Europe, followed the pathways to the maturation of their labour markets as charted by Kuznets. Their passages coincided with the evolution of labour market institutions that currently safeguard the rights and entitlements of workers in the industrial societies. The development of labour markets culminated in the establishment of a European social model that sought to guarantee most workers resident in the European Union secure employment based on open-ended contracts and improved terms and conditions of work together with minimal disparities in wages.

Some figures relating to the maturing of labour markets that build on earlier work (Jose, 2008) are presented in Tables 4.3 to 4.5. The indicators examined are: employment population ratios, age-specific and skill-specific unemployment rates, and the presence of atypical forms of employment. The data refer to a representative sample of five large countries of the European Union: France, Germany, Italy, Spain and the United Kingdom.

Table 4.3 gives the employment population ratios for men and women in the age group 15 to 64 years for selected years from 1990 to 2011. In most cases these ratios have been rising, especially for women, which shows that new income-earning opportunities have been opened to ever-growing numbers of people. Figures in Table 4.4 give a more detailed view of the employment and unemployment situation in 2011. The employment population ratios and unemployment rates among men and women in the working age groups, cross-classified by their educational attainments, are given in the table. The three levels of education taken into account – less than upper secondary, upper secondary and tertiary – are reasonable proxies for the skill content of

**Table 4.3: Employment population ratios (age 15–64 years) in selected European countries**

| | Male | | | | Female | | | |
|---|---|---|---|---|---|---|---|---|
| | 1990 | 1998 | 2006 | 2011 | 1990 | 1998 | 2006 | 2011 |
| France | 69.7 | 66.6 | 67.5 | 68.2 | 50.3 | 52.4 | 57.1 | 59.7 |
| Germany | 75.7 | 72.5 | 72.8 | 77.4 | 52.2 | 56 | 61.4 | 67.7 |
| Italy | 72 | 66.7 | 70.5 | 67.5 | 36.4 | 37.1 | 46.3 | 47.2 |
| Spain | 71 | 67 | 77.3 | 63.2 | 31.6 | 35.7 | 54 | 52.8 |
| UK | 82.1 | 78.1 | 78.4 | 75.4 | 62.8 | 64.2 | 66.8 | 65.3 |

*Source:* OECD Employment Outlook, 2002, 2004, 2007, 2010 and 2013, Statistical Annex, Table B

Table 4.4: Employment and unemployment rates among men and women aged 25–64 by educational attainment, 2011

| | France | | Germany | | Italy | | Spain | | UK | |
|---|---|---|---|---|---|---|---|---|---|---|
| | Men | Women | Men | Women | Men | Women | Men | Women | Men | Women |
| **Employment rates** | | | | | | | | | | |
| Less than upper secondary | 62.7 | 49.4 | 66.7 | 49.2 | 67.9 | 33.1 | 61.6 | 41.9 | 66.1 | 47.9 |
| Upper secondary education | 78.1 | 69 | 82.1 | 73.1 | 81.3 | 62.6 | 74.2 | 60.8 | 82.8 | 72.9 |
| Tertiary education | 87.2 | 81 | 91 | 84 | 84.9 | 74.3 | 82.1 | 75.8 | 87.7 | 78.9 |
| **Unemployment rates** | | | | | | | | | | |
| Less than upper secondary | 12.5 | 13.3 | 15.7 | 12.1 | 8.4 | 11.3 | 25.5 | 27.8 | 12.2 | 9.6 |
| Upper secondary education | 6.6 | 8.4 | 6.2 | 5.4 | 5 | 7.1 | 17.6 | 21.2 | 5.8 | 6 |
| Tertiary education | 4.6 | 5.1 | 2.3 | 2.7 | 3.9 | 6.3 | 10.7 | 12.6 | 4 | 3.8 |

*Source:* OECD 2013, Statistical Annex, Table D

workers. As we move up the educational scale, employment population ratios for both men and women are found to rise by significant margins. There is a pronounced decline in the rate of unemployment as we move up the skill categories. The figures show that progress made in industrial economies by way of extending higher education has drawn more skilled workers into the labour force and effectively minimised the probability of their unemployment.

People's perceptions of own employment status are clearly brought out by the reported rates of unemployment. There is a high probability of skilled workers – both men and women – operating in a sellers' market and thereby making voluntary choices to accept full-time or part-time employment. In this regard, there is a case for viewing the huge influx of part-time workers into the labour markets of industrial economies from a supply side optic. However, many of us, conditioned to accept the universality of the post-war construct of employment in industrial societies – full-time and life-time jobs – are inclined to see the ascent of atypical forms of employment, especially part-time jobs, with scepticism.

The figures presented in Table 4.5 on gendered patterns of part-time employment as a share of total employment and the share of women in total part-time employment suggest that among the countries under review, there has been a gradual increase in the share of part-time employment and that its incidence has always been higher among women by a factor of four to five over the average for men. However, we also observe that increases in part-time employment are more evident among men than women. This is related to another

**Table 4.5: Part-time employment as a percentage of total employment**

| | | 1990 | 1994 | 1998 | 2002 | 2006 | 2008 | 2012 |
|---|---|---|---|---|---|---|---|---|
| France | Male | 4.4 | 5.3 | 5.8 | 5.2 | 5.2 | 5.2 | 5.9 |
| | Female | 21.7 | 24.5 | 25 | 24.1 | 22.6 | 22.7 | 22.4 |
| Germany | Male | 2.3 | 3 | 4.6 | 5.5 | 7.6 | 7.9 | 8.7 |
| | Female | 29.8 | 28 | 32.4 | 35.3 | 38.8 | 38.3 | 37.8 |
| Italy | Male | 3.9 | 4.2 | 4.9 | 4.9 | 5.5 | 6.1 | 7.5 |
| | Female | 18.2 | 20.6 | 22.4 | 23.5 | 29.3 | 30.6 | 32.3 |
| Spain | Male | 1.4 | 2.4 | 2.9 | 2.5 | 3.8 | 3.8 | 6.1 |
| | Female | 11.5 | 14.3 | 16.6 | 16.4 | 21 | 21 | 22.9 |
| UK | Male | 5.3 | 7 | 8.2 | 9.1 | 9.9 | 10.2 | 12.2 |
| | Female | 39.5 | 41.2 | 41.2 | 40 | 38.7 | 37.7 | 39.4 |

*Source:* OECD Employment Outlook, 2002, 2004, 2007, 2009 and 2013 Statistical Annex Table E

observation that, over the years, women have accounted for more than three-quarters of the total volume of part-time employment.

Do these developments portend to a qualitative deterioration of labour market conditions? Perhaps it is too early to arrive at such a prognosis. Yet the data do point to the need for a structured analysis of the supply price of labour and time disposition of people who newly enter labour markets, particularly women workers. In this regard, we need to take into account the historical trend noted earlier of a continuous decline in the hours worked per person in the industrialised world. Quite possibly the gradual reduction of working time points to a situation where workers are gaining greater leverage over their work and leisure. Even if we make allowance for the extent to which this downward trend could have been influenced by a rising share of part-time work, we cannot underrate its importance as an indicator of qualitative improvements in the living standards of workers in industrial economies.

An important observation from the European experience is that the growth of GDP and worker productivity would remain prominent explanatory variables underlying the growth of employment and structural changes in labour markets. This in turn depends on how Europe would position itself in maintaining the momentum of growth in an era of rapid globalisation. The evidence suggests that by and large the industrial economies are placed at vantage points and endowed with sufficient resources and political consensus for policy responses that could take them to higher levels of productivity and employment.

With active labour markets policies embedded in policy responses, Europe is in a better position to offer labour market protection, which is conceptually a different kind of protection, to all its incumbents. It builds on the assumption that workers can acquire the wherewithal to operate in a sellers' market by combining their income security, employment flexibility and mobility in labour markets. The underlying European social model is premised on a pervasive presence of the state in public policy space, organising the material resource required to govern markets and to influence outcomes in terms of employment and incomes of the industrialised world.

## Developments in the Indian labour market

Our review of data on long-term structural changes in labour markets of industrialised economies in the preceding section provides a template for assessing similar changes, if any, in the Indian context. Here we will review the employment situation based on some comparable data, albeit for a shorter time horizon, generated through the quinquennial surveys of the National Sample Survey Organization (NSSO). Together these data cover a period of 28 years from the 38th round in 1983 to the 68th round in 2011–12. The period under review is too short to fully explore the related dimensions of long-term changes that occurred in the West. There have, however, been countries in Asian which experienced the entire gamut of changes in product and labour markets within shorter time horizons. The experience of South Korean is a case in point, where significant rises in output, employment and skill levels of the population together with steep falls in fertility and mortality rates have occurred in less than a third of the time taken for similar transition in the West (Oshima, 1994). As globalisation connects more people to the global markets, developing countries, notably India, are poised to undergo a similar transformation of their labour markets.

Following on from the earlier arguments about the importance of the changes in the composition of the labour market in the West, we will review the employment status data on the Indian population by comparing: 1) male and female workers and 2) those belonging to rural and urban areas. The emphasis placed on separating the data into rural and urban components is important as it draws attention to the overwhelmingly rural origins of the population in a country that has less than a 30% level of urbanisation. This is different from the situation noted in any industrially advanced country even in the early stages of industrialisation. We also take a look at changes in the composition of workers into three sectors – primary, secondary and tertiary – and their distribution into two status groups – own account workers and wage employees. We will look at changes in the age and educational composition of the workforce mainly to see what inference can be drawn on the manner in which the labour market is evolving in India. Ideally one should carry out a more disaggregated analysis of data at the level of major states in India, which would provide a rich mine of observations on patterns in the direction of changes under way in different regions.

Between 1983 and 2011–12 the employed workforce of India defined by workers' usual status in principal and subsidiary activities increased from 302 million to 473 million at an annual rate of approximately 1.7%. Between the last two survey rounds held in 2009–10 and 2011–12 the workforce increased by 14 million.[3] These are quite impressive

[3] The figures have been derived from Government of India (2010b) Figure 2, NSSO (Government of India, 2013) Table 8.

numbers judged by the sheer size of the population. However, it is important to further examine these developments by rural and urban locations. First, we take a look at the aggregative worker participation rates from successive rounds of the National Sample Survey (NSS). They seem to suggest a hazy picture and no definitive pattern or trend about the evolution of labour markets.

In terms of worker participation rates we are nowhere near the levels observed among the industrial economies as they came closer to the threshold of becoming mature labour markets (see Table 4.6). The rate for men both in rural and urban areas hover around 55%, which is nothing exceptional when compared with the levels of well over 70% noted in Europe during the 1970s. Nor has there been any discernible rise of the rates in rural areas over 25 years from 1983. In urban areas on the other hand there has been a gradual increase in participation rates of men. The differential worker participation rates noted among women between urban and rural areas point to an interesting pattern emerging in labour markets at an early stage of development. In general, urban areas have lower labour market participation rates. There is also a trend towards a consistent decline of women's participation rates in rural areas over successive rounds of the NSS, while no such trend is visible in urban areas. Put together they suggest that the current tendency towards greater urban migration in India is likely to bring about an overall reduction of worker participation rates among women in the near future.

The figures given in Table 4.7 on sector-wise changes in the distribution of the workforce over different rounds of the NSS give a somewhat more positive picture. There is a clear trend towards decline in the primary sector's share of both male and female workers in rural

**Table 4.6: Worker participation rates according to usual status in different NSS rounds**

| | | Rural | | Urban | |
|---|---|---|---|---|---|
| NSS round | Year | Male | Female | Male | Female |
| 38th | 1983 | 547 | 340 | 512 | 151 |
| 43rd | 1987–88 | 539 | 323 | 506 | 152 |
| 50th | 1993–94 | 553 | 328 | 521 | 155 |
| 55th | 1999–00 | 531 | 299 | 518 | 139 |
| 61th | 2004–05 | 546 | 327 | 549 | 166 |
| 64th | 2007–08 | 548 | 289 | 554 | 138 |
| 66th | 2009–10 | 547 | 261 | 543 | 138 |
| 68th | 2011–12 | 55 | 253 | 563 | 155 |

*Source:* NSSO (2010, Statement 11; 2013B, Statement 1)

**Table 4.7: Distribution (per 1,000) of usually employed people by industry divisions, by area of residence and gender**

| | Primary | | | | Secondary | | | | Tertiary | | | |
|---|---|---|---|---|---|---|---|---|---|---|---|---|
| | Rural | | Urban | | Rural | | Urban | | Rural | | Urban | |
| NSS round | Male | Female | Male | Female | Male | Female | Male | Female | Male | Female | Male | Female |
| 38th | 775 | 875 | 103 | 310 | 100 | 74 | 342 | 306 | 122 | 48 | 550 | 376 |
| 43rd | 745 | 847 | 91 | 294 | 121 | 100 | 340 | 317 | 133 | 52 | 564 | 385 |
| 50th | 741 | 862 | 90 | 247 | 112 | 83 | 329 | 291 | 147 | 56 | 580 | 463 |
| 55th | 714 | 854 | 66 | 177 | 126 | 90 | 328 | 294 | 161 | 58 | 608 | 529 |
| 61st | 665 | 833 | 61 | 181 | 155 | 102 | 344 | 324 | 180 | 66 | 595 | 495 |
| 64th | 665 | 835 | 58 | 153 | 162 | 97 | 343 | 323 | 173 | 68 | 597 | 524 |
| 66th | 628 | 793 | 60 | 139 | 193 | 130 | 346 | 333 | 178 | 76 | 593 | 528 |
| 68th | 594 | 749 | 56 | 109 | 220 | 167 | 353 | 340 | 187 | 83 | 591 | 551 |

*Note:* Primary = agriculture; secondary = mining and quarrying, manufacturing, electricity, water, construction; tertiary = hotel and restaurant, transport, storage and communication, other services.

*Source:* NSSO (2010) Statement 1 and NSSO (2013B) Table 5

and urban areas. Likewise, in the case of male workers in rural areas there is a tangible increase in shares, although in small numbers, of those engaged in the secondary and tertiary sectors. The service sector in urban areas too has shown a distinct tendency to absorb a larger share of the workforce over the years. It should also be noted that the sector is a heterogeneous mix of occupations with wide variation in the skill endowments of people engaged therein.

Tables 4.8 and 4.9 summarise the distribution per 1,000 male and female workers in rural and urban areas categorised into two main status groups: the self-employed and the wage employed, with the latter split into two subcategories: regular employees receiving wages or salaries and casual workers mostly on daily wages. Nothing spectacular emerges from this table and we are unable to identify any pattern of participation rates, except in the case of self-employed male workers in rural areas where there has been a notable decline in the relative numbers in this group. This suggests that they have moved into the ranks of wage employees and picked up jobs either as regular or causal workers. Self-employed women workers in rural areas also tend to move in and out of wage employment.

The data suggest that we are far from realising any sizeable reduction in the share of self-employed men and women in rural areas. Any change in the situation might come about along with extensive urbanisation and an expansion of non-farm employment opportunities in the countryside. However, it is difficult to envisage any major shift in the composition of workforce soon since there are several structural factors that impede such shift. One such factor that deserves closer attention is the presence of a sizeable share of women workers, especially in rural areas, who report subsidiary employment of less than a month's duration as their usual status. In 2011–12 as many as 29.7 million women and 3.6 million men in rural areas reported subsidiary employment status. In urban areas the numbers were comparatively smaller with 4 million women and 1 million men.[4] The social and economic background of the subsidiary status workers varies widely across the states depending on the nature of land distribution, crop pattern and non-farm employment. This remains an interesting area for research as it would provide us with considerable insights into the factors underlying the subsidiary workers' entry or withdrawal from economic activities within the national accounting framework.

---

[4] The figures have been worked out from the population estimates in NSSO (Government of India, 2013, Table 8).

**Table 4.8: Distribution (per 1,000) of usually employed by status in different NSSO rounds: rural areas**

| | Male | | | | Female | | | |
|---|---|---|---|---|---|---|---|---|
| | Self-employed | Regular wage/ salaried | Casual labour | Total wage workers | Self-employed | Regular wage/ salaried | Casual labour | Total wage workers |
| 38th | 605 | 103 | 292 | 395 | 619 | 28 | 353 | 381 |
| 43rd | 586 | 100 | 314 | 414 | 608 | 37 | 355 | 392 |
| 50th | 577 | 85 | 338 | 423 | 586 | 27 | 387 | 414 |
| 55th | 550 | 88 | 362 | 450 | 573 | 31 | 396 | 427 |
| 61st | 581 | 90 | 329 | 419 | 637 | 37 | 326 | 363 |
| 64th | 554 | 91 | 355 | 446 | 583 | 41 | 376 | 417 |
| 66th | 535 | 85 | 380 | 465 | 557 | 44 | 399 | 443 |
| 68th | 545 | 100 | 355 | 455 | 593 | 56 | 351 | 406 |

*Source:* NSSO (2013A) Statement 3 with similar data from earlier rounds and NSS) (2013B) Table S34

**Table 4.9: Distribution (per 1,000) of usually employed people by status in different NSSO rounds: urban areas**

| | Male | | | | Female | | | |
|---|---|---|---|---|---|---|---|---|
| | Self-employed | Regular wage/ salaried | Casual labour | Total wage workers | Self-employed | Regular wage/ salaried | Casual labour | Total wage workers |
| 38th | 409 | 437 | 154 | 591 | 458 | 258 | 284 | 542 |
| 43rd | 417 | 437 | 146 | 583 | 471 | 275 | 254 | 529 |
| 50th | 417 | 420 | 163 | 583 | 448 | 292 | 261 | 553 |
| 55th | 415 | 417 | 168 | 585 | 453 | 333 | 214 | 547 |
| 61st | 448 | 406 | 146 | 552 | 477 | 356 | 167 | 523 |
| 64th | 427 | 420 | 154 | 574 | 423 | 379 | 199 | 578 |
| 66th | 411 | 419 | 170 | 589 | 411 | 393 | 196 | 589 |
| 68th | 417 | 434 | 149 | 583 | 428 | 428 | 143 | 571 |

*Source:* NSSO (2013A) Statement 3 with similar data from earlier rounds and NSSO (2013B) Table S34

It is quite possible that the subsidiary workers form part of a vast reservoir of informal employment hidden in the countryside. The crux of the employment problem in India lies in bringing these workers, invisible in terms of the National Accounts Statistics – most of them women – into the paid labour force and enabling them to move into remunerative employment opportunities. An earlier generation of economists led by K.N. Raj (1957) had debated the problem and its solutions, placing emphasis on two aspects: 1) raising the productivity and thereby the reserve price of labour in the countryside; and

2) creating revolving employment leading to more 'sedimented' employment in the economy. These are the two types of policy interventions falling respectively on the supply and demand sides of the labour market. India's National Rural Employment Guarantee programme is the classic case of an intervention to deal with rural employment on the demand side of the market (Ministry of Rural Development. 2012).[5]

From 1990 onwards the economy registered faster growth, around 8% per annum, and such growth has had an impact on the employment situation. Initially, however, the growth of employment in secondary and tertiary sectors was not particularly impressive, so much so that the first decade of the new millennium was described as one of 'jobless growth' in India. In the light of an insightful analysis of the changing labour situation, Thomas (2015) argued that major structural changes occurred in the Indian economy from the early 2000s and these were reflected in some growth of employment mainly outside of agriculture. Between 2004–05 and 2011–12 the agricultural workforce of India declined by 33 million while the non-agricultural workforce increased by 48 million. A fall in the number of self-employed workers of 13 million was compensated by a rise in the number of regular and causal workers of 41 million.

Thomas (2015) lists two factors that contributed to a withdrawal of workers, both male and female, from agriculture. First is a marked acceleration in the growth of employment in construction in rural areas, a significant part of which occurred in states such as Rajasthan, Uttar Pradesh, Bihar and Madhya Pradesh. This in turn is linked to increased migration towards construction sites in urban areas, which is the case with male workers. Secondly the decline of employment in agriculture went hand in hand with a marked rise in the number of people attending educational institutions. The decline in employment between 2004–05 and 2011–12 was almost entirely among those who were younger than 35 years. These two observations point to what could possibly be done on the supply side of the market (and the limits too) for enhancing the participation and mobility of workers, especially women, in the emerging labour markets of India.

[5] Many analysts of India's employment situation praise the employment creation schemes launched under the auspices of the National Rural Employment Guarantee Act, 2005. The Act sought to guarantee 100 days of paid work to every rural household, which demanded wage employment. It has stipulated that at least a third of all jobs should go to women and women should be entitled to equal wages (2005, Schedule II).

First is the crucial importance of generating domestic migratory flows for which the chain of causation starts with an improvement in public health leading to a reduction in fertility rates. Since the 1990s there have been important developments among states in the heartland of India showing an early stage of demographic transition with a fall in fertility rates and modest rise in educational levels. As a result, relatively young workers are entering the workforce and accounting for a sizeable share of the domestic migrant workforce now visible across the entire country.[6]

Bihar is the typical example of an Indian state where the demographic transition is manifested through increased migration.[7] According to the NSS on Migration held in 2007–08, Bihar has the highest out-migration rate for employment-related reasons (565 per 1,000). Among male workers, who migrate for economic reasons, the proportion resident in other states of India is the highest for Bihar at 84% (NSSO, 2010, Statements 6.3.1, 6.2.1). The emerging pattern of migration, exemplified by Bihar, has important implications for the rest of India.

The NSS data shows that the rate of migration increases as we move up the quintile classes of monthly per capita consumption spending in both urban and rural areas. Concomitantly the rate of migration also increases as we move up the educational categories of people from primary to middle and secondary educational level.[8] Further improvement in income and educational standards of the

[6] Singh et al. (2011) argue that the volume of outmigration increases substantially from low income states towards states offering greater opportunities for employment in the informal economy. Using census data for 1991 and 2001, the authors point out that Bihar and Uttar Pradesh have emerged as the largest sources of net interstate migration for economic reasons. Czaika (2011) has pointed out that interstate migration is increasingly fulfilling the requirements for lesser-skilled labour in states and regions that already account for a larger share of international migrants, who in turn have better skills and higher earning strength.

[7] Literacy in Bihar, though lowest among Indian states, increased from 48% in 2001 to 64% by 2011; the gap with the national average reduced from 17% to 10%. The period saw dramatic improvement in school enrolment ratios. Total fertility rate in Bihar in 2005–06 at 3.9 was still high compared with the all India average of 2.5, indicating that the population is growing faster than in other states (Mukherji and Mukherji, 2012).

[8] The progression is striking among male migrant workers from urban areas where migrant workers are distributed in the following order based on their educational background: not literate – 9.5%; below primary - 13.2%; primary or middle – 20.1%; secondary and higher secondary – 29.1% (NSSO, 2010, Report 533, Table 21).

population is bound to occur, and that would invariably trigger greater migratory flows out of low income regions. Scholars that have studied the situation in Bihar share a view that migration has played an important role in shaping the economy of the state, and that remittances have been an important source of economic support to all migrant labour households.[9] It has been argued that migration resulted in a tightening of rural labour markets through creating labour shortages for agricultural operations. Rodgers and Rodgers (2011) draw attention to the fact that in Bihar, there has been a rise in rural wages, leading to a lowering of wage differentials from what prevailed in western India. Also, there has been an equalisation of rural wages between men and women in the aftermath of migratory flows. The experience of Bihar suggests that a rising worker participation in the non-farm sectors of the economy following demographic changes is liable to be repeated in all low-wage states of India.

The second policy intervention influencing the supply of workers would need to focus on shifting people into more remunerative jobs in the non-farm sector. This goal takes us back to the set of issues posed by Kuznets concerning potential changes in the age composition of workers and their shift towards improved skills and productivity. Here we seem to have a more upbeat picture with some promising developments in the horizon as indicated by the results of the NSSs. From 1993–94 onwards there has been a consistent decline in the worker participation rates of children in the age group 5–14 years. By 2011–12 the ratios came down from 62 to 11 per thousand for girls in rural areas and from 25 to 4 per thousand in urban areas. The corresponding figures for boys came down from 64 to 12 in rural areas and from 36 to 15 urban areas. The ratios still remain stubbornly high and far from an optimal level of zero.

However, there has been an improvement in literacy levels of the working population which indicates that the country as a whole is at an early stage of moving to a convergence in the skill levels of its working population. In 2012 the literacy levels of the population

[9] Thumbe (2011) pointed out that Uttar Pradesh and Bihar have been the top remittance-receiving states, respectively accounting for 20% and 12% of all domestic remittances. Together with Rajasthan, West Bengal and Odisha received more than half of the flow of domestic remittances in 2007–08. In Bihar, 19% of rural households and 10% of urban households received remittances, much of which came from interstate migrants. According to Mukherji and Mukherji (2012) an average remittance-receiving household thus became entitled to an additional income support of Rs. 4,500 per month. Such extra income accounted for as much as 7% of the state domestic product of Bihar.

stood at 717 per thousand for men and 555 per thousand for women in rural areas. The corresponding figures in urban areas were 842 and 747 respectively. The survey also suggests that India is nearer to realising some gains in the skill content of workers. By 2012 in rural areas, 198 per thousand literate men in the age group 15 years and above and 152 per thousand literate women of the same age group had acquired higher secondary and above levels of qualifications. The corresponding figures in urban areas were 420 and 348 respectively.[10] Another observation is that there has been a noticeable increase of female students of the age group 15–19 years, most of who are likely to be pursuing higher education. Between 1999 and 2012 the student–population ratio in that age group increased from 26% to 54% in rural areas and from 52% to 70% in urban areas (Thomas, 2015).

## Conclusion

This chapter attempts to understand the direction and magnitude of changes in key variables such as labour force and employment in relation to some historical antecedents specific to the experience of western industrial economies. The 19th century was a period when major changes affecting the size and composition of the labour force in the West took place together with urbanisation, a shift of workforce from agriculture towards more productive sectors of the economy, ever-increasing living standards and a reduction in the drudgery of work. We also listed some observations made by economic historians, notably Kuznets, on the chain of causation and synergy underlying various factors of production and factor incomes leading to the maturing of labour markets under the aegis of modern economic growth. Further, we reviewed some recent evidence from industrial economies pertaining to the evolution of labour markets that culminated in the establishment of a European social model.

The long-term structural changes that unfolded in the industrial economies are used as a template for assessing similar changes, if any, in the Indian context. We organised a review of the employment situation based on some comparable data for a shorter period from the NSSO. The findings show that India is at the very early stages of a qualitative transformation leading to improvement in worker participation rates along with structural changes in the distribution

[10] Likewise 68 per thousand of literate men and 46 per thousand of literate women in rural areas had qualifications above graduate level; in urban areas the corresponding figures were 231 and 196 respectively. See NSSO (2015, 26–28).

of the workforce into sectors, status groups, gender divisions and skill categories. Nonetheless, there have been some impressive gains in managing the labour market from the supply side by way of improving the age structure and skill content of the workforce. There is, however, a long way to go with the maturing of markets and development of appropriate labour institutions. At best one can only accelerate this process with the right mix of policy interventions.

## References

Czaika, M. (2011). 'Internal and International Migration as a Response to Double Deprivation: Some Evidence from India', Conference Paper, ECONSTOR, ZBW Leibniz Information Center for Economics.

Dreze, J. and Sen, A. (2014). *An Uncertain Glory: India and its Contradictions*. Penguin: London.

Government of India. (2010a). *Annual Report to the People on Employment*, Ministry of Labour and Employment.

Government of India. (2010b). *Migration in India: July 2007–June 2008*, Report No. 533, National Sample Survey Office, Ministry of Statistics and Programme Implementation.

Government of India. (2013). *Key Indicators of employment and Unemployment in India, 2011–2012*, NSS 68th Round, June.

Jose A.V. (2008). Labour Regulation and Employment Protection in Europe: Some Reflections for Developing Countries. *Economic and Political Weekly*, XLIII(22).

Kuznets, S. (1972). *Modern Economic Growth: Rate, Structure and Spread*. New Delhi: Oxford IBH Publishing Company.

Maddison, A. (2003). *The World Economy: A Millennial Perspective*. New Delhi: Overseas India Press Limited.

Ministry of Rural Development. (2012). *Sameeksha, An Anthology of Research Studies on the Mahatma Gandhi Rural Employment Guarantee Act 2005, 2006–2012*. Orient Black Swan.

Mukherji, A. and Mukherji, A. (2012). *Bihar: What Went Wrong? And What Changed?* Working Paper No. 2012-107, New Delhi: National Institute of Public Finance and Policy.

NSSO. (2010). *Employment and Unemployment Situation in India 2007–08, NSS 64th Round (July 2007–June 2008)*, National Sample Survey Office Ministry of Statistics and Programme Implementation Government of India.

NSSO. (2015). *India - Employment and Unemployment, (July 2011–June 2012), NSS 68th Round*, National Sample Survey Office Ministry of Statistics and Programme Implementation Government of India.

Oshima, H.T. (1994). The Impact of Technological Transformation on Historical Trends in Income Distribution of Asia and the West. *Journal of Developing Economies*, 32(3).

Raj K.N. (1957). Employment Aspects of Planning in Underdeveloped Economies, Fiftieth Anniversary Commemoration Lectures. Cairo: National Bank of Egypt.

Rodgers, G. and Rodgers, J. (2011). Inclusive Development? Migration, Governance and Social Change in Rural Bihar. *Economic and Political Weekly*, XLVI (23).

Singh, V.K, Kumar A, Singh R.D, and Yadava K.N.S. (2011). Changing Pattern of Internal Migration in India: Some Evidence from Census Data. *International Journal of Current Research*, 3(4), 289–295.

Thomas, J. (2015). India's Labour Market during the 2000s: An Overview. In K.V. Ramaswamy (Ed.) *Labour, Employment and Economic Growth in India*. Cambridge: Cambridge University Press.

Thumbe, C. (2011). *Remittances in India: Facts and Issues*, Working Paper No. 331, Bangalore: Indian Institute of Management.

FIVE

# Rural-urban and gender differences in time spent in unpaid household work in India

*Laishram Ladusingh*

## Introduction

The well-being of societies and households depends on the daily activities performed by every person, either for monetary compensation or not (Stiglitz et al., 2007). However, many countries do not acknowledge the contribution of unpaid work to human welfare. A clear example of this is that such unpaid work does not form part of the measurement of gross domestic product (GDP), the most commonly used measure to determine the economic performance of a country and to make international comparisons. This oversight has led to the neglect and discrimination of individuals engaged in activities which have no monetary compensation. This is felt particularly acutely among women. Common perceptions and feminist perspectives hold that women's economic contribution is equal to that of men, yet they enjoy less leisure and personal time. Moreover, the contribution they do make is not recognised as it is hidden from statistical accounts and seen as less valuable as it is unpaid. Discriminatory sociocultural practices are reflected in the uneven distribution of time spent on paid and unpaid work by gender. Gender-based divisions of roles and responsibilities in most societies mean that women are much more likely than men to engage in unpaid work. Most of this unpaid work is performed in the household by women and girls, often at the cost of schooling, with no remuneration and includes activities such as cleaning clothes, cooking, serving meals, shopping, caring for children, older people or sick household members, maintaining the garden and making minor household repairs to list but a few. Even when provided outside the household, the services are often at low or no remuneration. For those employed in caring roles such as nursery or school teachers, nurses and domestic workers, wages tend to be low or stagnant.

From the perspective of female empowerment, inequalities in education, health, nutrition, access and control over resources, it is imperative to value time spent by women on unpaid work. Goldschmidt-Clermont and Pagnossin-Aligisakis (1999) have argued that the economic dimension of human labour inputs into household work is of equal importance as labour inputs into market activities. Economists have also accepted for a long time that the monetary value of final consumption gives a misleading picture of real consumption when the goods and services produced by unpaid work of household members are excluded (Nordhaus and Tobin, 1972; Kende, 1975). Kuznets (1944) and Clark (1958) acknowledged that ignoring the income and wealth generated by housework introduces a bias in economic analysis. However, no significant progress has been made particularly in India to recognise and value the unpaid work of women despite the fact that the country is a party to international commitments to advance the goals of equality, development and peace for women (Fourth World Conference of Women in Beijing, 1995) and that women's rights are human rights (World Conference on Human Rights in Vienna, 1993). Ferrant et al. (2014) have argued that the gender gap in unpaid work has significant implications on women's ability to take part in the formal labour market and therefore to benefit from emerging opportunities.

The exclusion of household production from the System of National Accounts (SNA) dishonours women by ignoring the monetary value of their contribution from household work in the total value of market and non-market production. The SNA revisions (United Nations 1993, 2008) embraced the criticisms and suggested development of satellite accounts for household production. Goldschmidt-Clermont and Pagnossin-Aligisakis (1999) provided satellite accounts of SNA and non-SNA activities for seven European countries. Bridgman et al. (2012) using the American Time Use Survey adjusted GDP accounting for household production in 1965 and 2010 and found 39% and 26% inflation in GDP in 1965 and 2010 respectively. Landefeld and McCulla (2000), Holloway et al. (2002), Abraham and Mackie (2005) and Krueger et al. (2009) are other scholars who made important contributions in the development of satellite accounts. In China, Dong and An (2012), using the country's first large-scale time use survey conducted in 2008, found that the contribution of household production to GDP varies from 25% to 35% depending on the methods adopted for valuing unpaid household work. In the

Indian context Hirway (2015) advocates the integration of unpaid work in macroeconomic policy and suggests methods for valuing unpaid work.

The current study recognises time as the most precious and limited resource for economic empowerment of women and considers inputs of time spent by women in unpaid work crucial for empowerment of women in India. The key aim is to identify the gender gap in time spent in unpaid work and the differences in time spent in unpaid work by age and rural-urban location. Significant factors determining time spent for household maintenance and for the care of children, older people and the sick are also examined. Keeping in view that women are the main caregiver in households besides other unpaid household work, the study also provide estimates of monetary value of care for children, the sick and older people by age and sex.

## Methods and materials

The data used in this study are taken from the Time Use Survey (TUS) for India conducted in 1998–99 by the National Sample Survey Organization. This is the only TUS India has conducted and can be a benchmark for comparison with future TUSs. So, while we acknowledge that the data are somewhat old, they are the only reliable measures of time use in India on a national scale. In short, we feel that the limitation of the time since the data were collected is far outweighed by the importance of examining this subject as it has a tremendous impact on the situation of women and the wider economic performance of the country.

The survey covered 18,591 households spread over 52 districts and 6 states of India with each state representing one of the 6 major regions, namely, north, south, east, west, central and north-east. The sampling design used was three-stage stratified design. The population was first stratified into districts, then into villages/urban blocks within districts and finally households within villages/urban blocks. Hence districts were stratified by total population density and the relative size of the tribal population. Villages/urban blocks were then stratified by type of household to ensure the proportionate representation of all type of households.

The Indian TUS covers everyone aged 6 years and older. The activities were grouped into following categories: 1) SNA (productive and economic) activities: a) primary production activities, b) secondary production activities, and c) trade, business and services; 2) extended SNA activities: a) household maintenance, management and shopping in own households, b) care for children, the sick, older people and disabled in own household, and c) community services and help to other households; 3) non-SNA activities: a) learning, b) social and cultural activities and c) personal care and self-maintenance.

Data on time spent in SNA, non-SNA and extended SNA activities were collected for a one-week reference period. Data were collected for three types of days, 1) normal, 2) weekly variant and 3) abnormal. Abnormal days refer to days on which major events such as marriage, festivals and other celebrations days take place as people are highly likely to be engaged in special activities on these days and not in their day-to-day lives. Weekly variant days refer to weekend days where it is believed that people prefer to spend more time on leisure activities or maintenance activities. A new activity classification comparable with UN guidelines was developed for this TUS and interviewing methods rather than diary or observation methods were adopted for data collection. Household and individual questionnaires provide additional sociodemographic data such as age, sex and residence. In this analysis we have focused on the time spent on relevant activities on normal days as people are more likely to be engaged in their usual daily routine activities on these days. Hence we are able to get a better estimate of the dominate patterns of how people organise and use their time.

The TUS of 1998–99 used in this study as mentioned is the only authentic activities time diary data of its kind in India, and was conducted by National Sample Survey Organization under the Ministry of Statistics and Programme Implementation, Government of India (Central Statistical Organization, 2000). The study shall serve as a baseline reference for any future assessment of changing roles of women in India whenever such data become available. The burden and stress of performing non-remunerative household work reflected from this study can lead government and civil societies to initiate a fresh look and promote public policies for the welfare of women in India.

## Defining unpaid work

Unpaid work refers to activities in the household and community for providing services to its members that has no monetary compensation. Using the 'third party' criteria developed by Hill (1979) such activities are considered as work because if a third person were responsible for carrying out these activities then they would charge for providing such services. Hence activities that could be performed by a third party for pay can be deemed to meet the 'third person criterion'. This can then be further subdivided into two broad categories: 1) household maintenance and management and 2) care of children, the sick and older people. Household maintenance and management includes a broad range of activities:

1. Cooking food, preparing beverages and serving
2. Cleaning utensils, dwelling and surroundings
3. Washing clothes and ironing, scenting and ordering clothes and linen
4. Gardening and taking care of pets, servicing and repairing household appliances
5. Travelling related to household maintenance, managing and shopping for the household
6. Carrying out construction and repairs
7. Maintaining and improving the home

The activities included in the category of care of children, the sick and older members of the household are:

1. Taking physical care of children, bathing, dressing, feeding, playing, toileting
2. Teaching, training and instructing children
3. Taking physical care of sick, disabled and older members of households
4. Dressing, bathing, changing clothes, and care of sick, disabled and older members of households
5. Travelling related to care of children, sick, older people and other members
6. Carrying out any other activity related to the care of children, sick and older people not included elsewhere

For completeness and for comparison, analysis of time spent for primary and secondary production activities for monetary compensation are also included in the analyses. Primary production relates to agriculture, mining, forestry, animal farming, fishing, plantation and horticulture. Secondary production relates to construction, manufacturing, trade and business and service-providing activities. Both primary and secondary activities are for monetary compensation. On the other hand, watching television, sleeping, reading and personal care are not considered as work as these activities cannot be performed by a third party.

## Analysis of the data

Descriptive statistics, diagrammatic representations and cross-classifications are used for finding gender differentials in time spent on unpaid work by age, sex and place of residence. However, the nature of the data presents a methodological issue. Because a large proportion of the sample do not engage at all in these activities the amount of time spent for individuals not engaged in unpaid work is zero. Hence the distribution of time spent on such unpaid work is highly skewed. Because of this is it not possible to use ordinary least squares linear regressions as they would be likely to yield misleading results and interpretations (Brown and Dunn, 2011). Considering this it has been necessary to use a Tobit regression model[1] to explore which factors are associated with time spent on household maintenance and time spent on care of children, the sick and older people.

The collection of time use diary data in developing countries such as India can be problematic for various reasons. First it is very unlikely that households in India record activities on a daily basis but rather fill in the data in batches after a few days or even at the end of the week. Hence the data on time use is subjected to recall bias or omission. Moreover the data is usually collected by an available adult respondent, for instance the head of household, who may not know the activities of other members and time spent by them. This is likely to be particularly so for children and members of the household who most often stay outside. Also, it is important to be aware that the reported time spend on activities is usually rounded up. The interpretation and inference drawn from this study should bear these limitations of time use data in mind.

## Results and discussion

How people in India spent time engaging in daily activities with and without monetary compensation is shown in Figure 5.1. For the country as a whole, 58% of the total 24-hour period, which equates to around 14 hours, was spent on personal care and self-maintenance which includes sleeping, eating, recreation and listening to music. Following that around 11% of the time was spent on primary production activities and another 7% on secondary production activities. This shows that India was still a predominately agricultural

---

[1] A Tobit regression model is appropriate for dependent variables which cannot take values below or above a certain limit.

**Figure 5.1: The proportion of time spent on average on daily activities in India**

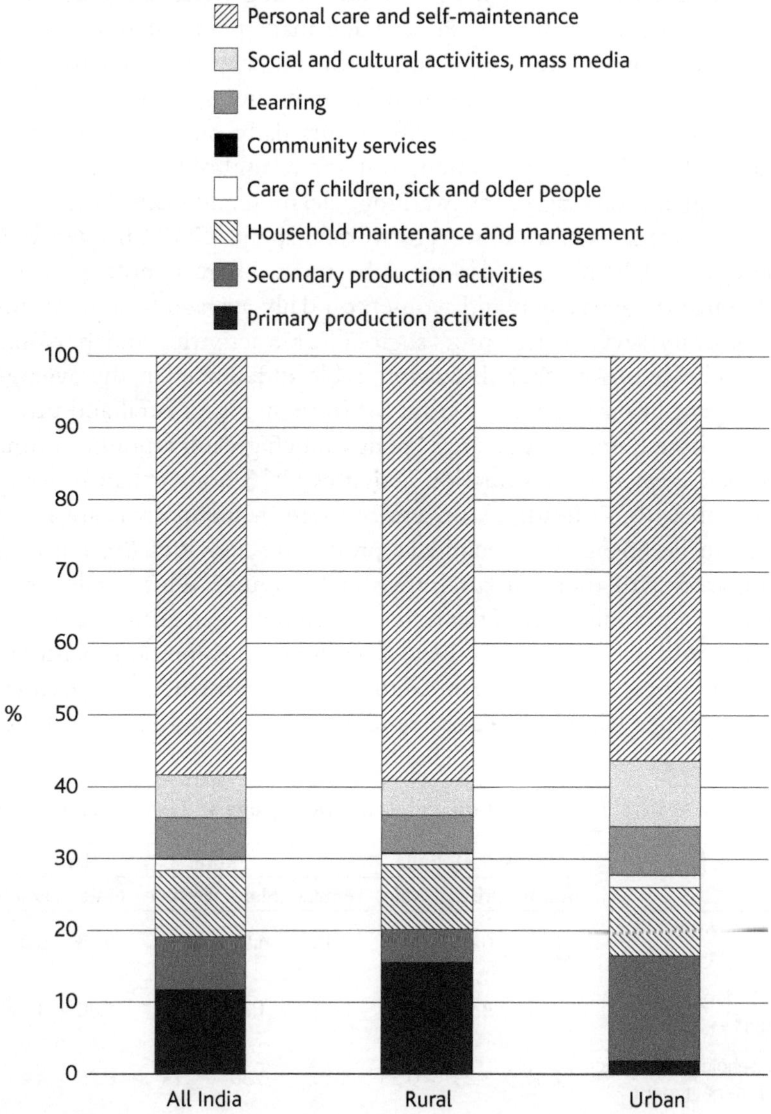


economy at the time that the data were collected. In terms of unpaid work Indians spend on average 9% of their time, around 2.2 hours a day, on household maintenance and management and a mere 1.6%, which is less than half an hour, on providing care for children, the sick and older people. Finally, participating in sociocultural activities, such as watching TV and reading newspaper, and learning activities each accounted for 6% of the total time spent.

Time spent in unpaid household work and economically productive activities differ by sex and place of residence in general (see Table 5.1). For the sample as a whole, the average man spent 3.4 hours a day on primary production activities, while the average woman spend 2.16 hours. However, the male-female gap in time spent on secondary production activities is wider, 2.89 hours daily on average by men and just 0.80 hours by women. But for household chores such as preparing and serving foods, washing, cleaning and other household maintenance activities on average women spent 4.23 hours a day in contrast to 0.30 hours a day spent by men. There is no significant difference between men and women on daily average time spent for community service, learning, sociocultural activities and personal care. The results further show noticeable differences in the average time spent in productive activities for those living in rural and urban areas. Those living in rural areas spent a much greater amount of time engaged in primary production activities (3.73 hours) than those in urban areas (0.45 hours). Conversely those in urban areas are more likely to be engaged in secondary productive activities (3.51 hours) compared with those in rural areas (1.10 hours). This rural–urban contrast is an indication of the difference in the occupational structure of rural and urban residents. Urban residents work predominantly in trade, business, services, manufacturing and construction activities. On the other hand, most rural residents are engaged in agriculture,

**Table 5.1: Average hours spent on daily activities by age and residence in India**

| | All India | | | | Rural | | Urban | |
|---|---|---|---|---|---|---|---|---|
| | Rural | Urban | Male | Female | Male | Female | Male | Female |
| Primary production activities | 3.73 | 0.45 | 3.40 | 2.16 | 4.56 | 2.86 | 0.53 | 0.36 |
| Secondary production activities | 1.10 | 3.51 | 2.89 | 0.61 | 1.72 | 0.44 | 5.80 | 1.03 |
| Household maintenance and management | 2.17 | 2.29 | 0.30 | 4.23 | 0.30 | 4.15 | 0.29 | 4.45 |
| Care of children, sick and older people | 0.38 | 0.41 | 0.16 | 0.33 | 0.13 | 0.64 | 0.13 | 0.72 |
| Community services | 0.02 | 0.01 | 0.02 | 0.02 | 0.02 | 0.02 | 0.01 | 0.01 |
| Learning | 1.26 | 1.61 | 1.53 | 1.17 | 1.47 | 1.03 | 1.70 | 1.52 |
| Social and cultural activities, mass media | 1.14 | 2.21 | 1.59 | 1.29 | 1.33 | 0.94 | 2.23 | 2.19 |
| Personal care and self-maintenance | 14.21 | 13.51 | 14.15 | 13.86 | 14.49 | 13.92 | 13.31 | 13.73 |

farming, forestry, mining and quarrying. However, outside these activities the pattern of time use was quite similar between the two groups. For example, the average amount of time spent on unpaid work in rural areas was 2.17 hours for household maintenance and management and a further 0.38 hours for caring activities. This is almost identical to those living in urban areas for which the figures were 2.29 hours and 0.41 hours respectively.

In contrast to the rural–urban comparison there are clear gender biases in the amount of time spent doing paid and unpaid work in these areas. Men spent more time engaged in paid activities while women spent much more time engaged in unpaid activities. On average women spent more than 4 hours a day on household maintenance and management, regardless of whether they lived in rural or urban areas, while men only spent about 20 minutes a day on these activities. Similarly, women spent more time than men caring for children, sick and older members of household. It is interesting that these gender differences are similar for both rural and urban areas. For example, women in rural areas spend an average of 4.15 hours a day on household chores while women in urban areas spent 4.45 hours on these activities.

Figure 5.2 disaggregates time spent in unpaid household work during an average week by major activities. Performing cooking-related activities is the major burden for women requiring 17.2 hours per week on average, which is more than half of the total time spent by women in a week on unpaid household work. Following this, women spent a further 4.8 hours per week on average cleaning. This

**Figure 5.2: Time spent in unpaid household work by activities by women in India**

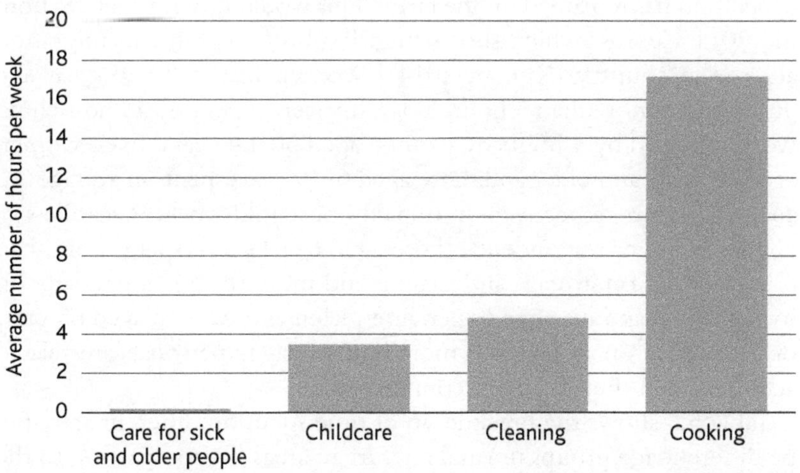

includes activities such as washing utensils, laundering and performing other household chores. The previous analyses have already shown that women perform much more of the caring duties in the household. However, these more disaggregated data allow us to look at whether this is due to care for children or for the sick and older members of the household. The data reveal that on average women spend a considerable amount of time, 3.5 hours per week, on the care of children in the household. In contrast care for the sick and older people accounts for a negligible proportion of unpaid household work performed by women, accounting for about a quarter of an hour per week on average.

Differences in the average time spent on daily activities for the different age groups and by sex are shown in Table 5.2. Looking across the different age and sex groups, it is clear that there are differences in the amount of time spent doing paid and unpaid work by age and sex. As might be expected those in the 'prime working age' groups, that is 20–34, 35–49 and 50–64 years, spend the most time doing paid work, that is, primary and secondary production activities. If we combine the average number of hours spend in both primary and secondary production activities, men in these age groups respectively spend 8.22, 8.83 and 7.49 hours a day on average in paid work and women spend 3.07, 3.82 and 3.3 hours a day on average. A distinctive feature for women is that they are more likely to be engaged in primary production activities and less in secondary production activities. However, there is an interesting age-related pattern within this broader trend with those in the older age group spending much less time in secondary productive activities. This suggests that those in the younger generations have migrated from the countryside into the cities for work while the older generation has remained on the farm. This would fit with analyses from the 2011 Census, which shows high levels of rural–urban migration across the country (Kumar, 2014). Women in the 30–49-year age group spent more than 5 hours a day, on average, in unpaid household work followed by 4 hours by women aged 50–64 years. Even women aged 65 years and older and those aged 6–19 years spent on average 2.2 and 1.82 hours respectively in unpaid household work. Regardless of gender younger respondents, those aged 6–19 years, spent more than 4 hours daily on average in learning and more than 2 hours daily on sociocultural and mass media activities. Men and women aged 65 years or older spent on average 4–5 more hours a day in personal care-related activities than their younger counterparts.

Table 5.3 shows the breakdown of time spent on different activities by different age groups in rural and urban areas. In comparison to the

**Table 5.2: Average hours spent on daily activities by sex and age in India**

| | Male | | | | | Female | | | | |
|---|---|---|---|---|---|---|---|---|---|---|
| | 6–19 | 20–34 | 35–49 | 50–64 | 65+ | 6–19 | 20–34 | 35–49 | 50–64 | 65+ |
| Primary production activities | 1.32 | 4.15 | 4.61 | 4.53 | 2.83 | 1.03 | 2.39 | 3.04 | 2.68 | 1.17 |
| Secondary activities | 0.90 | 4.07 | 4.22 | 2.96 | 1.10 | 0.40 | 0.68 | 0.82 | 0.62 | 0.20 |
| Household maintenance and management | 0.20 | 0.32 | 0.34 | 0.40 | 0.36 | 1.82 | 5.69 | 5.44 | 3.96 | 2.20 |
| Care of children, sick and older people | 0.07 | 0.16 | 0.16 | 0.10 | 0.19 | 0.24 | 1.16 | 0.49 | 0.58 | 0.54 |
| Community services | 0.01 | 0.02 | 0.02 | 0.03 | 0.02 | 0.02 | 0.01 | 0.01 | 0.02 | 0.03 |
| Learning | 4.83 | 0.30 | 0.01 | 0.01 | 0.00 | 4.19 | 0.13 | 0.02 | 0.01 | 0.00 |
| Social and cultural activities, mass media | 2.84 | 1.18 | 0.89 | 1.03 | 1.20 | 2.41 | 0.90 | 0.89 | 0.83 | 0.81 |
| Personal care and self-maintenance | 13.84 | 13.80 | 13.76 | 14.93 | 18.29 | 13.88 | 13.04 | 13.29 | 15.31 | 19.04 |

**Table 5.3: Average hours spent on daily activities by age and residence in India**

| | Rural | | | | | Urban | | | | |
|---|---|---|---|---|---|---|---|---|---|---|
| | 6–19 | 20–34 | 35–49 | 50–64 | 65+ | 6–19 | 20–34 | 35–49 | 50–64 | 65+ |
| Primary production activities | 1.60 | 4.36 | 5.25 | 4.67 | 2.61 | 0.14 | 0.54 | 0.56 | 0.74 | 0.34 |
| Secondary production activities | 0.47 | 1.51 | 1.44 | 1.09 | 0.49 | 1.17 | 4.37 | 5.22 | 4.01 | 1.21 |
| Household maintenance and management | 1.01 | 3.06 | 2.66 | 2.00 | 1.23 | 0.76 | 3.06 | 3.18 | 2.32 | 1.26 |
| Care of children, sick and older people | 0.17 | 0.64 | 0.30 | 0.34 | 0.35 | 0.10 | 0.74 | 0.38 | 0.31 | 0.38 |
| Community services | 0.02 | 0.02 | 0.02 | 0.02 | 0.03 | 0.01 | 0.01 | 0.01 | 0.02 | 0.02 |
| Learning | 4.27 | 0.13 | 0.01 | 0.01 | 0.00 | 5.22 | 0.42 | 0.02 | 0.02 | 0.01 |
| Social and cultural activities, mass media | 2.36 | 0.73 | 0.58 | 0.62 | 0.64 | 3.37 | 1.80 | 1.61 | 1.84 | 2.12 |
| Personal care and self-maintenance | 14.10 | 13.56 | 13.75 | 15.24 | 18.60 | 13.20 | 13.06 | 13.02 | 14.75 | 18.70 |

differences already noted in the amount of time spent in primary and secondary production activities in paid work between these two areas, there are only relatively minor differences in the age-related patterns of time spent doing unpaid work. In all but the youngest two age groups there is a slight tendency for those who live in urban areas to spend more time on average performing household maintenance and management tasks. However, there are no significant differences in the patterns of time spent providing care to children, the sick or older people between rural and urban residents.

Although the foregoing analyses clearly indicates gender and age differences in the providing unpaid work in India it is necessary to perform multivariate analyses to test to see which factors have greatest explanatory power once the effects if all factors are looked at simultaneously. This is because it is likely that several of the explanatory factors are strongly related to one another. To test what factors were significantly associated with doing unpaid work two Tobit regression analyses were performed, one for household management and maintenance as the outcome variable and one for caring for a child, the sick or an older person. The Tobit regression coefficients and standard errors are shown in Table 5.4.[2] It is clear that, even after controlling for the effects of all the other variables in the model, those who live in urban areas spend less time on household management and maintenance than their rural counterparts. However, this association is reversed for providing care as those in urban areas spend more time doing so. Gender differences are even starker. Women spend a statistically significantly greater amount of time on both types of unpaid work. Women spend over five and a half times more time on household management and maintenance than men and almost twice as much time on providing care. Following the earlier results that showed that those of working age had similar profiles in terms of the amount of time spent on performing unpaid work the analyses for age have been regrouped into three broader categories: 6–15 years old, 16–59 years old and 60+ years old. The results show that, compared with the youngest age group, those in the prime working age group and those in the older age group are much more likely to spend time doing either form of paid work. The results for the probability of

[2] The β coefficient should not be interpreted as the effect of $x_i$ on $y_i$, as with a linear regression model. Instead, it should be interpreted as the combination of 1) the change in $y_i$ of those above the limit, weighted by the probability of being above the limit; and 2) the change in the probability of being above the limit, weighted by the expected value of $y_i$ if above.

**Table 5.4: Tobit regression coefficients and standard errors for time spent on household management and maintenance and time spent on care for children, sick and older people**

| | Household management and maintenance | | Child, sick and older people care | |
|---|---|---|---|---|
| | β | SE(β) | β | SE(β) |
| Rural | 1 | | 1 | |
| Urban | **–0.10** | **0.045** | **0.17** | **0.045** |
| Male | 1 | | 1 | |
| Female | **5.56** | **0.046** | **1.92** | **0.047** |
| 6–15 years | 1 | | 1 | |
| 16–59 years | **4.5** | **0.064** | **2.22** | **0.065** |
| 60+ years | **2.51** | **0.099** | **1.5** | **0.099** |

*Note:* All analyses controlled for household size, whether in paid work and level of literacy. β-beta coefficients, SE-standard error. Figures in **bold** are statistically significant at the p<0.01 level

doing any household management and maintenance show that those of working age are 4.5 times more likely than those in the youngest age group to do this and those in the 60+ age group are 2.51 times more likely. The figures for the probability of providing care are respectively 2.22 times and 1.5 times more likely.

Finally, given the previous arguments about the importance of the hidden value of women's contribution to GDP and the national economy, Table 5.5 provides the estimated monetary value of labour inputs for cooking and childcare by sex and age groups. The value of labour inputs for cooking and childcare are worth Rs.1,142 crores[3] and Rs.948 crores respectively. The contributions of women to the total monetary values are 96% for cooking and 82% for childcare. Women aged 20–49 years contribute 69% to the total monetary value of labour inputs for cooking and women in the 6–19 years group contribute a similar share for childcare. The results on the time spent by women in unpaid household work exemplify the landscape of women's roles and market structure in India. During the 1970s the laudable objectives embodied in the constitution to improve the general working conditions for all and to achieve equality for men and women have only been partially met. Most working women are gradually moving into the informal sectors of the labour market as male employment moves to more market-based activities. This is partly due to male-dominated rural to urban migration and the marginalisation of the agriculture sector (Kumari, 2014). According

[3] A crore denotes 10,000,000 (ten million).

**Table 5.5: Monetary value of labour inputs for cooking and childcare by age and sex in Indian Rupees**

| | Male | Female | Total |
|---|---|---|---|
| **Cooking** | | | |
| 6–19 | 123,781,856 | 1,669,174,915 | 1,792,956,771 |
| 20–29 | 125,218,880 | 3,340,578,350 | 3,465,797,229 |
| 30–49 | 130,046,855 | 4,538,792,559 | 4,668,839,414 |
| 50–64 | 58,529,484 | 1,109,505,591 | 1,168,035,075 |
| 65+ | 27,449,030 | 297,165,917 | 324,614,947 |
| Total | 465,026,105 | 10,955,217,330 | 11,420,243,435 |
| **Childcare** | | | |
| 6–19 | 580,411,387 | 2,871,334,173 | 3,451,745,560 |
| 20–29 | 366,583,941 | 2,530,699,039 | 2,897,282,979 |
| 30–49 | 484,872,958 | 1,444,817,610 | 1,929,690,568 |
| 50–64 | 168,950,384 | 689,925,018 | 858,875,402 |
| 65+ | 100,412,853 | 240,773,452 | 341,186,304 |
| Total | 1,701,231,522 | 7,777,549,291 | 9,478,780,813 |

to the Economic Survey of India (2007–08), 93% of India's workforce was self-employed and in the informal sector. As of 2009–10 the total estimated employment in India was 465 million of which 280 million people are in the formal sector and the rest in the informal sector. The fact that a large proportion of women are still working in the informal sector suggests that women's burden of unpaid household work has not changed significantly over time.

## Conclusion

This chapter highlights the potential of time use data to explore gender and rural–urban differences in roles and responsibilities in households. In turn this gives us a vital insight into the burden that women in India bear for unpaid household tasks. The results clearly show that traditional gender roles prevail in India with women spending more time per week than men doing these tasks. Men on the other hand spent more time engaged in paid employment in the formal economy. Even where women are engaged in paid employment, unlike men, they must also often shoulder the dual burden of doing both paid work and unpaid household work. It is not an overstatement to say that if women do not prepare and serve food then everyone would go to bed with empty stomach as it is only women who spend time cooking in households

These figures compare poorly with other countries in the region. For example, women's labour market participation rate in Bangladesh is almost twice as high as it is in India (57% and 29%, respectively) even though Bangladesh is a much poorer country (Dreze and Sen, 2014). This is all-the-more alarming when one considers that it is women in their mid-20s who do the most unpaid household work in India. This coincides with the prime age of childbearing for women. There have been great strides in providing childcare services throughout India under the auspice of the Integrated Child Development Services scheme. This was launched in 1975 in pursuance of the National Policy for Children and is aimed at children under 6 years, pregnant and lactating women and women in the age group of 15–44 years. The beneficiaries of the scheme are to a large extent identical with those of the Maternal and Child Health Program. The programme provides an integrated approach for converging all basic services for improved childcare, early stimulation and learning, health and nutrition, water and environmental sanitation aimed at the young children, expectant and lactating mothers, other women and adolescent girls in a community (Kapil, 2002). Yet despite these developments it is clear that many women of child rearing age are excluded from the labour market due to having to take on all the childrearing responsibilities.

The situation is the same when we consider caregiving to older people and long-term care for those who are sick. Currently there are low levels of public provision for care in India. Hence intergenerational and intra-household time transfers are crucial for sustaining support to these groups. Yet it almost always falls on women to provide this care, which in turn takes them out of the paid workforce and condemns them to domestic servitude. Yet if we look at examples from other countries we can see that in countries like Denmark, Finland, Norway, Sweden and Italy, both parents are allowed to take paternal leave on full or part pay in the case of birth or adoption. In India it is becoming necessary to explore these state-funded options as a policy to reduce the burden of caregiving for women. Time use data can make explicit the actual care provided by individuals and help in refining the policy.

The contribution of unpaid household work to welfare goes beyond the household members because of the close link between home production and the market economy. The emergence of part-time work and the feasibility of home-based production as a source of viable income generation demonstrates that the monetary value of unpaid housework can be realised and should be integrated into macroeconomic and public policies. To boost the economy of a developing country like India it is important to assess the changing dynamics of unpaid and paid work over time and space. Time use data can make explicit the actual distribution of time spent on different activities and help policy makers in refining the policies to remove obstacles to paid employment and boost economic growth. However, rather than merely responding to the trend of greater female labour market participation, generally in low paid and low skilled jobs involving long hours of work, the government could support training programmes. Such programmes would provide avenues for women to move out of demanding but low paid work to work in better paid jobs with greater promotion prospects. Another key advance would be the introduction of regulated public policies for satellite accounting of household work to be fully integrated in the calculations for GDP. By so doing this would make visible the extent of the contributions made by women and challenge traditional stereotypes. Reshaping deep rooted attitudes towards gender roles and responsibilities in priority can boost the economy in the long run.

## References

Abraham, K.G. and Mackie, C. (2005). *Beyond the market: Defining non-market accounts for the United States.* Washington, D.C: National Academies Press.

Central Statistical Organization. (2000). *Report of the time use survey.* Ministry of Statistics and Programme Implementation, Government of India, New Delhi.

Clark, C. (1958). *The economics of house-work.* Bulletin of the Oxford University Institute of Economics and Statistics.

Dreze, J and Sen, A. (2014). *An Uncertain Glory: India and its Contradictions.* London: Penguin.

Bridgman, B., Dugan, A. Lal, M. and Osborne, M. (2012). Accounting for household production in the National Accounts, 1965–2010. *Survey of Current Business*, 92(5), 23–36.

Brown, J. and Dunn, P. (2011). Comparisons of Tobit, Linear, and Poisson-Gamma Regression Models. *Sociological Methods and Research*, 40(3), 511–535.

Dong, X.-Y. and An, X. (2012). *Gender patterns and value of unpaid work findings from China's first large-scale time use survey*, United Nations Research Institute for Social Development (UNRISD) Research Paper 2012–16. http://www.unrisd.org/80256B3C005BCCF9/(httpAuxPages)/7CE1453DB093FB41C1257A8E004D6A57/$file/Dong%20and%20An.pdf. Accessed 1 February 2013.

Ferrant, G., Pesando, L.M. and Nowacka, K. (2014). *Unpaid Care Work: The missing link in the analysis of gender gaps in labour outcomes*. OECD Development Centre. http://www.oecd.org/dev/development-gender/Unpaid_care_work.pdf. Accessed on 22/1/2016.

Goldschmidt-Clermont, L. and Pagnossing-Aligisakis, E. (1999), Households' Non-SNA Production: Labour Time, Value of Labour and of Product, and Contribution to Extended Private Consumption. *Review of Income and Wealth*, 45(40), 519–529.

Hill, T.P. (1979). Do-it-yourself and GDP. *The Review of Income and Wealth*, 25(1), 31–39.

Hirway, I. (2015). *Unpaid work and the economy: Linkages and their implications*. Working Paper No. 838, New York: Levy Economics Institute.

Holloway, S., Short, S. and Tamplin, S. (2002). *Household satellite account (experimental) methodology*. London: Office for National Accounts.

Kapil, U. (2002). Integrated Child Development Services (ICDS) scheme: a program for holistic development of children in India. *The Indian Journal of Pediatrics*, 69(7), 597–601.

Kende, P. (1975). Vers une evaluationde la consummation reelle desmenages. *Revue Consommation*, No.2, CREDOC, Paris.

Krueger, A.B., Kahneman, D. Schkade, D. and Stone, A.A. (2009). National time accounting: The currency of life. In Krueger, A.B.(Ed.). *Measuring the subjective wellbeing of nations: National accounts of time use and wellbeing*. Chicago: University of Chicago Press, 9–81.

Kumari, S. (2014). Rural-urban migration in India: determinants and factors. *International Journal of Humanities and Social Sciences*, 3(2), 161–180.

Kuznets, S. (1944). *National Income and its composition, 1919–1938*. National Bureau of Economic Research.

Landefeld, J.S. and Mc Culla, S.H. (2000). Accounting for nonmarket household production within a national accounts framework. *Review of Income and Wealth*, 46, 289–307.

Nordhaus, W. and Tobin, J. (1972). Is growth obsolete? In W. Nordhaus and J. Tobin (Eds) *Economic Research: Retrospect and Prospect, Volume 5: Economic Growth*, NBER: 1–80.

Stiglitz, J., Sen, A. and Fitoussi, J.P. (2007), *Report on the Commission on the Measurement of Economic Performance and Social Process*, Paris: Commission on the Measurement of Economic Performance and Social Process. http://www.stiglitz-sen-fitoussi.fr. Accessed on 22/1/2016.

United Nations (1993). System of National Accounts, Department for Economic and Social Information and Policy Analysis – Statistics Division, New York. https://unstats.un.org/unsd/nationalaccount/docs/1993sna.pdf. Accessed 22 January 2007.
United Nations (2008). System of National Accounts Department for Economic and Social Information and Policy Analysis – Statistics Division, New York. https://unstats.un.org/unsd/nationalaccount/docs/sna2008.pdf. Accessed 22 January 2007.

# SIX

# Activity status, morbidity patterns and hospitalisation in India

*Harihar Sahoo*

## Background

Trends in life expectancy across both developed and developing countries show that people are living longer. In line with these global developments mortality rates in India have decreased, which has led to significant gains in life expectancy. Figure 6.1 shows that the crude birth rate[1] has more than halved over the last century. There has also been a steady fall in crude death rates[2] from a high of 47 in 1911–21 to a low of just over 7 in 2010. This fall in mortality has driven a significant increase in life expectancy throughout India. In 1901–11 average life expectancy was just 22 years. This was doubtless caused by very high rates of infant mortality. Yet by 2006–10 this had risen to 66 years. As noted in earlier chapters in this volume these demographic changes have been accompanied by changes in the patterns of death and disease. This shift from communicable diseases to non-communicable diseases (NCDs) as the main causes of mortality and morbidity is referred to as the epidemiological transition (Omran, 1971). Hence, despite these great improvements in extending life expectancy there are concerns that healthy life expectancy has not always kept pace with these increases as many people are living with lifestyle-related chronic diseases like diabetes, heart diseases, impairments and mental illness. Evidence from studies conducted in developed countries indicates that morbidity rates will mean that a proportion of one's life expectancy is liable to be lost through disability (Ghosh and Arokiasamy, 2009).

[1] The crude birth rate is the number of live births among the population of a given geographical area during a given year, per 1,000 mid-year total population of the same area during the same year.

[2] The crude death rate is the number of deaths among the population of a given geographical area during a given year, per 1,000 mid-year total population of the same area during the same year.

**Figure 6.1: Trends in birth and death rates in India, 1901–2008**

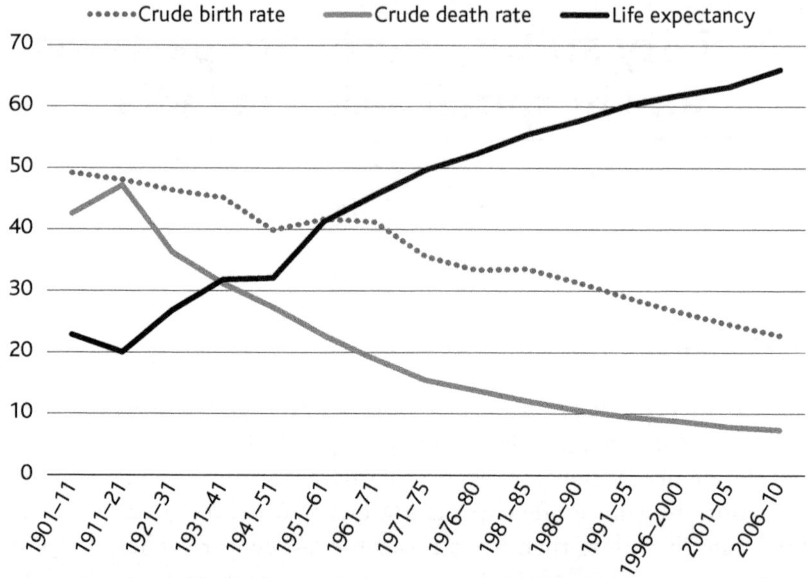


*Source:* Figures from 1901–71 are based on Census estimates extracted from India, Ministry of Health and Family Welfare (2007). Figures for 1971–2010 are based on averages computed from the Sample Registration System estimates.

Therefore, addressing and studying these changing morbidity patterns in India is of upmost importance in their own right but also because they have long been recognised as measurable indicators of well-being (Shariff, 1995).

India is not alone in experiencing this epidemiological transition. Since the 1970s, all of South Asia has experienced significant reductions in premature death and disability from communicable and nutritional diseases such as pneumonia, diarrheal diseases and malnutrition. At the same time NCDs have been emerging as leading causes of death and now NCDs account for between one-third and two-thirds of all deaths and disability in the region (Siegel et al., 2014). The situation in India is somewhere in the middle for the region as chronic diseases account for around 50% of annual deaths. Indeed these rates are estimated to be higher in India than in high income countries (Patel et al., 2011). A 2014 study reported that around 28.5% of the population in India had a NCD and 8.9% had multi-morbidities, with two or more NCDs present (Pati et al., 2014). The scale of the impact of these diseases is enormous. It has been estimated that 9.2 million productive years of life were lost to cardiovascular disease alone in India in 2000. This is expected to increase to 17.9 million years by 2030 (Mahal et al.,

2010). However, although NCDs are on the rise and communicable diseases are falling it is important to bear in mind that the latter still contribute about 30% of the disease burden in India and are a major risk to health and well-being (John et al., 2011).

Yet while these figures show what is happening at the national level they say little about regional or socioeconomic differences in morbidity patterns. One of the major features of social epidemiological research in Europe and North America has been on inequalities in health (Marmot, 2005). Overall the evidence from high income countries is that there is a social gradient in health, such that those in the more advantageous positions in society tend to have better health. In India, however, some studies have found the opposite to be true. In their study on multi-morbidity, Pati and colleagues (2014) found that the prevalence of NCDs increased with increasing household wealth. Just under 7% of residents in households in the lowest wealth quintile reported two or more NCDs compared with 11% in the highest wealth quintile. In contrast, a study in Bangalore in the south of the country reported much lower rates of chronic disease (13.8%) and found a socioeconomic gradient of health with people living below the poverty line much more likely to report chronic conditions than people living above the poverty line (Bhojani et al., et al., 2013). This suggests not only that socioeconomic inequalities in morbidity exist in India but that the strength and direction of those inequalities might differ by region.

Not only do these diseases have an obvious impact on the health and well-being of individuals and groups who are most affected by them they can also incur huge financial costs. Poor health and illness lead to people having to leave work either temporarily or permanently. As Basariya (2015) observes sickness is the most important cause of absenteeism in the Indian industrial sector. Long-term sickness absence or disability can also result in the loss of income from work and a reliance on social security or insurance payments. Aside from this becoming ill can necessitate medical expenses (Lee et al., 2015; Pati et al., 2014). This is a particular concern in India as it is estimated that over 70% of healthcare is financed through out-of-pocket payments by households at the time and point of healthcare use (Government of India, 2009). These expenses are a key barrier to accessing healthcare services in India among the less advantaged groups in society (Bhojani et al., 2012). Moreover, they can plunge people into poverty leading to a vicious cycle of cumulative disadvantage. It was estimated that in 2004 around 63 million people in India, roughly 7% of the total population, may have fallen below the poverty line due to health spending. (Berman et al., 2010; Shahrawat and Rao, 2011). A 2010 World Bank study showed that cardiovascular disease alone leads to catastrophic spending for 25% of Indian families and drives 10% of families into poverty (Mahal et al., 2010). As the Ministry of Health and Family Welfare notes this does not just impact on the individual but has serious ramifications for the family, community and wider society:

> 'incidence of catastrophic expenditure due to health care costs is growing and is now being estimated to be one of the major contributors to lack. The drain on family incomes due to health care costs can neutralize the gains of income increases and every Government scheme aimed to reduce poverty.' (Government of India, 2014)

Although researchers and health planners have expressed concerns about whether the burden of disease due to morbidity follows the secular trend of mortality, relatively few studies have examined the pattern of morbidity prevalence across Indian regions. Yet there are substantial regional and socioeconomic differences in standards of living, quality of life and health, including disparities in health seeking behaviour and access to the healthcare facilities across India.

Health status is determined by a range of factors such as having a healthy environment (including the work environment), especially having access to a safe drinking water supply, sanitary disposal of excreta and other wastes, and pollution-free housing and work places. Adequate nutrition is also a key factor. This in turn depends on the production, accessibility, affordability and intra-familial distribution of food. Finally, limiting exposure to risk factors for communicable diseases and lifestyles that influence the occurrence of NCDs is important for ensuring good health (Nongkynrih et al., 2004). Due to the increase in industrialisation and urbanisation as well as the demographic and lifestyle changes noted in Chapter 3 in the current volume, India is facing a growing double burden of NCDs alongside the persistent threat of communicable diseases. In India, NCDs account for around 40% of all hospital stays and 35% of all outpatient visits (Mahal et al., 2010). Therefore, it is essential to study the pattern of communicable and NCDs across the different regions and groups in India.

This study aims to examine inequalities in disease by economic activity status in India. A person's economic activity status is considered to be an important social determinant of their health. Much of one's life is spent in work. Not only do individuals work for many years over their lifetime but they also work for many hours per day. Therefore, one's activity status has the potential to impact on health. However, worldwide, but especially in India, activity status has received relatively little attention in the literature on the determinants of health, relative to other measures such as education, wealth and occupation. This chapter seeks to redress this lacuna. Moreover, as it is likely that the relationship between disease and socioeconomic status in Indian population groups is influenced by the stage of health transition of the region in which they live. Because different regions of India are at different stages of epidemiological transition it is highly likely that the relationship between economic activity status and disease will vary by region.

## Data and methods

The National Sample Survey Organization has conducted three nationwide surveys on the use of medical services by various sections of population in 1986–87 (42nd round), 1995–96 (52nd round) and 2004 (60th round). This chapter analyses data from the 60th round as it is the latest in the series. The data were collected through a survey on 'Morbidity and Health Care'. Alongside this subject, surveys were undertaken separately on 'Household Consumer Expenditure' and 'Employment and Unemployment'. The survey on morbidity and health care covered morbidity and use of healthcare services including immunisation and maternity care, problems of older people, and household spending on healthcare services (Government of India, 2006).

Morbidity can be measured in two ways: self-perceived and observed. Self-perceived morbidity is that which is perceived and reported by an individual and largely depends on their perception and awareness of different health conditions. Observed morbidity refers to the health conditions which are observed by a trained and independent observer through diagnosis/clinical test (Murray and Chen, 1992; Schultz and Tansel, 1996). The enquiry on self-perceived morbidity was conducted with a reference period of 15 days. All spells of poor health suffered by each member, both present as well as the deceased, of the sample household, during the 15 days preceding the date of enquiry, whether or not the patient was hospitalised for treatment, were covered in the survey.

Economic activity status was measured using 14 categories that cover a wide range of statuses from employers to beggars. These are:

1) Worked in household enterprise (self-employed)/own account worker; 2) Employer; 3) Worked as helper in household enterprise (unpaid family worker); 4) Worked as regular salaried/wage employee; 5) Worked as casual wage labour: in public works; 6) In other types of work; 7) Did not work but was seeking and/or available for work; 8) Attended educational institution; 9) Attended domestic duties only; 10) Attended domestic duties and was also engaged in free collection of goods; 11) Rentiers, pensioners, remittance recipients and so on; 12) Not able to work due to disability; 13) Beggars, prostitutes; and 14) Other activity.

## Prevalence of ailments

The data presented in Figure 6.2 show that the prevalence of ailments in the day before the survey is 57 persons per 1,000 people in the population in India. However, this national average masks a great deal of regional variation ranging from 34 in the north-eastern region to 76 in the southern region. Taking the long reference period, we can see that the prevalence of ailments during last 15 days is 91 per 1,000 population. Again there are regional differences ranging from 75 in the northern region to 112 in the southern region. The prevalence of ailments is much higher in the southern regions. However, it is important to be aware that this may be because of cultural differences in the willingness to report the occurrence of health problems, rather

**Figure 6.2: Prevalence of ailments per 1,000 people by regions of India, 2004**

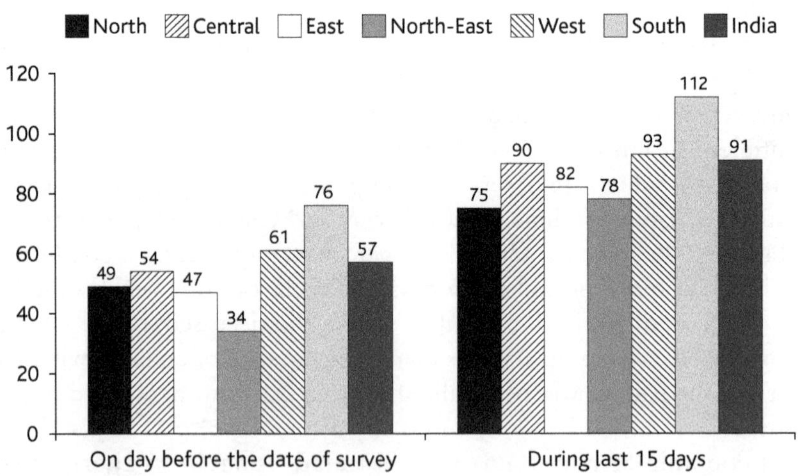


*Source:* Computed from NSS individual data

than necessarily reflecting differences in the objective levels of health between these regions.

Table 6.1 presents a more fine-grained analyses of the health of the nation by looking at the prevalence of ailments per 1,000 persons for each of the states in India. The prevalence rates are much higher in southern states like Kerala and Pondicherry. Among the northern states Punjab shows the highest prevalence and Delhi shows the lowest prevalence while among eastern states West Bengal shows the highest prevalence and Jharkhand shows the lowest prevalence. With respect to communicable and NCDs, a similar pattern is observed: Kerala shows the highest prevalence of NCDs among the states of India.

Table 6.2 presents the results for the reported rate of different diseases during the last 15 days by the different regions in India. It is evident that among the categories of communicable diseases, fever of unknown origin, respiratory ailments including ear/nose/throat and diarrhoea/dysentery are much higher compared with other diseases. However, regional differences are again evident. Overall the prevalence of communicable disease in India is 39 per 1,000 persons. It varies from 31.8 in the northern region to the maximum of 48 in the north-eastern region. The prevalence of NCD in India is 28.9 per 1,000 persons. Across the regions, NCDs are much higher in southern regions (44.8) followed by the western region (34.5) and are lowest in the north-eastern region (17.3). Among the different categories of NCDs, the prevalence of disorders of the joints and bones is the highest (5.6 per 1,000) followed by hypertension (4.5), bronchial asthma (3.3), gastric or peptic ulcers (3.3) and diabetes (2.7). With respect to the disabilities and injuries, the prevalence is 5.7 in India ranging from 3.2 in north-eastern states to 7.1 in southern states. Within the category of disabilities and injuries, accidents/injuries/ burns/factures/poisoning account for the highest prevalence.

## Prevalence of ailments by activity status and by age group

Activity status varies by age groups which in turn affects the occurrence of different diseases. Therefore, it is essential to study the prevalence of ailments by activity status and by age group. Figure 6.3 shows the prevalence rate for reporting any disease by activity group for the day immediately before the survey and for the previous 15 days. There is clearly a wide disparity in the rates of disease among the different groups. As might be expected those who are unable to work due to disability have the highest rate of illness. Following those there is the rather diverse group which comprises rentiers, pensioners and

**Table 6.1: Prevalence of ailments per 1,000 people by states of India, 2004**

| | Day before survey | During last 15 days | | | |
|---|---|---|---|---|---|
| | | All | CDs | NCDs | Ds and Is |
| **North** | 49 | 75 | 32 | 25 | 5 |
| Jammu and Kashmir | 46 | 71 | 36 | 24 | 3 |
| Himachal Pradesh | 62 | 85 | 24 | 38 | 8 |
| Punjab | 86 | 127 | 53 | 46 | 5 |
| Chandigarh | 41 | 69 | 24 | 22 | 1 |
| Uttaranchal | 31 | 55 | 28 | 14 | 8 |
| Haryana | 58 | 94 | 41 | 31 | 5 |
| Delhi | 7 | 14 | 3 | 6 | 1 |
| Rajasthan | 41 | 60 | 26 | 17 | 5 |
| **Central** | 54 | 90 | 47 | 20 | 6 |
| Uttar Pradesh | 63 | 102 | 53 | 22 | 6 |
| Chhattisgarh | 38 | 70 | 38 | 15 | 5 |
| Madhya Pradesh | 36 | 62 | 33 | 16 | 5 |
| **East** | 47 | 82 | 36 | 23 | 4 |
| Bihar | 27 | 54 | 31 | 12 | 2 |
| West Bengal | 83 | 125 | 44 | 42 | 8 |
| Jharkhand | 7 | 36 | 19 | 8 | 1 |
| Orissa | 34 | 75 | 39 | 14 | 4 |
| **North-East** | 34 | 78 | 48 | 17 | 3 |
| Sikkim | 33 | 50 | 27 | 13 | 4 |
| Arunachal Pradesh | 22 | 60 | 40 | 7 | 2 |
| Nagaland | 13 | 59 | 48 | 3 | 2 |
| Manipur | 14 | 28 | 17 | 7 | 1 |
| Mizoram | 12 | 19 | 10 | 3 | 1 |
| Tripura | 43 | 122 | 88 | 24 | 1 |
| Meghalaya | 29 | 51 | 32 | 5 | 6 |
| Assam | 37 | 82 | 49 | 20 | 4 |
| **West** | 61 | 93 | 37 | 35 | 7 |
| Gujarat | 50 | 72 | 31 | 28 | 6 |
| Daman and Diu | 12 | 23 | 13 | 6 | 1 |
| Dadra and Nagar Haveli | 8 | 16 | 13 | 4 | 0 |
| Maharashtra | 66 | 104 | 40 | 38 | 8 |
| Goa | 94 | 124 | 66 | 50 | 3 |
| **South** | 76 | 112 | 38 | 45 | 7 |
| Andhra Pradesh | 67 | 97 | 27 | 42 | 7 |
| Karnataka | 40 | 62 | 22 | 25 | 5 |
| Lakshadweep | 86 | 128 | 48 | 50 | 14 |
| Kerala | 179 | 252 | 91 | 100 | 12 |
| Tamil Nadu | 60 | 96 | 37 | 35 | 6 |
| Pondicherry | 138 | 173 | 27 | 65 | 34 |
| Andaman and Nicobar Islands | 32 | 54 | 23 | 18 | 9 |
| **India** | 57 | 91 | 39 | 29 | 6 |

*Notes:* The sum of prevalence of communicable diseases (CDs), non-communicable diseases (NCDs), disabilities and injuries (Ds and Is) may not add up to 1,000 because of comorbidity and diagnosed and undiagnosed ailments.

*Source:* Computed from NSS individual data

Table 6.2: Reported rates of different diseases (per 1,000) during last 15 days by regions of India, 2004

| | North | Central | East | North-east | West | South | India |
|---|---|---|---|---|---|---|---|
| **Communicable diseases** | **31.9** | **46.5** | **36.1** | **48.1** | **37.4** | **38.4** | **39.3** |
| Diarrhoea/dysentery | 2.7 | 6.5 | 5.2 | 10.3 | 3.7 | 2.6 | 4.6 |
| Worm infestation | 0.4 | 0.3 | 0.3 | 0.5 | 0.6 | 0.4 | 0.4 |
| Amoebiasis | 0.2 | 0.4 | 0.5 | 0.8 | 0.2 | 0.2 | 0.3 |
| Hepatitis/jaundice | 0.6 | 0.4 | 0.5 | 0.5 | 0.1 | 0.4 | 0.4 |
| Respiratory including ENT ailments | 7.1 | 5.5 | 5.2 | 5.8 | 6.9 | 8.5 | 6.5 |
| Tuberculosis | 1.2 | 1.5 | 0.9 | 0.3 | 1.0 | 0.9 | 1.1 |
| Conjunctivitis | 0.5 | 0.4 | 0.2 | 0.2 | 0.5 | 0.4 | 0.4 |
| Diseases of skin | 2.0 | 2.4 | 1.8 | 0.8 | 2.0 | 2.1 | 2.0 |
| Sexually transmitted diseases | 0.1 | 0.1 | 0.0 | 0.0 | 0.0 | 0.0 | 0.1 |
| Malaria | 1.8 | 1.7 | 1.1 | 3.0 | 3.6 | 0.6 | 1.7 |
| Eruptive xanthoma | 0.2 | 0.6 | 0.7 | 0.0 | 0.2 | 0.4 | 0.4 |
| Mumps | 0.3 | 0.5 | 0.1 | 0.4 | 0.1 | 0.2 | 0.3 |
| Diphtheria | 0.1 | 0.1 | 0.1 | 0.8 | 0.2 | 0.1 | 0.1 |
| Whooping cough | 0.9 | 3.3 | 2.7 | 2.6 | 3.1 | 1.2 | 2.3 |
| Fever of unknown origin | 12.9 | 21.8 | 15.4 | 20.4 | 14.0 | 19.5 | 17.6 |
| Tetanus | 0.0 | 0.0 | 0.1 | 0.0 | 0.0 | 0.0 | 0.0 |
| Filariasis/elephantiasis | 0.0 | 0.2 | 0.2 | 0.0 | 0.0 | 0.1 | 0.1 |
| Diseases of mouth/teeth/gum | 0.9 | 0.9 | 1.0 | 1.7 | 1.0 | 0.8 | 0.9 |
| **Non-communicable diseases** | **24.8** | **20.1** | **23.2** | **17.3** | **34.5** | **44.8** | **28.9** |
| Gastritis/gastric or peptic ulcer | 2.6 | 3.7 | 4.7 | 6.4 | 1.4 | 2.9 | 3.3 |
| Heart disease | 2.0 | 1.5 | 2.1 | 1.6 | 3.6 | 3.5 | 2.4 |

(continued)

**Table 6.2: Reported rates of different diseases (per 1,000) during last 15 days by regions of India, 2004 (continued)**

| | North | Central | East | North-east | West | South | India |
|---|---|---|---|---|---|---|---|
| Hypertension | 3.8 | 1.7 | 3.1 | 1.8 | 6.0 | 8.8 | 4.5 |
| Bronchial asthma | 3.4 | 3.0 | 2.8 | 1.1 | 3.8 | 4.0 | 3.3 |
| Disorders of joints and bones | 4.5 | 3.4 | 3.2 | 2.2 | 8.6 | 9.5 | 5.6 |
| Diseases of kidney/urinary system | 1.2 | 0.7 | 0.6 | 0.3 | 1.2 | 0.9 | 0.9 |
| Prostatic disorders | 0.1 | 0.1 | 0.1 | 0.1 | 0.1 | 0.1 | 0.1 |
| Gynaecological disorders | 1.2 | 1.2 | 1.3 | 0.8 | 0.7 | 1.2 | 1.1 |
| Neurological disorders | 1.5 | 1.5 | 1.3 | 0.6 | 1.7 | 3.1 | 1.8 |
| Psychiatric disorders | 0.5 | 0.4 | 0.4 | 0.1 | 0.6 | 1.2 | 0.6 |
| Glaucoma | 0.1 | 0.4 | 0.2 | 0.0 | 0.2 | 0.2 | 0.2 |
| Cataract | 0.6 | 0.8 | 0.9 | 0.5 | 1.3 | 2.1 | 1.2 |
| Goitre | 0.1 | 0.1 | 0.1 | 0.0 | 0.0 | 0.1 | 0.1 |
| Diabetes mellitus | 1.8 | 0.9 | 1.2 | 0.7 | 4.1 | 6.2 | 2.7 |
| Under-nutrition | 0.1 | 0.0 | 0.2 | 0.1 | 0.3 | 0.1 | 0.1 |
| Anaemia | 0.6 | 0.2 | 0.5 | 0.8 | 0.6 | 0.3 | 0.4 |
| Cancer and other tumours | 0.6 | 0.4 | 0.5 | 0.1 | 0.4 | 0.6 | 0.5 |
| **Disabilities and injuries** | **4.5** | **5.8** | **4.3** | **3.2** | **7.0** | **7.1** | **5.7** |
| Locomotor | 1.4 | 1.8 | 1.4 | 1.1 | 1.9 | 1.8 | 1.6 |
| Visual including blindness | 0.3 | 1.0 | 0.3 | 0.5 | 1.1 | 1.0 | 0.7 |
| Speech | 0.1 | 0.1 | 0.1 | 0.3 | 0.3 | 0.4 | 0.2 |
| Hearing | 0.4 | 0.5 | 0.3 | 0.8 | 1.3 | 0.8 | 0.6 |
| Accidents/injuries/burns/fractures/poisoning | 2.3 | 2.4 | 2.2 | 0.6 | 2.5 | 3.2 | 2.5 |
| Other (un/diagnosed) ailments | 12.0 | 14.5 | 16.8 | 7.4 | 13.8 | 20.9 | 15.7 |
| **Total** | **74.5** | **89.5** | **82.2** | **78.0** | **93.3** | **112.0** | **91.1** |

*Note:* ENT: ear, nose and throat.

*Source:* Computed from NSS individual data

**Figure 6.3: Prevalence of ailments per 1,000 people on the day before the date of survey and for the previous 15 days by activity status, 2004**

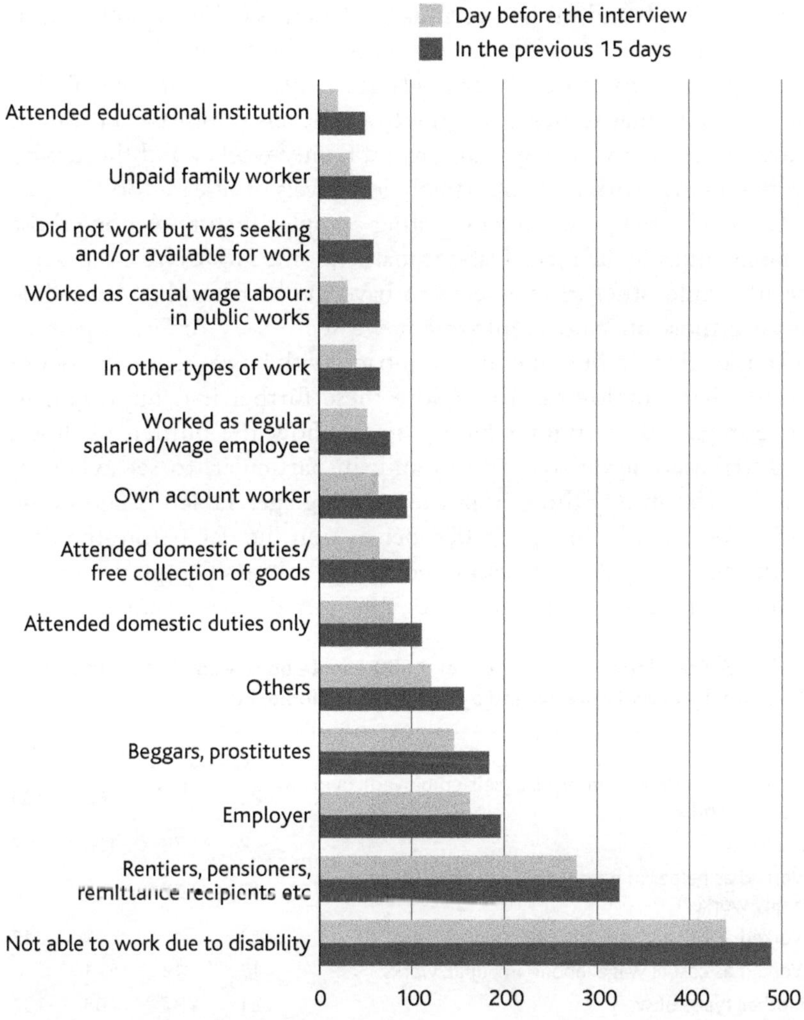


*Source:* Computed from NSS individual data

those who rely on remittances. However, as this group is outside of the formal labour market and reliant on forms of personal or social security transfers for their financial well-being this is not surprising and fits with the findings from the studies mentioned above. Moreover, it is likely that those in this group are older and that these figures are picking up normal age-related disease patterns. This is investigated more thoroughly later in this chapter. Perhaps it is more surprising, at least for a European or North American audience, that those in the employer class have the next highest rate of disease. In the day before the interview the prevalence of ailments among this group was 163/1,000 and in the previous 15 days it was 196/1,000. This is a higher prevalence rate than was reported by those who identified as beggars or prostitutes. Conversely at the other end of the scale the figures show that students had the lowest levels of disease. However, those who were working as an unpaid family worker and those who were seeking work had comparably low levels of disease too.

Overall these figures present a rather complex picture. Among those who are outside the formal labour market, some groups have the worst health while other groups seem to have the best health. Meanwhile among those in paid employment we see a very different pattern than is evident in high income countries, with bosses reporting worse health than employees. To explore these further it is important to disaggregate these figures by age to see how the burden of illness is distributed across age groups and, in particular, to see where it falls hardest among those of prime working age. Table 6.3 shows the prevalence of ailments per 1,000 persons on the day before the date of the survey by activity status and by age group. The prevalence of ailments increases as age increases. We can also see socioeconomic

**Table 6.3: Prevalence of ailments per 1,000 people on the day before the date of survey by activity status and by age group of India, 2004**

| | 15–29 | 30–44 | 45–59 | 60+ |
|---|---|---|---|---|
| Worked in household enterprise (self-employed): own account worker | 25 | 44 | 68 | 186 |
| Employer | 2 | 78 | 160 | 387 |
| Worked as helper in household enterprise (unpaid family worker) | 17 | 37 | 69 | 153 |
| Worked as regular salaried/wage employee | 23 | 41 | 99 | 242 |
| Worked as casual wage labour: in public works | 17 | 19 | 71 | 0 |
| In other types of work | 21 | 37 | 63 | 137 |
| Did not work but was seeking and/or available for work | 22 | 72 | 193 | 173 |
| Attended educational institution | 22 | 26 | 157 | 96 |
| Attended domestic duties only | 31 | 69 | 128 | 270 |
| Attended domestic duties and was also engaged in free collection of goods | 36 | 67 | 89 | 164 |
| Renters, pensioners, remittance recipients and so on | 125 | 77 | 155 | 335 |
| Not able to work due to disability | 302 | 460 | 482 | 490 |
| Beggars, prostitutes | 81 | 91 | 178 | 270 |
| Others | 55 | 143 | 156 | 303 |
| Total | 26 | 51 | 93 | 258 |

*Source:* Computed from NSS individual data

variations in the prevalence rates across the different economic activity groups. The data show that, again as would be expected, those who cannot work due to a disability have the highest prevalence of ailments across all age groups. Aside from this group, among those aged 15–29 years it is the most socially and financially vulnerable groups, those reliant on income transfers and beggars and prostitutes, who also report the highest rates of disease. It is of great concern that younger people in these groups suffer from multiple forms of disadvantage. However, apart from these groups there is relatively little variation in the prevalence of ailments among this age group. This is a similar picture for the next oldest age group, the 30–44 year olds. Although we begin to see the emergence of inequalities in this age group, for example employees in public works have the lowest prevalence rate at 17/1,000 while the rate among employers has risen to 78/1,000, the rates are still relatively low (save for those with a disability which prevents them from working). However, as we move to the next age group we can see that the inequalities become much more pronounced. In this age group, there are a number of groups who have relatively high rates of disease, such as those seeking work, employers, those in educational institutions, beggars and so on, and another group, including the self-employed, unpaid family workers and employees in public works who have relatively low levels of disease. This pattern is largely repeated in the older age group. To see whether these patterns differed for longer-term ailments, that is those that had occurred within the past 15 days, the analyses were repeated for the prevalence of ailments per 1,000 persons during the last 15 days by activity status and by age group (see Table 6.4). The data show a very similar pattern. Again, it is those who are out of the labour market due to a disability who have the highest rates for all age groups. Looking beyond this group though we see the same pattern that the prevalence of ailments increases with age but that inequalities appear to widen too. However, when looking at the groups who do more or less well it is difficult to see a clear pattern or social gradient across the activity categories. As with the more proximate incidence of disease we see a mix of groups who have suffered from some sort of ailment in the past 15 days. For example, among those aged 45–59 years the prevalence rate for all aliments for those who are seeking work is 273/1,000. Yet the rate for employers is not far behind at 194/1,000. Conversely, in the same age bracket, those engaged in causal labour in public works have a rate of 79/1,000 and for unpaid family workers it is 102/1,000.

To see whether certain activity statuses are still associated with a higher risk of morbidity after controlling for the effect of other

**Table 6.4: Prevalence of ailments per 1,000 people during last 15 days by activity status and by age group of India, 2004**

| | 15–29 | 30–44 | 45–59 | 60+ |
|---|---|---|---|---|
| Worked in household enterprise (self-employed): own account worker | 49 | 68 | 102 | 244 |
| Employer | 20 | 101 | 194 | 443 |
| Worked as helper in household enterprise (unpaid family worker) | 35 | 59 | 102 | 196 |
| Worked as regular salaried/wage employee | 49 | 64 | 125 | 278 |
| Worked as casual wage labour: in public works | 32 | 99 | 79 | 1 |
| In other types of work | 40 | 64 | 99 | 185 |
| Did not work but was seeking and/or available for work | 43 | 107 | 273 | 298 |
| Attended educational institution | 47 | 33 | 157 | 129 |
| Attended domestic duties only | 56 | 102 | 167 | 320 |
| Attended domestic duties and was also engaged in free collection of goods | 63 | 101 | 131 | 216 |
| Renters, pensioners, remittance recipients and so on | 133 | 127 | 182 | 387 |
| Not able to work due to disability | 346 | 507 | 516 | 553 |
| Beggars, prostitutes | 81 | 142 | 204 | 350 |
| Others | 77 | 167 | 201 | 355 |
| Total | 49 | 79 | 128 | 310 |

*Source:* Computed from NSS individual data

variables, a logistic regression analyses was performed. As the later Table 6.8 shows it is evident that the likelihood of having any morbidity during the last 15 days before the survey compared with those who are self-employed is lower among those whose activity status is unpaid family worker, worked as regular salaried/wage employee, worked as casual wage labour: in public works, and in other types of work, compared with those whose activity status is own account worker. The likelihood of having any morbidity is substantially higher among those who are not able to work due to disability followed by beggars and prostitutes, rentiers, pensioners, remittance recipients and so on, and employers.

## Types of disease by activity status during the 15 days before the survey

Although these analyses show some interesting socioeconomic differences in the prevalence and likelihood of reporting an ailment across the different activity status groups in India, they tell us relatively little about the types of ailments that different groups suffer from. As we have already seen in Table 6.2 the types of ailments that are recorded differ widely in their severity and treatability. For example, while conditions such as anaemia and conjunctivitis are widespread and unpleasant they are relatively easy to treat compared with conditions such as malaria and heart disease. Hence it is possible that although one group may appear to have higher rates of disease the types of disease they have might be less severe and/or more easily treatable. Thus it is important to examine the types of ailments that are most commonly reported across these activity status groups to see if we are comparing like with like. Moreover, such fine-grained analysis might help us to identify conditions that are particularly prevalent among certain groups which might aid the development of policies or interventions to reduce them.

The top five diseases reported during the last 15 days for the different economic activity groups are reported in Table 6.5. From the analysis, we can see that there are a number of common diseases that occur across all the groups. However, there are also some notable differences. In the majority, the fevers of unknown origin and other diagnosed ailments are ranked as either the first or the second most common complaint. Indeed, these are the most commonly reported conditions among the population as a whole. Yet the relative combined burden of these health problems differs between the groups, ranging from 28 per 1,000 among own account workers to 50 per 1,000 for those who were in education. Following these rather general and unspecified conditions it appears that disorders of the joints and bones, respiratory ailments and hypertension are the next most prevalent set of diseases. Again these are relatively common across almost all of the economic activity groups, although the relative ranking of the diseases differs between them. However, there were a number of groups who had somewhat different disease profiles which might reflect specific risk factors that people in these groups face. For example, the main cause of illness for casual workers in public works was respiratory illnesses but they were also the only group which had high levels of reported conjunctivitis and eruptive xanthoma. This suggests that they are exposed to pollutants or irritants through their work. Conversely those who are registered as disabled are the only group to report high rates of locomotive, neurological and psychiatric disorders. Overall these figures show that there is a fairly common set of health problems experienced across all economic activity groups in India, but that certain groups have rather distinct patterns of disease which might reflect particular exposures. Lastly, they provide further evidence for the double burden of disease by showing that both communicable and NCDs are prevalent.

**Table 6.5: Top five diseases during last 15 days by economic activity groups (total)**

| Usual activity status | 1 | 2 | 3 | 4 | 5 |
|---|---|---|---|---|---|
| Self-employed worker | Fever of unknown origin (14.6) | Other diagnosed ailments (13.5) | Disorders of joints and bones (7.8) | Respiratory including ear/nose/throat ailments (6.6) | Bronchial asthma (6.1) |
| Employer | Other diagnosed ailments (12.9) | Diabetes mellitus, Heart disease (11.9) | Disorders of joints and bones (10.5) | Hypertension (9.1) | Gastritis/gastric or peptic ulcer (5.5) |
| Worked as unpaid family worker | Fever of unknown origin (19.1) | Other diagnosed ailments (17.3) | Disorders of joints and bones (7.4) | Gastritis/gastric or peptic ulcer (6.1) | Diarrhoea/dysentery (5.4) |
| Worked as regular salaried/wage employee | Other diagnosed ailments (19.3) | Fever of unknown origin (13.3) | Hypertension (20.2) | Respiratory including ear/nose/throat ailments (7.5) | Diabetes mellitus (6.7) |
| Worked as casual wage labour: in public works | Respiratory including ear/nose/throat ailments (30.9) | Other diagnosed ailments (28.4) | Fever of unknown origin (16.1) | Conjunctivitis (8.2) | Eruptive xanthoma (6.1) |
| In other types of work | Fever of unknown origin (18.4) | Other diagnosed ailments (18.2) | Disorders of joints and bones (7.5) | Respiratory including ear/nose/throat ailments (6.3) | Gastritis/gastric or peptic ulcer (6.2) |
| Did not work but was seeking and/or available for work | Fever of unknown origin (26.2) | Other diagnosed ailments (16.1) | Respiratory including ear/nose/throat ailments (10.1) | Diabetes mellitus (6.2) | Gynaecological disorders (3.8) |
| Attended educational institution | Fever of unknown origin (35.1) | Other diagnosed ailments (15.8) | Respiratory including ear/nose/throat ailments (11.3) | Diarrhoea/dysentery (5.9) | Diseases of skin (3.4) |

(continued)

| Usual activity status | 1 | 2 | 3 | 4 | 5 |
|---|---|---|---|---|---|
| Attended domestic duties only | Other diagnosed ailments (16.2) | Fever of unknown origin (13.0) | Hypertension (10.0) | Disorders of joints and bones (9.7) | Respiratory including ear/nose/throat ailments (5.2) |
| Attended domestic duties and free collection of goods | Fever of unknown origin (16.5) | Other diagnosed ailments (16.4) | Disorders of joints and bones (6.7) | Gastritis/gastric or peptic ulcer (6.6) | Gynaecological disorders (5.8) |
| Rentiers, pensioners, remittance recipients and so on | Hypertension (16.6) | Disorders of joints and bones (11.5) | Heart disease (9.6) | Other diagnosed ailments (9.3) | Diabetes mellitus (9.0) |
| Not able to work due to disability | Locomotor (14.6) | Neurological disorders (10.6) | Other diagnosed ailments (8.2) | Psychiatric disorders (7.7) | Disorders of joints and bones (6.4) |
| Beggars, prostitutes | Other diagnosed ailments, diseases of skin (15.5) | Respiratory including ear/nose/throat ailments (9.6) | Fever of unknown origin (9.0) | Diarrhoea/dysentery (6.5) | Hypertension (5.9) |
| Others | Disorders of joints and bones (10.8) | Other diagnosed ailments (10.7) | Fever of unknown origin (10.5) | Hypertension (8.0) | Bronchial asthma (7.7) |
| Total | Fever of unknown origin (19.6) | Other diagnosed ailments (14.9) | Respiratory including ear/nose/throat ailments (7.3) | Disorders of joints and bones (6.2) | Diarrhoea/dysentery (5.1) |

*Source:* Computed from NSS individual data

## Hospitalisation

The rates of hospitalisation during the past year for India as a whole and the main regions are presented in Figure 6.4. The national average is 24 people per 1,000 population; however, there are wide variations across the regions. The lowest levels of hospitalisation are found in the central and north-eastern regions (15) with the highest rates in the southern region (38). The average duration of hospitalisation in India is 9 days, varying from 11 days in public hospitals to 8 days in private hospitals (Figure 6.5). The north-eastern states show the longest duration of stay (18 days) in the public hospitals. The rates of hospitalisation per 1,000 persons during the last 365 days by activity status and by age groups are presented in Table 6.6. It is evident that the rate of hospitalisation is higher among those who have a disability (140), followed by the rentiers/pensioners (79) and then employers (72). There is clear-cut variation in the rate of hospitalisation by the age groups of the population.

Average duration of stay in the hospital is higher among patients with disabilities or injury compared with those with either communicable or NCDs (Table 6.7). Among those who suffer from communicable diseases, the average duration of stay is highest for those with tuberculosis (16.7 days) followed by those with skin diseases (16.2 days).

To test whether activity status is still associated with a higher risk of hospitalisation after controlling for the effect of other variables, a logistic regression analyses was performed. As Table 6.8 shows it is

**Figure 6.4: Hospitalisation rate per 1,000 population during year before the survey by regions of India, 2004**

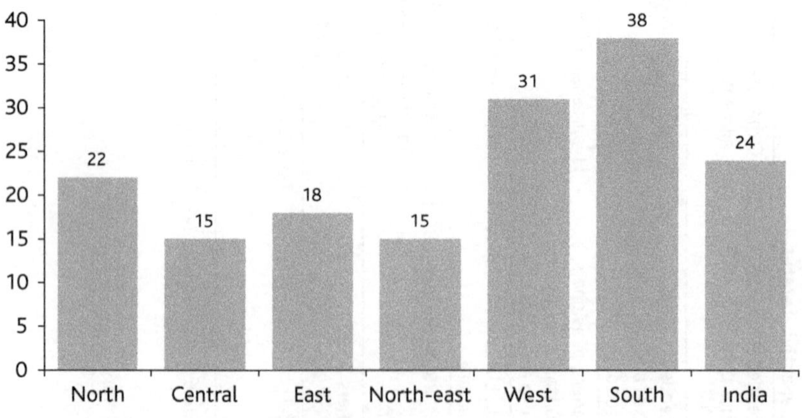


*Source:* Computed from NSS individual data

evident that the likelihood of being hospitalised during the year before the survey is substantially higher among the disabled, those whose usual activity status is rentiers, pensioners or remittance recipients.

**Figure 6.5: Average duration of stay (in days) in the hospital by type of hospital and regions of India, 2004**

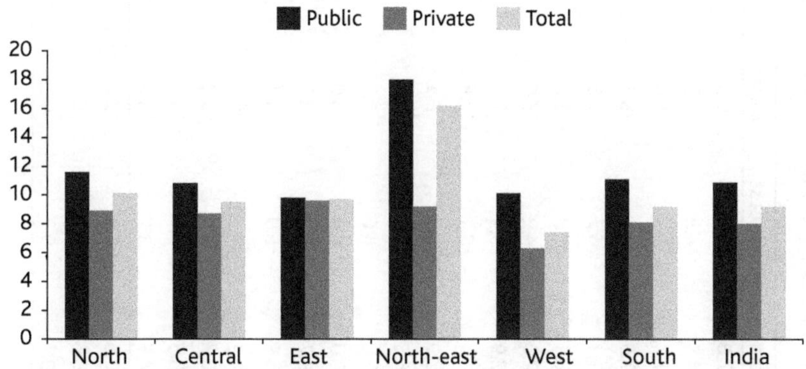


*Source:* Computed from NSS individual data

**Table 6.6: Hospitalisation rate per 1,000 people during last year by activity status and by age group of India, 2004**

| Usual activity status | 15–29 | 30–44 | 45–59 | 60+ | Total |
|---|---|---|---|---|---|
| Worked in household enterprise (self-employed): own account worker | 17 | 22 | 35 | 47 | 28 |
| Employer | 38 | 55 | 51 | 149 | 72 |
| Worked as helper in household enterprise (unpaid family worker) | 15 | 20 | 26 | 34 | 18 |
| Worked as regular salaried/wage employee | 21 | 29 | 52 | 62 | 32 |
| Worked as casual wage labour: in public works | 8 | 27 | 51 | 100 | 29 |
| In other types of work | 17 | 23 | 31 | 32 | 22 |
| Did not work but was seeking and/or available for work | 35 | 48 | 85 | 38 | 38 |
| Attended educational institution | 14 | 5 | 3 | 22 | 11 |
| Attended domestic duties only | 26 | 31 | 46 | 49 | 33 |
| Attended domestic duties and was also engaged in free collection | 19 | 23 | 27 | 28 | 22 |
| Rentiers, pensioners, remittance recipients and so on | 55 | 39 | 58 | 89 | 79 |
| Not able to work due to disability | 105 | 167 | 184 | 138 | 140 |
| Beggars, prostitutes | 11 | 15 | 40 | 20 | 19 |
| Others | 35 | 115 | 93 | 75 | 34 |
| Total | 19 | 26 | 40 | 61 | 24 |

*Source:* Computed from NSS individual data

**Table 6.7: Average duration of stay in the hospital during last year prior to the survey by nature of ailment and by regions of India, 2004**

| Nature of ailments | North | Central | East | North-east | West | South | Total |
|---|---|---|---|---|---|---|---|
| **Communicable** | **8.7** | **7.9** | **7.8** | **6.8** | **6.3** | **7.1** | **7.4** |
| Diarrhoea/dysentery | 5.3 | 7.2 | 4.3 | 4.8 | 3.8 | 4.1 | 4.7 |
| Worm infestation | 7.7 | 6.4 | 7.4 | 8.5 | 5.4 | 4.4 | 6.0 |
| Amoebiasis | 6.9 | 13.0 | 7.9 | 4.1 | 8.7 | 5.7 | 8.5 |
| Hepatitis/jaundice | 7.9 | 10.6 | 11.1 | 6.7 | 7.6 | 8.0 | 8.6 |
| Respiratory including ENT ailments | 6.6 | 6.9 | 8.1 | 7.3 | 5.6 | 7.1 | 6.9 |
| Tuberculosis | 14.4 | 12.4 | 22.0 | 24.9 | 13.6 | 20.7 | 16.7 |
| Conjunctivitis | 8.4 | 4.7 | 7.9 | 9.4 | 7.1 | 3.7 | 6.5 |
| Diseases of skin | 10.1 | 7.6 | 11.4 | 15.1 | 32.3 | 13.7 | 16.2 |
| Sexually transmitted diseases | 11.8 | 7.0 | 22.0 | 8.0 | 2.5 | 14.8 | 9.8 |
| Malaria | 5.5 | 7.4 | 6.3 | 7.3 | 5.2 | 6.9 | 6.1 |
| Eruptive xanthoma | 12.0 | 6.9 | 7.0 | 4.6 | 3.2 | 3.8 | 4.5 |
| Mumps | 3.0 | 4.8 | 18.0 | 4.4 | 3.0 | 11.4 | 4.9 |
| Diphtheria | 7.4 | 8.9 | 6.7 | 7.8 | 3.7 | 6.2 | 5.4 |
| Whooping cough | 20.5 | 6.9 | 5.1 | 5.9 | 4.1 | 7.0 | 5.9 |
| Fever of unknown origin | 8.9 | 6.3 | 6.5 | 6.1 | 4.5 | 6.4 | 6.3 |
| Tetanus | 16.5 | 8.9 | 10.7 | 7.0 | 9.8 | 29.3 | 14.7 |
| Filariasis/elephantiasis | 2.0 | 9.4 | 10.5 | 7.4 | 4.5 | 6.3 | 7.9 |
| Diseases of mouth/teeth/gum | 11.3 | 10.7 | 14.5 | 3.7 | 8.7 | 9.1 | 10.4 |
| **Non-communicable diseases** | **10.2** | **9.8** | **10.6** | **10.2** | **7.6** | **9.9** | **9.5** |
| Gastritis/gastric or peptic ulcer | 9.8 | 8.2 | 8.6 | 7.8 | 6.7 | 7.4 | 8.0 |
| Heart disease | 9.5 | 11.9 | 10.1 | 9.7 | 9.2 | 9.7 | 9.9 |

(continued)

| **Nature of ailments** | **North** | **Central** | **East** | **North-east** | **West** | **South** | **Total** |
|---|---|---|---|---|---|---|---|
| Hypertension | 6.0 | 8.3 | 10.0 | 10.9 | 4.0 | 7.8 | 6.8 |
| Bronchial asthma | 8.6 | 6.9 | 10.9 | 9.8 | 6.9 | 9.1 | 8.5 |
| Disorders of joints and bones | 13.7 | 19.3 | 13.8 | 15.0 | 9.8 | 11.3 | 12.7 |
| Diseases of kidney/urinary system | 11.6 | 10.2 | 11.5 | 12.3 | 8.4 | 8.8 | 9.7 |
| Prostatic disorders | 7.7 | 7.6 | 9.2 | 5.8 | 9.3 | 14.1 | 9.6 |
| Gynaecological disorders | 8.2 | 8.4 | 8.9 | 7.4 | 6.4 | 8.7 | 8.2 |
| Neurological disorders | 11.2 | 10.1 | 10.5 | 10.1 | 11.3 | 14.3 | 12.3 |
| Psychiatric disorders | 15.6 | 11.7 | 12.8 | 30.0 | 14.6 | 18.0 | 15.3 |
| Glaucoma | 9.0 | 5.6 | 6.2 | 7.9 | 3.4 | 3.6 | 5.2 |
| Cataract | 2.9 | 5.3 | 5.1 | 8.9 | 4.0 | 5.0 | 4.7 |
| Goitre | 6.7 | 3.5 | 5.4 | 5.0 | 4.1 | 13.5 | 8.9 |
| Diabetes mellitus | 14.0 | 7.7 | 11.9 | 10.7 | 8.2 | 10.2 | 9.9 |
| Under-nutrition | 6.0 | 6.3 | 15.0 | 9.3 | 6.8 | 8.7 | 8.3 |
| Anaemia | 9.2 | 10.2 | 8.7 | 11.9 | 4.8 | 5.4 | 7.2 |
| Cancer and other tumours | 15.9 | 16.3 | 21.4 | 17.7 | 8.5 | 15.1 | 15.2 |
| **Disabilities and injuries** | **12.9** | **11.8** | **12.2** | **18.6** | **10.2** | **13.6** | **12.4** |
| Locomotor | 12.1 | 9.8 | 13.8 | 15.3 | 9.5 | 17.3 | 12.8 |
| Visual including blindness | 4.4 | 6.5 | 11.7 | 6.1 | 5.8 | 10.2 | 7.8 |
| Speech | 9.3 | 11.2 | 7.8 | 0.0 | 15.0 | 18.4 | 10.4 |
| Hearing | 5.7 | 10.3 | 8.7 | 14.7 | 4.0 | 6.2 | 6.4 |
| Accidents/injuries/burns/fractures/poisoning | 13.5 | 12.5 | 12.1 | 20.0 | 10.7 | 13.4 | 12.7 |
| Other (un/diagnosed) ailments | 9.9 | 9.7 | 9.7 | 54.5 | 7.1 | 7.8 | 9.4 |
| Total | 10.1 | 9.5 | 9.7 | 16.2 | 7.4 | 9.2 | 9.2 |

*Source:* Computed from NSS individual data

**Table 6.8: Odds ratio showing the effect of usual activity status on any morbidity during the last 15 days and hospitalisation during the year before the survey, India, 2004: results from logistic regression analysis**

| Usual activity status | Any morbidity | Hospitalisation |
|---|---|---|
| Worked in household enterprise (self-employed): own account worker (R) | | |
| Employer | 1.711*** | 1.476*** |
| Worked as helper in household enterprise (unpaid family worker) | 0.876*** | 0.846*** |
| Worked as regular salaried/wage employee | 0.952 | 0.972 |
| Worked as casual wage labour: in public works | 0.735 | 0.972 |
| In other types of work | 0.857*** | 0.893*** |
| Did not work but was seeking and/or available for work | 1.162** | 1.263*** |
| Attended educational institution | 1.114*** | 1.116*** |
| Attended domestic duties only | 1.270*** | 1.233*** |
| Attended domestic duties and was also engaged in free collection | 1.288*** | 1.221*** |
| Rentiers, pensioners, remittance recipients and so on | 1.845*** | 1.970*** |
| Not able to work due to disability | 7.933*** | 5.535*** |
| Beggars, prostitutes | 2.674*** | 1.510* |
| Others | 1.819*** | 1.868*** |
| Constant | 0.017*** | 0.022*** |

*Note:* Variables controlled in the model are age group, sex, marital status, place of residence, educational level, caste, religion, household type, safe drinking water, monthly per capita consumption expenditure and region; (R): Reference category; ***p<0.01, **p<0.05, *p<0.10

Meanwhile it is lower among unpaid family workers, those who worked as regular salaried/wage employees, casual wage labourers and those who are engaged in other types of work compared with own account workers.

## Conclusion

The study provides a comprehensive picture of the relationships between activity status, morbidity patterns and level of hospitalisation in India and across its six main geographical regions. Regional differences are striking, as the reported prevalence of ailments is higher in southern regions than other regions in India. The greater social and economic development, coupled with greater accessibility of healthcare services, could be responsible for the regional variations observed during the study. Analysis of reported morbidity indicates that the potential risk of ailments is much higher in Kerala than in other states. Reported morbidity prevalence rates are highest in Kerala, Punjab, West Bengal, Goa and Maharashtra and lowest in Bihar, Rajasthan and Madhya Pradesh. Alongside these regional patterns there are wide differences in morbidity rates among different socioeconomic groups. The results also show a social pattern in health which is quite different from that usually observed in high income countries. Contrary to research in Europe, North America and Japan, the results do not show a clear social gradient in health. One principle distinction among the groups in these data appears to be between those who are in the formal labour market and those who are out of the formal labour market. Still even among those who are working for pay there are notable socioeconomic differences between the different groups. This contrasts with the high degree of similarity in the main causes of illness that are reported across these groups. Hence it appears that although members of these different groups suffer from similar illnesses, the rates and severity of these illnesses differs between them. However, in contrast to findings from studies in Europe and North America, these figures appear to show that it is those in the most advantageous socioeconomic positions, notably employers, who suffer the greatest burden of ill health.

Some researchers, commenting on this, have suggested that there may be serious flaws in the healthcare surveys, which primarily depend on the self-reported illness of the respondents (Sen 2002; Dilip 2002; Murray and Chen, 1992). A significant limitation to the currently available evidence on the magnitude and direction of socioeconomic inequalities in NCDs is the widespread use of self-reported cases of physician diagnoses as source data. Wealthier and more educated people tend to have relatively better access to healthcare as well as greater knowledge about disease conditions, compared with those in lower socioeconomic status groups. As a result, the use of self-reported measures of NCDs may systematically underestimate the true NCD prevalence and could lead to an artificial inequality that makes social gradients appear positive, especially in low and middle income countries. In a study based on six low and middle income countries, Vellakkal and colleagues (2014) compared prevalence rates of NCDs derived from symptom/criterion-based measures to self-reported doctor diagnosed conditions. They found marked differences in the prevalence levels based on these two measures from which they concluded that:

> 'Socioeconomic inequalities in NCD prevalence tend to be artefactually positive when using self-report compared with symptom-based or criterion-based diagnostic criteria, with greater bias occurring in low-income countries.' (Vellakkal, Millett, Basu, et al., 2014:1)

The other common argument for the rise in reported morbidity prevalence is that the people with higher levels of education and media exposure are more conscious in these states, which may lead to better reporting of ailments. These findings and the arguments warrant an immediate attention of the survey designers to adopt more appropriate methodologies to address these issues. It is observed that prevalence of illness increases with age. The high prevalence rate of NCDs among the older population points to the need for special targeting of healthcare services for older people. Surprisingly, it is found that the burden of the ailments is reported to be higher among some of the better-off sections than poor people. Aside from the aforementioned methodological issues it is possible that the higher reported prevalence of NCDs is a result of the higher prevalence of poorer health behaviours, such as higher calorie diets and the consumption of high fat foods, among the rich people. It is imperative that health budgets target these populations with very different patterns of disease profiles and healthcare access.

Notwithstanding these methodological issues, the key message from these results strongly echoes that of Bhojani and colleagues (2013), that there is a real need to improve healthcare services and information on the prevention and management of chronic conditions for many groups in India. However, as they note, the National Urban Health Mission that was due to be implemented between 2008–12 by the federal government to improve health systems has not yet been fully implemented.

## References


Basariya, S.R. (2015). Employee Absenteesim in Indian Industries. *International Journal of Science and Research*. 4(10), 141–156.

Berman, P., Ahuja, R. and Bhandari, L. (2010). The impoverishing effect of healthcare payments in India: new methodology and findings. *Economic and Political Weekly*, 45, 65–71.

Bhojani, U., Thriveni, B.S., Devadasan, R. et al. (2012). Out-of-pocket healthcare payments on chronic conditions impoverish urban poor in Bangalore, India. *BMC Public Health*, 12(1), 1.

Bhojani, U., Beerenahalli, T.S., Devadasan, R., Munegowda, C.M. et al. (2013). No longer diseases of the wealthy: prevalence and health-seeking for self-reported chronic conditions among urban poor in Southern India. *BMC Health Services Research*, 13(1), 1.

Dilip, T.R. (2002). Understanding Levels of Morbidity and Hospitalisation in Kerala, India. *Bulletin of World Health Organisation*, 80 (9), 746–751.

Ghosh, S amd P. Arokiasamy. (2009). Morbidity in India: Trends, Patterns and Differentials, *Journal of Health Studies*, II: 136–148.

Government of India. (2006). *Morbidity, health care and the condition of the aged, NSS 60th round (January-June 2004)*, National Sample Survey Organization Report No 507 (60/25.0/1), New Delhi: Ministry of Statistics and Programme Implementation.

Government of India. (2009). *National Health Accounts Cell: National Health Accounts India 2004–05.* New Delhi: Ministry of Health and Family Welfare, Government of India.

Government of India. (2014). *National Health Policy 2015 Draft.* Ministry of Health and Family Welfare.

Government of India, Ministry of Health and Family Welfare. (2007). *Family Welfare Statistics in India 2006.* New Delhi: Ministry of Health and Family Welfare.

John, T.J., Dandona, L., Sharma, V.P. and Kakkar, M., 2011. Continuing challenge of infectious diseases in India. *The Lancet*, 377(9761), p252–269.

Lee, J.T., Hamid, F., Pati, S. et al. (2015). Impact of noncommunicable disease multimorbidity on healthcare utilisation and out-of-pocket expenditures in middle-income countries: cross sectional analysis. *PloS one*, 10(7), e0127199.

Mahal, A., Karan, A., Engelgau, M. (2010). *The Economic Implications of Non-Communicable Disease for India.* Washington: The World Bank.

Marmot, M. (2005). Social determinants of health inequalities. *The Lancet*, 365(9464), 1099–1104.

Ministry of Health and Family Welfare. (2014). *National Health Policy 2015 Draft.* (Government of India, 2014).

Murrey, C.J.L. and Chen, L.C. (1992). Understanding Morbidity Change, *Population and Development Review*, 18(3), 481–503.

Nongkynrih, B., Patro, B.K., and Pandav, C.S. (2004). Current status of communicable and non-communicable diseases in India, *JAPI*, Vol. 52: 118–123.

Omran A. (1971). The epidemiologic transition: A theory of the epidemiology of population change. *The Milbank Memorial Fund Quarterly*, 49(4), 509–538.

Patel, V., Chatterji, S., Chisholm, D. et al. (2011). Chronic diseases and injuries in India. *The Lancet*, 377(9763), 413–428.
Pati, S., Agrawal, S., Swain, S. et al. (2014). Non communicable disease multimorbidity and associated health care utilization and expenditures in India: cross-sectional study. *BMC Health Services Research*, 14(1), 1.
Schultz P.T. and Tansel, A. (1996). Wage and Labor Supply Effects of Illness in Cote D'Ivoire and Ghana: Instrumental Variable Estimates for Days Disabled. *Journal of Development Economics*, 53(2), 251–86
Siegel, K.R., Patel, S.A. and Ali, M.K. (2014). Non-communicable diseases in South Asia: contemporary perspectives. *British Medical Bulletin*, 111(1), 31–44.
Sen, A. (2002). Perception versus Observation – Self reported morbidity has Severe limitations and can be extremely misleading; *British Medical Journal*, 324(7342), 860–861.
Shahrawat, R. and Rao, K.D. (2011). Insured yet vulnerable: out-of-pocket payments and India's poor. *Health Policy Plan*. 1–9. doi:10.1093/heapol/czr029
Shariff, A. (1995). *Health Transition in India*, NCAER Working Paper No. 57, New Delhi: NCAER.
Vellakkal, S., Millett, C., Basu, S. (2015). Are estimates of socioeconomic inequalities in chronic disease artefactually narrowed by self-reported measures of prevalence in low-income and middle-income countries? Findings from the WHO-SAGE survey. *Journal of Epidemiology and Community Health*, 69(3), 218–225.

SEVEN

# Occupational class and chronic diseases in India

*Sanjay K. Mohanty and Anshul Kastor*

## Introduction

The aim of this chapter is to examine the differentials in chronic diseases among occupational classes in India. Our rationale for this study is as follows. Firstly, the Indian economy has become increasingly diversified with the growth of new forms of occupation, notably in the rapidly growing service sector. This raises questions about whether this change in employment structure is associated with a change in the nature of chronic illness among those in work. The nature of employment is increasingly contractual and less stable. There is evidence from small-scale studies that there has been an increase in work-related stress at work. This has a direct impact on the health and well-being of the working population. However, these studies are unrepresentative and therefore it is crucial that we use nationally representative data from large-scale surveys to test these findings. Secondly there is evidence that non-communicable diseases (NCDs) are on the rise and that work-related morbidity is also increasing. Third, though some attempts have been made in identifying the risk factors of NCDs, no study has examined the links between occupation and diseases pattern in India. Thus, understanding the role of occupational differentials in NCDs is essential for reducing inequalities in health.

In Chapter 6, Dr Sahoo examined the association between activity status, morbidity patterns and hospitalisation in India. He found differences in disease patterns and rates of hospitalisation across regions and by economic activity status using the 60th round of National Sample Survey (NSS) data. One of his key findings is that there is a higher burden of poor health among the socially and economically better off groups. In this chapter, we further examine the association of occupational class with chronic diseases using the second round of India Human Development Survey, 2011–12.

According to Omran (1971) as countries develop they pass through a series of epidemiological transitions. In the third of these transitions mortality due to infectious diseases declines and is replaced by chronic NCDs such as cardiovascular diseases, cancer and dementia as the main killers. Evidence from a wide number of countries has shown that industrialisation brought with it new threats to health, such as occupational hazards and psychosocial factors. Yet the eradication of infectious diseases and the reduction of mortality in infancy and mid-life have allowed many more people to survive into older ages (Horiuchi and Wilmoth, 1998). Populations are ageing and life expectancy continues to increase throughout most of the world as both death rates at older ages and fertility rates decline. As Sahoo shows in Chapter 6, India has also experienced a steep fall in death rates and a steady rise in life expectancy over the last few decades. However, some argue that industrial societies have passed through a third (or fourth or even a fifth) epidemiological transition which, by eliminating many acute and occupational illnesses, has shifted the burden of disease on to chronic conditions in later life (Olshansky and Ault, 1986; Olshansky et al., 1997; Smallman-Raynor and Phillips, 1999).

India, with a population of over 1.3 billion, is of global interest due to its size, diversity, socioeconomic inequality and the stages of demographic and epidemiological transition. With 17% of the world's population, the total fertility rate is close to replacement level and the growth of the older population (60+) is twice as fast as the overall population. Longevity has steadily increased and infant and child mortality have reduced. However, evidence suggests an expansion of morbidity across age and socioeconomic groups, unlike the compression of morbidity observed in some developed countries (Crimmins and Beltrán-Sánchez, 2010; Arokiasamy and Yadav, 2014). Thus, although people in India are living longer they are increasingly likely to be living with major health problems.

The conventional classification distinguishes between two main types of disease: communicable diseases and NCDs. The latter includes the cardiovascular diseases, diabetes, cancers and chronic respiratory diseases, arthritis, digestive diseases neuro-psychiatric conditions, genitourinary conditions and skin diseases. NCDs are the leading cause of death in India accounting for 50–60% of total deaths in the country (WHO, 2014). These diseases have long spells of illness, slow recovery and are often fatal. Furthermore, their treatment can be very expensive. The commonly identified risk factors for NCDs are tobacco use, obesity, high blood pressure, high glucose level, physical inactivity, high cholesterol (Sugathan et al. 2008; WHO,

2014). The economic, social and psychological benefits associated with the prevention and control of these illnesses are large at both the micro and macro level. At the micro level, people suffering from these diseases can experience a sort of multiple jeopardy as they face increased healthcare and self-care costs, and diminishing productivity and health. On the other hand, the loss of household productive labour time for patients and caregivers (which is a major indirect cost) presents a serious economic challenge for the families of those with such a condition. As a result, many families risk being driven into poverty. Whitehead and colleagues (2001) have termed this the 'medical poverty trap'. Evidence suggests that health spending due to NCDs can be catastrophic for poor households (Huffman et al. 2011; Engelgau et al., 2012). In the absence of insurance coverage households often have to resort to cutting back on non-health expenditure, mobilising cash/savings, selling assets, taking loans, diversifying income, wage labour and so on to cope with the financial loss due to illness. The macro-level estimate of the economic impact of the top five NCDs in India by 2012–30 was estimated at US$6.2 million (in 2010 US dollars) (Bloom et al. 2013)

Against this backdrop studies on health inequalities in India and developing countries more widely are crucial to inform public health priorities of national and local governments. However, the ability to examine these issues varies across the world and is linked to the availability of data and to the stage of the demographic and epidemiological transition of the country. Hence there are many studies from the more developed countries that have examined the socioeconomic gradient in health and relatively few from the low and middle income countries (LMICs) (Burström, 2012). The availability of death registration, high quality and representative cross sectional and longitudinal surveys have all facilitated health inequalities research in these countries. In developing countries, the availability of reliable data is primarily from Demographic Health Surveys that focus on maternal and child health. Hence using these surveys, there is a significant and growing literature from developing countries focused on inequalities in maternal and child health across wealth, caste, religion and related attributes between and within the countries (Braveman and Tarimo, 2002; Fatso and Kuate-Defo, 2005; Houweling et al. 2007; Poel and Speybroeck, 2009; Arokiasamy and Pradhan, 2010). Results from these studies show that the extent of health inequality varies over space and time and by the type of variables studies and methods used. However, unlike in the developed countries, NCDs mostly affect those of prime working age in India, as opposed to those in later life, and the onset of chronic diseases is earlier than that in developed countries. While there has been some attempt to understand the risk factors associated with chronic diseases, there is no nationally representative study that examined the differences in morbidity patterns among the different occupational groups in India.

## Review of the literature on occupational inequalities in health

The famous Black Report in the UK (1980) that examined class inequalities in health became a milestone in health inequality research worldwide (Macintyre, 1997; Arber and Khlat, 1997; Adler and Newman, 2002; Mackenbach et al., 2008). Following the Black Report, empirical studies on health inequality largely focused on socioeconomic gradient in health and healthcare. Measures such as infant and child mortality, adult mortality, life expectancy at birth, mental health, morbidity, function health, and self-reported health are used to measure health outcomes. The social and economic gradients are examined using education, income/consumption/wealth and occupation of the population (Adler et al. 1994; Mackenbach et al. 1997; Karlsson et al. 2010]. Alongside this, inequalities in healthcare use across socioeconomic groups have also been the subject of considerable research attention across countries. In addition, methods have been developed to measure the extent of health inequality in a population (Wagstaff, 1991; Mackenbach and Kunst 1997).

Occupation is a strong marker of social class because it provides financial reward, social status and easily measurable. Most of the studies on occupational health are in the broader domain of social inequalities in health. The majority of these have been conducted in developed countries in Europe, Japan and North America (Mackenbach et al., 1997; WHO, 2005; Mackenbach et al., 2008; Kagamimori, 2009; Mackenbach, 2012). As noted earlier the first systematic study on occupational differential on morbidity, mortality and healthcare was carried out under the chairmanship of Sir Douglas Black in the UK (Macintyre, 1997). The Black Report, as it became known, paved the way for numerous subsequent studies on the causes and consequences of inequalities in health. The report's authors considered occupational class as a form of social inequality and attributed adverse social, economic and environmental circumstances to health inequality. For their analyses they used the then current Registrar General's classification of social class that allocated occupations into one of five hierarchically organised categories; professionals – class I (such as doctors, lawyers, accountants), intermediate – class II (such as teachers, nurses, managers), skilled non-manual – class III n (such as bus drivers, carpenters), skilled manual – class III (such as clerical, shop assistants), partly skilled – class IV (such as bus conductors, agricultural workers) and unskilled workers – class V (such as labourers, cleaners, dock workers) (Rose and Pevalin 2005). The report assessed four possible explanations for socioeconomic inequalities in health: 1) artefact, 2) natural/social selection, 3) materialist/structural and 4) cultural/behavioural (Davey et al. 1990; Macintyre, 1997). The report concluded that material deprivation was seen as the main determinant of poor health under a materialist/structural explanation, although they acknowledged that cultural/behavioural factors could play a role through the adoption of poor health behaviours, such as smoking and poor diet.

Since the publication of the Black Report there has been a steady growth in the number of studies published on health inequalities. The development of large-scale, representative cross-national surveys has allowed researchers to examine the existence and extent of these inequalities across many different countries. For example, in a study of 13 developed countries, health inequality has been attributed to adverse socioeconomic circumstances (WHO, 2005). These findings have been supported by a study of 22 European countries in which Mackenbach et al. (2008) found a positive association of mortality and poor self-assessed health with low socioeconomic status. Similarly, Dalstra et al. (2005), found a higher prevalence of chronic diseases among the lower educational groups in eight European counties. Using longitudinal data for Britain Hattersley (1997) found lower life expectancy among lower grade professionals. This was supported by a later study which found that occupational differences explain a fifth of overall health inequality among women and a quarter among men in Britain (Borooah, 1999). This accords with the work by Neidhammer et al. (2008), using data from French SUMER survey, which found that blue collar workers were more likely to report poor self-reported health, long sickness absence and work injury. Studies on occupational health also focus on the specific industry where workers are vulnerable to good health. Borg and Kristensen (2000), using a prospective study of 18–59 year olds from Denmark, found lower health status among low social class. Work-related environment factors were the largest contributor to the worsening self-rated health. As was outlined in Chapters 2 and 3 in the current volume there is a large body of research from high income countries that has documented the adverse impact of stress on the physical and mental health of the population worldwide. This is supported by a systematic review of psychological, behavioural and biological determinants of stress and health (Schneiderman et al., 2005). In this model stress, which can be defined as negative events, chronic strain and traumas arising at or through work, can have adverse effects on physical and mental health and in the long-run weaken the bodily defence and become a risk factor for elevated blood pressure, heart diseases and other chronic diseases (Thoits, 2010).

However, as instructive as these studies have been for focusing attention on socioeconomic inequalities in Europe, some question the extent to which they can be generalised to LMICs due to their different historical and social circumstances (Sen, 2002; Reddy et al., 2007; Vellakkal et al., 2015). As Patel and colleagues (2011, 417) observe:

> 'Whereas socioeconomic development tends to be associated with healthy behaviours, rapidly improving socioeconomic status in India is associated with a reduction of physical activity and increased rates of obesity and diabetes. The emerging pattern in India is therefore characterised by an initial uptake of harmful health behaviours in the early phase of socioeconomic development. Such behaviours include increased consumption of energy-dense foods and reduced physical activity... After the early phase of socioeconomic development, increased health literacy and public awareness of chronic diseases will lead to richer people adopting healthier lifestyles more quickly than less educated and poorer population groups.'

Nonetheless there are a number of studies that have looked at socioeconomic inequalities in health in India (see Bhan et al., 2016 for a review). In their study of women's health in Kerala, in the south of India, Mohindra and colleagues (2006) found that those in the most disadvantaged positions, by caste and socioeconomic indicators, reported the worst health. Data from the 1998–99 India National Family Health Survey showed that there are not only inequalities in health between indigenous and non-indigenous tribes in India but also a socioeconomic gradient in health among indigenous tribes, such that those who have the best living standards also have the best health (Subramanian et al., 2006). These findings are corroborated by data from a large cross-national study on chronic illness and multi-morbidities in LMICs that showed a social gradient in chronic disease by education in India (as well as other LMICs) (Arokiasamy et al., 2015). In Chapter 6 of this book Sahoo provides empirical evidence of differences in the prevalence of disease and the risk of hospitalisation among different economic activity status groups. While these studies have been important in highlighting socioeconomic inequalities in health in India, most of these studies have tended to use wealth/poverty or education as their key measure of socioeconomic position (Bhan, Rao. and Kachwaha, 2016). To date, to the best of our knowledge, there has been no representative study carried out on health status by occupational class. This chapter seeks to redress that.

## Data and methods

Data for the present study is drawn from the India Human Development Survey-II, 2011–12, a large-scale population-based survey conducted by the University of Maryland and the National Council of Applied Economic Research, New Delhi. The survey covered a nationally representative sample of 42,152 households and 204,569 individuals in all states and union territories of India except Andaman Nicobar and Lakshadweep. The details of the survey design and sample coverage are available.[1] This is the most recent round of the survey that provides comprehensive information on household economic well-being (wealth, income and consumption expenditure), work and employment, type of occupation, short term morbidity, major morbidity and so on. The chronic diseases that are covered are diabetes, heart diseases, high blood pressure, diabetes, cancer and asthma. A variable of any chronic disease is computed using any of these diseases.

In the pre-colonial period, the occupational stratification in India was mainly based on caste structure. However, post-independence, the occupational segregation by caste has weakened considerably. The National Classification of Occupations 2004 classifies occupations in one, two, three and five-digit codes (similar to the International Labour Organization classification).[2] These classifications are used in various large-scale surveys. With respect to occupation, the survey collected data for 101 occupational categories and we have grouped these into seven broad divisions. These are: 1) professional, technical and related workers, 2) administrative, executive and managerial workers, 3) clerical and related workers, 4) sales workers, 5) service

[1] See http://www.icpsr.umich.edu/icpsrweb/DSDR/studies/36151

[2] See http://dget.nic.in/upload/uploadfiles/files/publication/Code%20Structure.pdf

workers, 6) farmers, fisheries, hunters, loggers and related workers, and 7) production and related workers, transport equipment operators and labourers.

The prevalence of each disease across each of the occupational classes is examined using both descriptive statistics and multivariate logistic regression analysis. Descriptive analyses are used to understand differentials in chronic diseases by type of occupation. A set of logistic regression models are used to understand the significant determinants of chronic diseases. The general specification of the regression model is:

$$Y = \beta_0 + \beta_1 X_1 + \beta_2 X_2 + \beta_3 X_3 + \beta_4 X_4 + \beta_5 X_5 + \beta_6 X_6 + \beta_7 X_7 + \beta_8 X_8$$

Where the Y is dichotomous and equal to 1 if the respondent has been diagnosed with any of the four chronic diseases (high blood pressure, heart disease, diabetes and any chronic diseases). The independent variables (X) are age, sex, place of residence (rural or urban), monthly per capita consumption spending quintile (poorest quintile as reference), educational attainment (non-literate, primary, secondary, higher secondary and graduation and above), marital status (currently married, unmarried and widowed, divorced or separated), religion (Hindu, Muslims and Others) and occupational class. Adjusted odds ratio of occupational class along with a 95% confidence internal are presented. The analysis is limited to the population in the age group 20–65 years who had some form of wage or salary income. A schematic presentation of samples is shown in Figure 7.1.

## Results

We begin the discussion by presenting the percent distribution of deaths by cause in broad age groups in India (Figure 7.2). In 2001–03, NCDs accounted for 42% of all deaths in the country. A closer look at the cause of death by age group suggests that NCDs are the leading cause of death in prime working age group. About half of the deaths in the 35–44 age group are due to NCDs, rising to 67% by age 55–69. In other words, most deaths in India in the prime working age group are due to communicable diseases

Table 7.1 presents the descriptive statistics for age, annual income and years of schooling across the different occupational classes and India as a whole. There is relatively little variation in the average age across the different social classes, although those in the higher

**Figure 7.1: Schematic presentation of working adults by type of occupation in India, 2011–12**

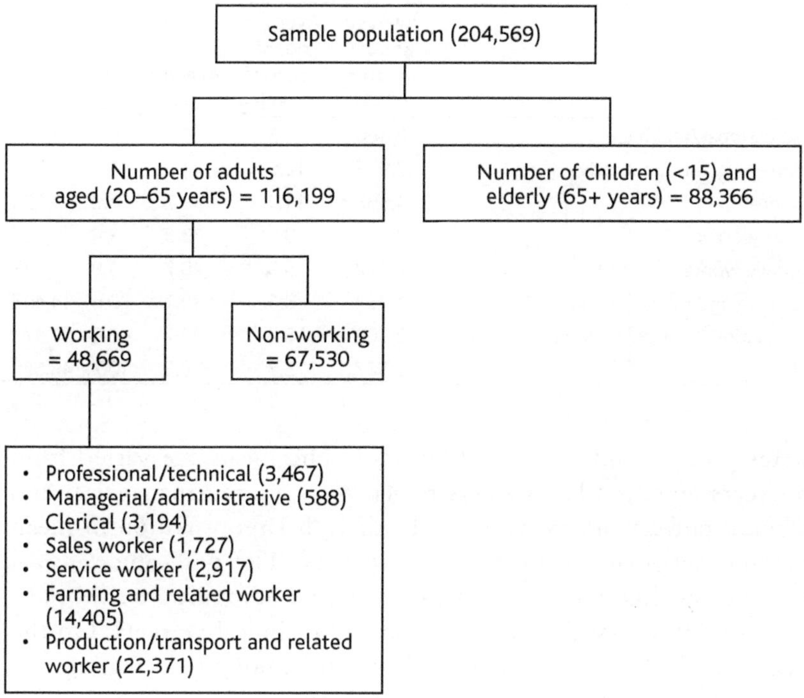


**Figure 7.2: Age pattern of cause of death in India, 2001–03**

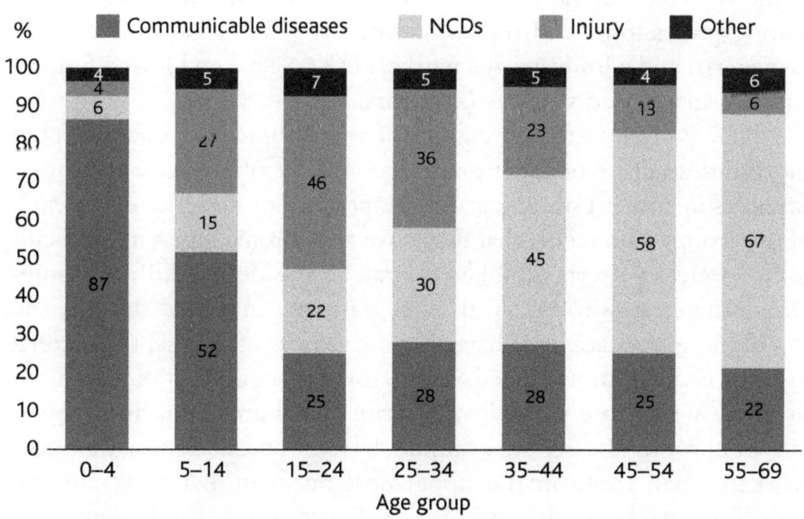


*Source:* ORGI and Center for Global Health Research (2009)

**Table 7.1: Sample characteristics of occupation group in 20–65 age group in India, 2011–12**

| | Average annual Income (US$) | Average no. of years of schooling | Average age | % | N |
|---|---|---|---|---|---|
| Professional/technical | 6,460 | 13.3 | 37.7 | 6.4 | 3,467 |
| Managerial/administrative | 7,972 | 12.6 | 41 | 1.1 | 588 |
| Clerical | 4,993 | 11.4 | 39.7 | 6.2 | 3,194 |
| Sales worker | 3,454 | 9.5 | 33.9 | 3.4 | 1,727 |
| Service worker | 2,972 | 5.9 | 40.7 | 5.8 | 2,917 |
| Farming and related worker | 1,454 | 3.1 | 39.7 | 30.6 | 14,405 |
| Production/transport and related workers | 2,109 | 5.2 | 37.7 | 46.6 | 22,371 |
| All | 2,527 | 5.7 | 38.5 | 100 | 48,669 |

status groups tend to be a little older. The mean age varied from 34 years among sales workers to 41 years among managerial and administrative workers. Conversely, there is large variation in mean income between the occupational classes. The per capita annual income was highest among managerial and administrative workers (US$7,972) followed by professional and technical workers. On the other hand, the per capita annual income among the farming and related worker was lowest (US$1,454); about one-sixth of that of those in the managerial and administrative group. The annual per capita income also corresponds strongly with the educational level of those in the working population. The mean years of schooling was highest among professional and technical workers (13.3 years) followed by managerial and administrative workers (12.6 years) and lowest among farming and related workers (3.1 years).

Table 7.2 presents the prevalence of any chronic illness and selected morbidities across occupational class and by other socioeconomic variables in India. Looking at the proportion of respondents in each of the groups who report that they have any chronic illness it is difficult to see a clear pattern. Unlike research in the developed economies where there tends to be an 'inverse gradient', such that those at the top of the social class scale have the lowest rates of disease, the pattern in India is much more mixed. There is some suggestion of a gradient in health with those in the lower occupational groups having a lower rate of chronic disease, for example 4.1% of production or transport workers, than those in the uppermost occupational class, but the overall pattern is much more varied. For example, the highest rates of chronic disease are among those in managerial or administrative

**Table 7.2: Differences in selected morbidity among working population in 20–65 age group in India, 2011–12**

| | Any chronic disease | | | Hypertension | | Heart disease | | Diabetes | | Asthma | |
|---|---|---|---|---|---|---|---|---|---|---|---|
| | Men | Women | All | Men | Women | Men | Women | Men | Women | Men | Women |
| Professional/technical | 7.3 | 7.9 | 7.5 | 4.4 | 4.9 | 1.0 | 0.7 | 3.1 | 2.7 | 0.2 | 1.1 |
| Managerial/administrative | 12.6 | 4.5 | 12.0 | 6.7 | 2.0 | 1.7 | 0.0 | 6.0 | 4.5 | 0.5 | 0.0 |
| Clerical | 8.8 | 8.1 | 8.7 | 4.8 | 3.8 | 0.7 | 0.6 | 4.1 | 3.4 | 0.7 | 1.2 |
| Sales worker | 4.6 | 5.7 | 4.7 | 2.7 | 2.4 | 0.8 | 2.4 | 2.1 | 2.0 | 0.2 | 0.0 |
| Service worker | 8.1 | 9.3 | 8.7 | 3.9 | 6.5 | 0.8 | 0.8 | 4.1 | 2.3 | 0.8 | 0.6 |
| Production/transport | 3.8 | 4.4 | 4.1 | 1.4 | 2.6 | 0.4 | 0.4 | 1.1 | 0.5 | 1.0 | 1.0 |
| Farming and related worker | 3.9 | 6.9 | 4.5 | 1.6 | 4.4 | 0.6 | 0.9 | 1.4 | 1.4 | 0.7 | 1.3 |
| *Total* | *5.9* | *7.7* | *6.8* | *2.8* | *4.8* | *0.9* | *1.0* | *2.3* | *2.1* | *0.9* | *1.1* |

jobs. However, this latter result might be explained by the clear gender differences in morbidity rates for this group with 12.6% of men in managerial/administrative positions reporting a chronic illness compared with only 4.5% of women in the same class. This varied socioeconomic pattern of prevalence rates in morbidity is also evident when we look at individual diseases. Among men the prevalence of hypertension was 4.4% among professional/managerial workers, 6.7% among managerial/administrative workers, 4.8% among clerical and related workers, 1.6% among farming and related workers and a lowest of 1.4% among production/transport workers. However, there appear to be some interesting gender differences as women in the higher social class groups tend to have lower rates of hypertension than men while those in the lower classes have higher rates. In the case of heart disease there is very little difference across the social class groups with the exception of women working in sales occupations (2.4%) and men in managerial/administrative jobs (1.7%). The social class patterning of diabetes is similar to that for hypertension. The gender differences are somewhat different insofar as the pattern is very similar for men and women with those in managerial/administrative reporting the highest prevalence. Likewise, the pattern for asthma was similar to that for heart disease with relatively low rates in the population and small differences between the occupational classes.

Table 7.3 presents result of logistic regression models for each of the chronic diseases as the outcome measure as well as a model looking at whether the respondent reported any chronic illness. For each model those who work in farming and related jobs are taken as the reference category as they are seen to best represent agricultural workers, who, if we follow the epidemiological transition model, should be more likely to suffer from communicable diseases. Meanwhile the others represent industrial or service sector jobs, and should therefore be more likely to suffer from NCDs. All models are controlled for age, sex, rural-urban, income quintile, educational level, level of literacy, religion and marital status. The results for the likelihood of reporting high blood pressure show that compared with those who work in farming and related trades people in each of the other occupational groups are much more likely to report high blood pressure. Moreover, there is some evidence of an inverse gradient in health as those in the managerial and administrative occupations had the greatest likelihood of reporting high blood pressure, almost twice as likely as those in farming and related trades, while those in production/transport jobs had the lowest likelihood. The results for heart disease show a very different pattern with none of the groups being more or less likely,

**Table 7.3: Results of the logistic regression analyses for the likelihood of being diagnosed with a chronic illness for different occupational groups in India, 2011–12**

| | High blood pressure | | Heart disease | | Diabetes | | Asthma | | Any chronic disease | |
|---|---|---|---|---|---|---|---|---|---|---|
| | OR | 95% CI | OR | 95% CI | OR | 95% CI | OR | 95% CI | OR | 95% CI |
| Professional/technical | **1.48** | (1.14–1.92) | 1.01 | (0.60–1.69) | **1.60** | (1.14–2.25) | 1.22 | (0.67–2.22) | **1.41** | (1.16–1.72) |
| Managerial/administrative | **1.73** | (1.17–2.57) | 1.13 | (0.52–2.45) | **2.27** | (1.46–3.53) | 1.48 | (0.56–3.88) | **1.86** | (1.39–2.51) |
| Clerical | **1.37** | (1.07–1.75) | 0.76 | (0.45–1.26) | **1.70** | (1.25–2.32) | 1.56 | (0.97–2.50) | **1.38** | (1.15–1.65) |
| Sales worker | **1.63** | (1.15–2.30) | 1.60 | (0.89–2.87) | **1.71** | (1.11–2.63) | 0.55 | (0.20–1.51) | **1.40** | (1.08–1.82) |
| Service worker | **1.63** | (1.30–2.04) | 1.11 | (0.70–1.76) | **1.87** | (1.37–2.55) | 0.96 | (0.60–1.53) | **1.48** | (1.25–1.76) |
| Production/transport | 1.15 | (0.98–1.35) | 1.06 | (0.78–1.43) | **1.33** | (1.05–1.69) | 1.20 | (0.94–1.53) | **1.17** | (1.04–1.31) |
| Farming and related worker | 1 | | 1 | | 1 | | 1 | | 1 | |

*Notes:* Figures in **bold** are statistically significant at the $p<0.05$ level. All models are controlled for age, sex, rural-urban, income quintile, educational level, level of literacy, religion and marital status. Farming and related workers are taken as the reference category.

on average, of reporting heart disease compared with those in the reference category. However, the pattern for diabetes is very similar to that for high blood pressure. All occupational groups have an elevated risk of reporting diabetes compared with those in farming and related trades. Again, we see some evidence of this inverse gradient with those in the managerial and administrative occupational group more than twice as likely to report diabetes than those in the reference category while those in production/transport jobs are only a third more likely. However, this is not a true gradient as the odd ratios for the other groups are. For asthma, the results are even less clear. There is no clear pattern with some groups, for instance sales workers, appearing to have a lower likelihood while others, such as managerial and administrative workers, are more likely to report asthma. Yet only those in the clerical occupational group have a statistically significantly higher likelihood of reporting asthma. Finally, the results for the likelihood of reporting any chronic illness present a mixed picture. On the one hand, we can clearly see that all the other occupational groups are more likely to report a chronic illness than those who work in farming and related trades. On the other hand, there is no clear pattern across these occupational groups. While those in managerial and administrative occupations are most likely to report any chronic illness and those in production and transport jobs are least likely the odds ratios for the other groups are remarkably similar, ranging from 1.38–1.48.

## Conclusion

Using data from a large-scale population based survey, this chapter examines the role of occupation in explaining the chronic diseases in India. The advantages of using this data is the comprehensive information on occupational class as classified in National Classification of Occupations and the inclusion of health-related variables from a population-based representative survey. We have used the morbidities that are chronic in nature, namely hypertension, diabetes, heart diseases, asthma. A series of regression models were run controlling for occupational class, confounders, socioeconomic and lifestyle factors. We found that the prevalence of chronic diseases is significantly higher among professional/technical workers followed by managerial/administrative and clerical workers. This is also true for diabetes and high blood pressure. Second, the odds ratio of suffering from these morbidities declines by adjusting for other socioeconomic variables. Third, the odds of these diseases increase with the age of the household.

The findings of lower incidence of NCDs among farming and related workers are possibly due to undiagnosed diseases among these groups and the higher levels of physical labour in these occupations. Also, it needs to be remembered that only diagnosed illnesses are recorded in the survey. Hence it is quite possible that many people in the lower socioeconomic strata had never gone for diagnosis even though they might be carrying the disease. Recent studies have shown that poorer and less educated groups, who are also those most likely to be engaged in farm activities, are more likely to remain undiagnosed of chronic diseases (Aroikasamy et al., 2012). The recent launch of Longitudinal Aging Study in India (LASI) that aimed to follow over 60,000 older adults and use extensive biomarkers will provide insight on true prevalence of NCDs among poor, less educated and farming and related workers. Lack of knowledge of the adverse effects of NCDs and limited ability to pay for the health services are possible explanations for these undiagnosed diseases. Also, these workers are more likely to be engaged in physical labour compared with others. Second, the higher prevalence of NCDs among managerial/administrative workers followed by service workers is not surprising in the Indian context. Working in the private sector in India, in which there is a large proportion of managerial and administrative jobs, often involves working long hours and stressful conditions. The findings from Chapter 6 also support our findings that there are higher rates of NCDs among those working in the private sector than the public sector. Third, the recent initiative by the Government of India to extend health insurance to the whole population is a very welcome step. Given the fact that the NCDs primarily affect those in the working population and treatment of NCDs are expensive and often catastrophic, increased insurance coverage can mitigate the impact of health spending of the population.

These findings are in contrast to developed countries but in line with other studies in India. In developed countries, the prevalence of these diseases is higher among lower socioeconomic groups. However, studies from India documented higher prevalence of these diseases among economically better off groups. Our analyses were primarily among the working population. A comparative study among working and non-working population and industry specific studies will be helpful. In the next chapter (Chapter 8), Vijayantee and Kameanabhan examine a typical industry study of stress and health drawing from Indian police. That poor work conditions are detrimental to health is also shown in Chapters 9 and 11.

It should also be noted that there are some limitations with the current study. Despite the large nationally representative sample this is a cross-sectional study. Therefore there is no chance to assess the direction of the relationship between occupational position and health. Although there is ample evidence from occupational cohort studies in Europe that suggests that having a good job promotes health, rather than vice versa, it is not possible to rule out the possibility that social selection is responsible for this pattern of health inequalities in these data. However, this seems improbable given that those in the most advantageous positions report the worst health. It is unlikely that people would be selected into the top jobs based on having poorer health. Another limitation is that despite having a large sample the number of cases was not sufficiently large to undertake more disease-specific analyses. Such analyses would be useful for targeting specific interventions or policies to tackle diseases that were associated with certain occupational groups. Finally, the survey did not include variables that measured stress in general and work-related stress in particular.

In conclusion, based on the analyses, we suggest that there is a need for more industry-specific studies to shed light on the work environment and health in India. Some of the industry-specific studies that need attention are the armed forces and the police (see Chapter 8). Second, we suggest policies to protect employees from excess working hours and provisioning regular health check-ups to reduce work-related stress.

## References

Adler, N.E., Boyce, T., Chesney, M.A. et al. (1994). Socio-economic status and health. *American Psychologist*, 49(1), 15–24.

Adler, N.E. and Newman, K. (2002). Socioeconomic disparities in health: pathways and policies. *Health Affairs*, 21(2), 60–76.

Arber, S. and Khlat, M. (2002). Introduction to 'social and economic patterning of women's health in a changing world. *Social Science & Medicine*, 54(5), 643–647.

Arokiasamy, P. and Pradhan, J. (2010). Measuring wealth-based health inequalities among Indian children: the importance of equity and efficiency. *Health Policy and Planning*, 26(5), 429–40, czq075.

Arokiasamy, P. and Yadav, S. (2014). Changing age patterns of morbidity vis-à-vis mortality in India, *Journal of Biosocial Science*, 46(04), 462–479.

Arokiasamy, P., Uttamacharya, U., Jain, K. et al. 2015. The impact of multimorbidity on adult physical and mental health in low-and middle-income countries: what does the study on global ageing and adult health (SAGE) reveal?. *BMC Medicine*, 13(1), 1.

Bhan, N., Rao, K.D. and Kachwaha, S., 2016. Health inequalities research in India: a review of trends and themes in the literature since the 1990s. *International Journal for Equity in Health*, 15(1), 166.

Bloom, D., Cafiero, E.T., McGovern, M.E. et al. (2013). *The Economic Impact of Non-communicable disease in China and India: Estimates, Projection and Comparisons*. NBER, working paper No 19335, Cambridge MA.

Borg, V. and Kristensen, T.S. (2000). Social class and self-rated health: can the gradient be explained by differences inlife style or work environment?. *Social Science & Medicine*, 51, 1019–1030.

Borooah, V.K. (1999). Occupational class and the probability of long-term limiting illness. *Social Science & Medicine*, 49, 253–266.

Braveman, P. and Tarimo, E. (2002). Social inequalities in health within countries: not only an issue for affluent nations. *Social Science & Medicine*, 54, 1621–1635.

Burström, B., 2012. Commentary: self-rated health and mortality in low income settings. *International Journal of Epidemiology*, 41(6), 1727.

Crimmins, E.M and Beltrán-Sánchez, H. (2010). Mortality and morbidity trends: is there compression of morbidity?. *The Journals of Gerontology: Series B (Psychological Sciences and Social Sciences)*, 66(1), 75–86, p.gbq088.

Dalstra, J.A.A., Kunst, A.E., Borrell, C. et al. (2005). Socioeconomic differences in the prevalence of common chronic diseases: an overview of eight European countries. *International Journal of Epidemiology*, 34, 316–326.

Davey Smith, G., Bartley, M. and Blane, D. (1990). The Black Report on socioeconomic inequalities 10 years on. *British Medical Journal*, 301, 373–377.

Engelgau, M.M., Karan, A. and Mahal, A. (2012). The Economic Impact of Non-communicable Diseases on Households in India. *Globalization and Health*, 8(1), 1.

Fatso, J.C. and Kuate-Defo, B. (2005). Socioeconomic inequalities in early childhood malnutrition and morbidity: modification of the household-level effects by the community SES. *Health and Place*, 11, 205–225.

Hattersley, L. (1997). Expectation of life by social class. In Driver, F. and Whitehead, M. (Eds). *Health Inequalities*, Series DS, 15. London: TSO.

Horiuchi, S and Wilmoth, R. (1998). Deceleration in the age pattern of mortality at olderages. *Demography*, 35(4), 391–412.

Houweling, T.A.J., Ronsmans, C., Campbell, O.M.R. and Kunst, A.E. (2007). Huge poor-rich inequalities in maternity care: an international comparative study of maternity and child care in developing countries. *Bulletin of the World Health Organization*, 85(10), 745–754.

Huffman, M.D., Rao, K.D., Riveriere, A.P. et al. (2011). A cross sectional study of the microeconomic impact of cardiovascular disease hospitalization in four low and middle income countries. *PLoS ONE*, 6(6), e20821.

Karlsson, M., Nilsson, T., Lyttkens, C.H. and Lesson, G. (2010). Income inequality and health: Importance of a cross-country perspective. *Social Science & Medicine*, 70, 875–885.

Kagamimori, S., Gaina, A. and Nasermoaddeli, A. (2009). Socioeconomic status and health in the Japanese population. *Social Science & Medicine*, 68(12), 215–60.

Macintyre, S. (1997). The Black Report and Beyond: What are the issues? *Social Science & Medicine*, 44(6), 723–745.

Mackenbach, J.P. (2012). The persistence of health inequalities in modern welfare states: the explanation of a paradox. *Social Science & Medicine*, 75(4), 761–769.

Mackenbach, J.P. and Kunst, A.E. (1997). Measuring the magnitude of socio-economic inequalities in health: an overview of available measures illustrated with two examples from Europe. *Social Science & Medicine*, 44(6), 757–771.

Mackenbach, J.P., Kunst, A.E., Cavelaaras, A.E.J.M, et al. (1997). Socioeconomic inequalities in morbidity and mortality in western Europe. *The Lancet*, 3(49), 1655–1659.

Mackenbach, J.P., Stirbu, I., Roskam, A. et al. (2008). Socioeconomic inequalities in health in 22 European Countries. *The New England Journal of Medicine*, 358(23), 2468–2481.

Mohindra, K.S., Haddad, S. and Narayana, D. (2006). Women's health in a rural community in Kerala, India: do caste and socioeconomic position matter?. *Journal of Epidemiology and Community Health*, 60(12), 1020–1026.

Niedhammer, I., Chastang, J.F., David, S. and Kelleher, C. (2008). The contribution of occupational factors to social inequalities in health: Findings from the national French SUMER survey. *Social Science & Medicine*, 67(11), 1870–1881.

Olshansky, J. and Ault, B. (1986). The fourth stage of the epidemiological transition: the age of delayed degenerative diseases. *The Milbank Quarterly*, 64, 355–391.

Olshansky, S.J., Carnes, B., Rogers, R.G., Smith, L. (1997). Infectious diseases: new and ancient threats to world health. *Population Bulletin*, 52, 1–52.

Omran, A. (1971). The epidemiologic transition: A theory of the epidemiology of population change. *The Milbank Memorial Fund Quarterly*, 49(4), 509–538.

ORGI and Center for Global Health Research. (2009). *Report on cause of death in India 2001–2003*. Office of the Registrar General of India, New Delhi.

Patel, V., Chatterji, S., Chisholm, D. et al. (2011). Chronic diseases and injuries in India. *The Lancet*, 377(9763), 413–428.

Poel, E.V.D. and Speybroeck, N. (2009). Decomposing malnutrition inequalities between Scheduled Castes and Tribes and the remaining Indian population. *Ethnicity and Health*, 14(3), 271–287.

Reddy, K.S., Prabhakaran, D., Jeemon, P. et al. 2007. Educational status and cardiovascular risk profile in Indians. *Proceedings of the National Academy of Sciences*, 104(41), 16263–16268.

Rose, D. and Pevalin, D.J. (2005). *The National Statistics Socio-economic Classification: Origins, Development and Use*. Institute for Social and Economic Research, University of Essex, Palgrave Macmillan.

Schneiderman, N., Ironson, G., and Siegel, S.D. (2005). Stress and health: psychological, behavioral, and biological determinants. *Annual Review of Clinical Psychology*, 1, 607.

Sen, A. (2002). Health: perception versus observation. *BMJ*, 324, 860–61.

Smallman-Raynor, M. and Phillips, D. (1999). Late stages of epidemiological transition: health status in the developed world. *Health & Place*, 5(3), 209–222.

Subramanian, S.V., Smith, G.D. and Subramanyam, M. (2006). Indigenous health and socioeconomic status in India. *PLoS Med*, 3(10), e421.

Sugathan, T.N., Soman, C.R. and Sankaranarayanan, K. (2008). Behavioural risk factors for non-communicable diseases among adults in Kerala, India. *Indian Journal of Medical Research*, 127(6), 555–563.

Thoits, P.A. (2010). Stress and health major findings and policy implications. *Journal of Health and Social Behavior*, 51(1 suppl), S41-S53.

Vellakkal, S., Millett, C., Basu, S. et al. (2015). Are estimates of socioeconomic inequalities in chronic disease artefactually narrowed by self-reported measures of prevalence in low-income and middle-income countries? Findings from the WHO-SAGE survey. *Journal of Epidemiology and Community Health*, 69(3), 218–225.

Wagstaff, A., Paci, P. and Van Doorslaer, E. (1991). On the measurement of inequalities in health. *Social Science & Medicine*, 33(5), 545–557.

Whitehead, M., Dahlgren, G. and Evans, T. (2001). Equity and health sector reforms: can low-income countries escape the medical poverty trap?. *The Lancet*, 358(9284), 833–836.

World Health Organization. (2005). *Closing the Health Inequalities Gap: An International Perspective.* Gevena.

World Health Organization. (2014). *Non-Communicable Disease Country Profile 2014.* Geneva.

EIGHT

# Stress and health among the Indian police

*Vaijayanthee Kumar and T.J. Kamalanabhan*

## Introduction

This chapter examines the predictors of psychological stress among police personnel in India. In particular, we are interested in the role that emotional intelligence (EI) might play in moderating the relationship between the determinants of psychological stress, that is potential police stressors, and the subjective experience of stress itself.

A popular Indian proverb says work is worship. However, today work is more often than not seen as a source of stress rather than spiritual fulfilment. Excessive demands, lack of control and unrealistic expectations at work have made the lives of many employees unmanageable. This in turn presents some risks to employee mental health such as stress, burnout and depression. As discussed by the authors of Chapter 2 of this book, stress has been conceived in several ways, however, contemporary definitions recognise stress as a personal experience caused by pressures or demands on an individual which impact on their ability to cope (Blaug et al., 2007). In line with Chapter 2, there is a well-established body of research that has looked at the impact of stress at work on the health of the workforce. However, these studies tend to look at the workforce as a whole rather than at specific occupations.[1] Yet every line of work comes with its own stressors and job demands which raise their own problems. Therefore, if we are to advance our understanding of the mechanisms that cause stress and that, in turn, lead from stress to poor health it is important that we begin to look more closely at individual occupations. This chapter aims to do just that by looking at the role that EI might play in moderating the impact of stress among police officers in India. The police are an obvious choice for this type of research as it is widely

[1] A notable exception is nurses, as there has been a lot of occupation specific research among this group.

acknowledged that they have one of the most stressful occupations in the world (Anshel, 2000). With reference to the previous chapter, stress-related studies on the armed forces and the police are clearly needed in India. Being a police officer demands constant attention and alertness to maintain law and order in society. Alongside the usual occupational demands, the job comes with the responsibility of ensuring a safe and civilised society. Furthermore, along with the military and the other emergency services, police officers are unusual among other occupations as they are routinely engaged in activities that are dangerous, even life threatening, or which lead them to be feared, hated and at times reviled by members of the public, in the ordinary performance of their duties (Symonds, 1970; Ransley and Mazerolle, 2009). They are required to interact with citizens without emotional involvement and professionally intervene in situations which could generate instability, emotional pain or suffering (Valeria-Liliana-Amelia, 2013). Additionally, Ranta and Sud (2008) suggested that law enforcement officers are killed more often by job-related stress than by crime. As testament to this in 2014, 731 police officers in India lost their lives while on duty and a further 3,324 were injured in their line of work (National Crime Record Bureau, 2015). In fact, psychologists have argued that police officers experience levels of stress and pressure that are unequalled by any other profession (Somodevilla, 1978). Moreover, the job carries threats to officers emotional well-being and psychological health. A common trope within crime fiction is the socially isolated, depressed detective who has problems connecting with others and often relies on self-destructive coping mechanisms, such as excessive alcohol consumption. However, this is not just a fiction. Studies have shown that to carry out their job of maintaining law and order and engaging in investigations, police officers are required to be detached, unemotional, scientific and cautious (Mathur, 1995). Considering the nature and demands of their work, police personnel are certainly prone to experience stress.

Given the foregoing evidence it is imperative to address the causes and consequences of stress among police personnel as research indicates that stress leads to deleterious consequences (Maslach et al., 2001). The debilitating effect of stress impacts not only on individuals and organisations but has far-reaching effects on the wider community as well. At an individual level, studies have indicated that police officers experiencing stress reported poor physical and subjective health (Kirkcaldy et al., 1995; Berg et al., 2005) and burnout (Brown et al., 1996) and showed symptoms of depression, anxiety and drug and alcohol use (Richmond et al., 1998; Anderson et al., 2002; Harpold and Feenster, 2002; Violanti, 2004). In some extreme cases, chronic stress has led to attempted suicide among police officers (Anshel, 2000). The work-related consequences of stress in the police force include absenteeism from work (Wright and Saylor, 1991), job dissatisfaction (Norvell et al., 1998) and early retirement (Kop et al., 1999). Apart from the losses faced by the organisation from these outcomes, in terms of lost human capital and productivity, it is the society at large which suffers. Work-related stress can lead police officers to become cynical and engage in misconduct especially with the public (Niederhoffer, 1967; Vadackumchery, 1998). Police stress has been identified with destructive outcomes such as use of force towards the public (Burke and Mikkelsen, 2005) and immoral and callous behaviour towards civilians and victims. A stressed police force may therefore directly or indirectly lead to a decline in law and order and an increase in crime rates. In light of this evidence it is imperative to identify the sources of stress among the police force to mitigate the negative effects of stress. Moreover, to date there is small but growing body of evidence on the causes and consequences of stress among the police force in India. Hence this study aims to add to our knowledge in this field.

## The structure and organisation of the police in India

There are been records of police forces operating in India since the pre-colonial Kingdom era. However, during the reign of British India, the police force was organised with a clearer set of responsibilities modelled on the British Police force. In 1861, the Police Act was introduced, bringing about changes in the reforms of police organisation. This act, passed during the British rule, laid the foundation for the police set-up in the country. Interestingly, this Act is still followed in India with few reforms and amendments. Like many federal nations, the nature of the Constitution of India mandates law and order as a subject of the state, therefore the bulk of the policing lies with the respective states and territories of India. The police are state subjects and its organisation and work are governed by rules and regulations framed by the state government. However, in India's union territories, such as Delhi, the police organisation is governed by the central government Ministry of Home Affairs.

The state government has oversight over the police force in the state. The head of the police force in the state is the Director General of Police, who is responsible to the state government for administering the police force in the state and advising the government on police matters. A state is divided under several zones, further districts, circles and finally police stations. The police station is the basic unit of police administration in a district. The head of the police station is the Inspector. During the period of British rule, the commissionerate system was introduced in metropolitan cities such as Calcutta, Bombay, Hyderabad and Madras for an efficient working of police. However, today this system is prevalent in several other cities of India and is followed in the Union territories. In this system, the Commissioner is the most senior police officer. Down the hierarchy, there are several Deputy Commissioners, Assistant Commissioners, Inspectors and Sub-Inspectors. Delhi, one of the several Union Territories in India, is the capital and centre of the administrative functioning of the nation. The police in Delhi were first established in 1803 under the British rule. In 1978, Delhi started to follow the commissionerate system of policing. Delhi Police is one of the largest metropolitan police forces in the world and has 181 police stations.

The Indian police force can be broadly categorised into constables, inspectors, and officers. The constables belong to the lowest strata; they obey commands of inspectors/sub-inspectors and impart assigned duties as part of police work. The inspectors are placed at the intermediate level; they are expected to investigate cases. They are also responsible for the law and order situation in their area of jurisdiction and for supervising work at the police station. The officers (such as Circle Officers, Superintendent of Police, Assistant Superintendent of Police, and Senior Superintendent of Police) are responsible for administrative control over law and order in the town. They also take care of public complaints and grievances and supervise the work of policemen subordinate to them.

The rationale for the current study may be supported by the statistics of recorded suicide rates of police personnel and the complaints/cases registered against police personnel in India. The 2001 statistics revealed that there were 114 cases of police suicide across different states in India while the 2016 record disclosed 167 suicide cases (National Crime Records Bureau, 2016a). This increase in suicide cases may be attributed to the levels of stress among police personnel (Burke and Mikkelsen, 2007). Complaints against the police by civilians about their cynical behaviour have also considerably increased over the years. The number of complaints recorded in 2001 was 12,345. This increased dramatically in 2016 to 18,876 reported cases (National Crime Record Bureau, 2016b) which may be a result of chronic stress experienced by the personnel. These statistics convinced us to examine the stressors prevalent among Inspectors and Sub-Inspectors.

## Sources of stress among the police

There exists a substantial body of research on what causes stress among police officers that stretches back to the mid-1970s (Aaron, 2000). Acute stress responses are most likely to occur in response to critical incidents such as violent or difficult arrests (Anderson et al., 2002; Liberman et al., 2002), gruesome crime scenes (Violanti and Aron, 1993), unpredictable incidents in police work (He et al., 2002) and shift work (Brown and Campbell, 1994; Hart et al., 1995). More recently research has identified organisational factors, such as lack of influence over work activities and bias against one's racial, gender or ethnic group, which were found to be better predictors of police stress than the factors that represented the nature of police work (Morash et al., 2006). Morash and Harr (1995) have highlighted the significance of workplace problems as distinct stressors. This argument is supported by the results of a study by Buker and Weicko (2007) which aimed at assessing the effects of commonly examined police stressors in the Turkish National Police force. They revealed that organisational issues were the most important causes of stress in policing. Of all the several variables studied, job satisfaction, especially satisfaction with one's supervisor, was found to be the strongest predictor of stress. Alongside this the authors also identified excessive workload, inadequate staff, inadequate specific policies and an excess of 'red tape' as other key sources of stress for police officers. Similarly, other studies have identified a lack of supervision, unfair practices at work (Ayres and Flanagan, 1994), lack of participation in decision making (Morash et al., 2006; Slate et al., 2007) as possible stressors. Similarly, lack of recognition and insufficient administrative support was found to influence stress (Ayres and Flanagan, 1992). Morash and Harr (1995) highlighted the significance of workplace problems as distinct stressors, which included negative interactions with officers, feelings about status, opportunities and physical abilities and practice of bias and harassment. Furthermore, Morash et al. (2006) showed that bias among co-workers strongly predicted stress among police officers, which in turn led to a feeling of a lack of influence on how police work is accomplished. When police officers perceived themselves as having a strong work-related peer support system, they had lower stress levels and were much more likely to be able to cope with stressful situations (Ellison and Genz, 1983; Graf, 1986).

Research in India on police stress began to develop from the late 1980s. Early work in this area concluded that long and unpredictable working hours, dealing with people who broke the law and antisocial elements, threats of being injured or killed, bureaucratic structure, rigidly allocated work pattern, high disciplinary procedures and regimentation, lack of respect from public and work shifts were sources of stress among police personnel (Bhaskar, 1986; Mathur, 1995). More recent work has shown that many of these stressors persist. For example, Bano (2011) found that political pressure, lack of time for family, negative public image and low salaries were the primary causes of stress among police personnel in Uttar Pradesh. Similarly, Selokar and colleagues (2011), in an attempt to identify the stressors among police personnel in Wardha, Maharashtra, found that the majority of the personnel experienced stress due to various reasons such as criticism by superiors, excessive workload, lack of rewards, inadequate value given to abilities and commitments and no satisfaction from work. In line with research from other countries Suresh and colleagues (2013) found that among the Chennai police stress was due to organisational factors rather than physical hazards involved in police work. These factors included round clock duty, no time for family, inadequate salaries/facilities, negative interaction with other police staff, poor equipment, a lack of recognition, too many cases, insufficient staff and harassment. Similarly, in their study of constables in the northern part of Tamil Nadu, Srinivasan and Ilango (2013) found that lack of superior's interest in their subordinates, irregular office work, heavy workload and dealing with criminals were the main stressors. Finally, a more recent study by Singh and Kar (2015) showed that although stress was high among all police personnel, different ranks in the police force in Uttar Pradesh reported different stressors. For example, while Inspectors identified work overload, organisational structure, interpersonal, private and personal stressors as the main causes of stress, police officers found managing people and the ambiguity of the multiple roles they had to fulfil to be most stressful. Hence the existing research on police stress in India indicates that there are a wide range of job and organisational stressors faced by police personnel. These stressors vary across cities, rank and over time. Thus it is imperative to periodically survey the level and sources of stress among such professionals.

## Emotional intelligence

Emotions play a pivotal role among the police. A police officer is expected to deal with a wide and varied range of people including criminals, victims, the media and the public. Police officers are faced with emotionally exhausting events daily and are required to control negative emotions in an effort to conduct their jobs effectively. This requires them to maintain a state of emotional equilibrium. Policing requires the mastering of emotions and the effective application of psychological principles such as EI to understand and cope with the challenges of the job (Aremu, 2009).

EI has gained significant attention in the fields of psychology and management. EI may be described as a set of interrelated abilities for identifying, understanding and managing emotions, both in the self and in others (Mayer et al., 2000). It has been reliably linked to improved mental health, success at work and better performance (Martins et al., 2010). Studies have shown that employees with good ability to manage their own and their colleagues' emotions can more easily cope with physio-psychological job stressors (Hourani et al., 2006). In the context of police studies, Bar-On et al. (2000) have shown that those police officers who scored significantly higher on EI were less vulnerable to experiencing stress and coped better with it if they did experience it. Similarly, Chhabra and Chhabra (2009) found that EI was a significant predictor of occupational stress among Indian Border Security Force personnel. Based on their results they recommended that employers and employees work to develop emotional competencies to better manage stress at work. Most of other studies have revealed that policing involved a lot of emotional labour which can lead to emotional dissonance (Bhowmick and Mulla, 2016). To deal with emotional dissonance and manage the demands of emotional labour, studies have suggested that EI can act as a buffer, implying that those with high EI would be better able to manage emotional dissonance and will not end up with job strain such as burnout (Austin et al., 2008).

Stressors are stimuli that have the potential to create negative outcomes for individuals (Lazarus and Folkman, 1984). These stressors can create perceptions of stress, and eventually lead to negative psychological, behavioural, and physical outcomes. Lazarus and Folkman (1984) argued that perception is a necessary component of this type of psychological stress process. That is, stress and strain will only occur if the person perceives the situation as negative or stressful. They posited that emotions aid in appraising the situation as threatening or and stressful (Lazarus and Folkman, 1984). Subburaj and colleagues (2012) in their study on personality and stress among police constables clearly identified EI as a research gap in the process of stress among police personnel. Following these arguments, it is plausible that EI could act as a moderator, buffering the relationship between stressors and the experience of stress. Hence, our study aims to identify the antecedents of perceived psychological stress amongst police officers and to explore the potential buffering role of EI.

## The study

Data for the study were collected through a structured self-completion questionnaire from 493 police personnel which included Inspector and Sub-Inspector ranks, employed in police station unit situated in Delhi, the capital city of India. The two ranks were considered for the study as they have been largely overlooked in Indian studies which have tended to focus on those at the lower level of occupational hierarchy, Constables and Head Constables, while neglecting those in the middle of the hierarchy. This oversight is especially problematic given the findings from a recent study in Uttar Pradesh that found that inspectors had the highest level of stress among all police grades (Singh and Kar, 2015). Purposive sampling was employed for the current study to ensure that we selected participants who had completed two years of service in the police station unit. This was to ensure that they had been working for a sufficiently long time to have experienced any potentially stressful events and for the impact of those to have had an effect. The survey booklet containing a cover letter explaining the purpose of the study, instructions for completing the questionnaire, the study measures, and the demographic details were distributed personally to the samples in each organisation. To minimise social desirability participants were assured of anonymity and confidentiality of their responses.

## Measures

The two key variables in the study were perceived stress and EI. Perceived stress was measured using a 10-item perceived stress scale developed by Cohen and colleagues (1983). The respondents indicated their experience of stress past one year on a 5-point Likert scale ('strongly disagree to strongly agree') where high score indicated high stress experienced. Emotional intelligence was measured using a 33-item scale developed by Schutte et al. (1998). Respondents indicated their agreement or disagreement to each statement on a 5-point Likert scale ('strongly disagree' to 'strongly agree'). The high score indicated high EI while a low score meant lower EI.

To identify possible stressors that these Inspectors and Sub-Inspectors might face we developed a new set of survey questions for the purpose of this study. These questions were derived from an earlier qualitative study, using semi-structured interviews, with police inspectors (Kumar and Kamalanabhan, 2014). Thematic analysis (Braun and Clarke, 2006) was employed to draw themes (potential stressors) from the interview responses. These were then operationally defined and survey questions were generated from multiple sources such as already existing scales, literature review and verbatim responses gathered during the interviews. All the items were then subjected to scale development procedures. Items were anchored on a 5-point Likert scale ('strongly disagree to strongly agree'). The items along with operational definitions were first subjected to expert validity followed by factor reduction technique. The technique used was principal components analysis. Factor analysis yielded a 11-factor structure. Each factor was tested for reliability, using Cronbach alpha co-efficient. It was observed that all eleven factors exhibited reliability coefficients above 0.7. Further data were collected and confirmatory factor analysis was performed to test model fit.[2] After the data reduction and model fit assessments 45 items were retained. The final set of factors which represented potential stressors were labelled and operationally defined with the aid of subject matter experts as role ambiguity (RA), lack of career growth and development (CGD), perceived unfairness (PU), inflexible work schedule (IWS), work-family conflict (WFC), family-work conflict (FWC), lack of interpersonal trust (IP), public (P), work overload (WO), political interference (PI) and lack of feedback (LF). Examples of some of the question wording (by factor) are: I know exactly what is expected of me (RA), Training opportunities provided are relevant to my profession (CGD), The allocation of work is fair (PU), Even during an off day I am required to be on duty (IWS), The amount of time your job takes up makes it difficult to fulfil family responsibilities (WFC), You have to put off doing things at work because of demands from home (FWC), I trust my co-workers (IP), I receive negative comments from public (P), I take work home or receive work related calls at home (WO), Political involvement hinders the police work (PI).

## Results and analysis

Of the 493 participants, 81.7% were male, 79.1% were married and 64.9% were living in a nuclear family. Out of married employees, 39%

[2] All the measures indicated a good fit for the model: $\chi^2/df = 2.81$; Comparative Fit Index (CFI) = 0.95; Goodness of Fit index (GFI) = 0.93; Bentler Bonett Normed Fit Index (BBNFI) = 0.91; root mean square error of approximation (RMSEA) = 0.03.

had children. The sample consisted of 54.7% who were Sub-Inspectors and 45.3% who were inspectors. Over half (56.7%) of the sample were graduates and 22.7% were postgraduates while the rest had completed only school education. The mean age of the respondents was 29.61 (SD = 6.73) years and mean tenure in the organisation was 3.8 years. Average working hours per week was reported as 110.39 (SD = 3.11). Means and standard deviations for measures of stress, EI and the sources of stress were calculated and are shown in the first two columns in Table 8.1. As well as this we created a correlation matrix for all the variables to examine the extent to which they were associated at the bivariate level. This suggests that the relationship between the independent/predictor variables which represent potential stressors among police, and the dependent/outcome variable perceived psychological stress, share a positive relationship. However only few predictors, for example work overload and inflexible work schedule, were found to have a significant relationship. There were a number of significant correlations between the predictor variables. However, the strength of the relationships was only moderate at best which suggests that each factor is measuring something different, but related. The correlation matrix provides only a glimpse of the degree and direction of association among variables.

Multiple and hierarchical regression were performed to test the main and interaction effects of the antecedents (predictor variables) and the moderator variable (EI) on perceived psychological stress. To test interaction effects, multiplicative terms were created for the standardised independent variables. The standardised independent variables were then introduced into the equation in three successive steps (Aiken and West, 1991). In the first step, the independent variables (role ambiguity, lack of career growth and development, lack of fairness, inflexible work schedule, work-family conflict, family-work conflict, lack of interpersonal trust, public, work overload, political interference and lack of feedback) were introduced followed by the moderator variable (EI), and finally the two-way interactions were performed (each independent variable x moderator variable). Table 8.2 shows that the predictor variables alone accounted for 12% of the variance associated with perceived stress ($F=6.084$, $p<0.001$). Results of regression analyses (Table 8.2) shows that work-family conflict ($\beta=0.31$, $p<0.001$) contributes the most to the development of perceived psychological stress, followed by inflexible work schedule ($\beta=0.21$, $p<0.001$), work overload ($\beta=0.21$, $p<0.001$), perceived unfairness ($\beta=0.19$, $p<0.01$), family-work conflict ($\beta=0.17$, $p<0.01$) and political interference ($\beta=0.15$, $p<0.01$).

**Table 8.1: Correlation table for study constructs**

| | Mean | SD | 1 | 2 | 3 | 4 | 5 | 6 | 7 | 8 | 9 | 10 | 11 | 12 | 13 |
|---|---|---|---|---|---|---|---|---|---|---|---|---|---|---|---|
| 1. Lack of feedback | 1.77 | 0.70 | 1 | | | | | | | | | | | | |
| 2. Political interference | 3.16 | 0.83 | 0.12*** | 1 | | | | | | | | | | | |
| 3. Emotional intelligence | 3.43 | 0.10 | –0.17*** | –0.08 | 1 | | | | | | | | | | |
| 4. Work overload | 2.34 | 0.86 | 0.10** | 0.13*** | –0.30*** | 1 | | | | | | | | | |
| 5. Perceived psychological stress | 3.43 | 0.91 | 0.06 | 0.07* | 0.46*** | **0.22***** | 1 | | | | | | | | |
| 6. Public attitude toward police | 3.24 | 0.60 | 0.00 | 0.59*** | –0.04 | 0.06 | 0.04 | 1 | | | | | | | |
| 7. Lack of interpersonal trust | 2.30 | 0.74 | –0.55*** | –0.06 | –0.22*** | –0.14*** | **0.10**** | 0.16*** | 1 | | | | | | |
| 8. Perceived unfairness | 1.52 | 0.70 | –0.30*** | 0.00 | –0.06 | –0.03 | 0.05 | 0.01 | 0.39*** | 1 | | | | | |
| 9. Lack of career growth opportunities | 1.99 | 0.87 | 0.27*** | 0.17*** | –0.16*** | 0.10** | 0.02 | 0.07 | –0.41*** | –0.51*** | 1 | | | | |
| 10. Family–work conflict | 3.38 | 0.99 | 0.32*** | 0.17*** | –0.25*** | 0.12*** | 0.05 | 0.06 | –0.49*** | –0.38*** | 0.51*** | 1 | | | |
| 11. Work–family conflict | 3.28 | 0.76 | 0.30*** | –0.01 | –0.12*** | 0.07 | **0.07*** | 0.11** | –0.31*** | –0.53*** | 0.34*** | 0.73*** | 1 | | |
| 12. Inflexible work schedule | 3.9923 | 0.77 | 0.09 | 0.24*** | –0.09** | 0.03 | **0.15***** | 0.50*** | 0.22*** | –0.07 | 0.11*** | 0.14*** | 0.27*** | 1 | |
| 13. Role ambiguity | 1.6281 | 0.75 | 0.32*** | 0.12*** | –0.22*** | 0.15*** | 0.04 | –0.01 | –0.37*** | –0.32*** | 0.63*** | 0.52*** | 0.29*** | –0.02 | 1 |

*Note:* p<0.10*, p<0.05**, p<0.01***, p<0.001

**Table 8.2: Results of regression analysis predicting perceived psychological stress**

| Variable | Standardised beta | *t* value |
|---|---|---|
| Lack of feedback | 0.03 | 0.583 |
| Political interference | 0.15 | 2.164*** |
| Public attitude toward police | 0.06 | 0.313 |
| Work overload | 0.21 | 4.844**** |
| Lack of interpersonal trust | 0.03 | 0.461 |
| Perceived unfairness | 0.19 | 3.303*** |
| Lack of career growth opportunities | 0.07 | 1.161 |
| Family–work conflict | 0.17 | 2.162** |
| Work–family conflict | 0.31 | 3.987**** |
| Inflexible work schedule | 0.21 | 3.881**** |
| Role ambiguity | 0.01 | 0.311 |
| $R^2$ | 0.122 | |
| Adjusted $R^2$ | 0.102 | |
| F statistic | 6.084*** | |

*Note:* p<0.10*, p<0.05**, p<0.01***, p<0.001****.

Table 8.3 displays the results of the moderation analyses. The results indicate that EI (moderator) (Table 8.3, Model 2) is a significant predictor of perceived stress ($\beta$=0.433, $p<0.001$). On the interaction effects, the change of $R^2$ did not meet the conventional level of significance. Nevertheless, there is a significant interaction effect of lack of interpersonal trust ($\beta$=–0.100, $p<0.10$) and EI. Figure 8.1 represents the interaction effect following the method recommended by Aiken and West (1991). Figure 8.1 shows that lack of interpersonal trust is associated with stress in the case of personnel with low levels of EI. For personnel with high levels of EI, increase in the stressor is not related to decrease in stress. The results also show that EI significantly moderates the relationship between lack of career growth opportunities ($\beta$=–0.104, $p<0.05$) and stress. Figure 8.2 shows the graphical representation of the interaction effect. It indicates that stress reduces for personnel with high EI when the stressor, lack of career growth and development increases. It can be inferred that for personnel with low EI, stress increases with increase in the stressor.

## Discussion and conclusion

In this chapter we aimed to study the significant factors that contributed to stress experienced by police personnel in Delhi, the capital city of India. As stated in the previous section, political

**Table 8.3: Summary of hierarchical regression analysis for variables predicting perceived psychological stress**

| | Model 1 | Model 2 | Model 3 |
|---|---|---|---|
| | β | β | β |
| Lack of feedback | 0.009 | 0.012 | 0.020 |
| Political interference | 0.149 | **0.139** | **0.132** |
| Public attitude toward police | 0.060 | 0.050 | 0.041 |
| Work overload | **0.206** | **0.101** | **0.099** |
| Lack of interpersonal trust | 0.011 | 0.004 | 0.009 |
| Perceived unfairness | **0.254** | 0.076 | 0.070 |
| Lack of career growth opportunities | 0.082 | 0.023 | 0.025 |
| Family–work conflict | 0.198 | 0.236 | 0.201 |
| Work–family conflict | 0.313 | 0.246 | 0.236 |
| Inflexible work schedule | 0.241 | 0.161 | 0.162 |
| Role ambiguity | 0.020 | 0.038 | 0.046 |
| Emotional intelligence | | **0.433** | **0.437** |
| Lack of feedback × EI | | | –0.061 |
| Political interference × EI | | | 0.012 |
| Public attitude toward police × EI | | | –0.038 |
| Work overload × EI | | | –0.091 |
| Lack of interpersonal trust × EI | | | –0.100 |
| Perceived unfairness × EI | | | –0.039 |
| Lack of career growth opportunities × EI | | | **–0.104** |
| Family–work conflict × EI | | | 0.029 |
| Work–family conflict × EI | | | 0.077 |
| Inflexible work schedule × EI | | | 0.042 |
| Role ambiguity × EI | | | 0.092 |
| $R^2$ | 0.127 | 0.270 | 0.295 |
| F for change in $R^2$ | **5.825** | **93.530** | 1.502 |

*Note:* All variables were mean centred, EI: Emotional Intelligence; figures in bold are significant at the $p<0.05$ level.

interference, work overload, lack of perceived fairness, family to work conflict, work-family conflict and inflexible work schedule were found to be significant predictors of psychological stress. Politicians and bureaucrats are viewed as critically important agents for economic growth and public welfare. However, constant interruption and interference may lead to counter-intuitive results. In a democratic state like India, political parties and bodies play a significant role in state governance. In various states of the country, the police force is a state governance issue which is controlled by the ruling party of the state. However, the current study was carried out in the capital city, which is a union territory, where the police force is governed

**Figure 8.1: Two-way interaction effect of lack of interpersonal trust and emotional intelligence on perceived stress**

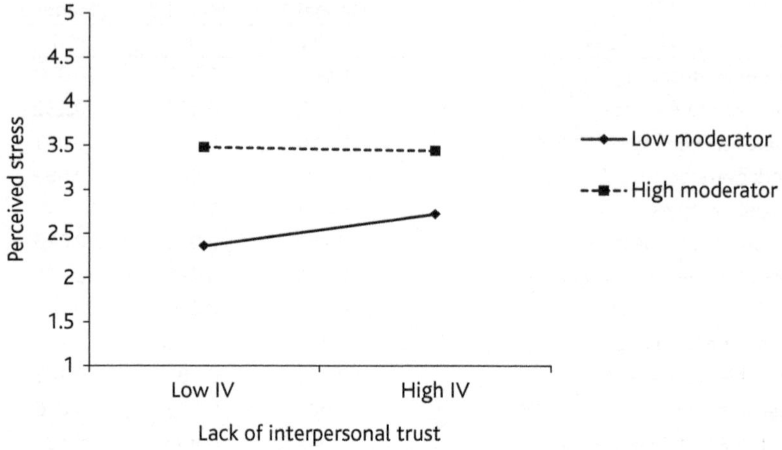


*Note:* moderator = emotional intelligence.

**Figure 8.2: Two-way interaction effect of lack of career growth opportunities and emotional intelligence on perceived stress**

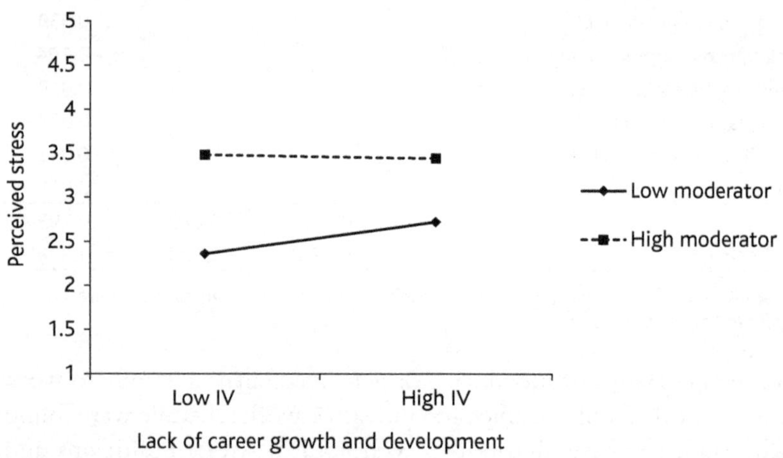


*Note:* moderator = emotional intelligence.

by the union party, minimising the role of state political party. It is an interesting finding that interference from political parties contributes to stress among the Inspectors and Sub-Inspectors in a city which is governed by the union/central government. Toch (2002) in examining stressors among the police, suggested that police officers believe that political connections play an important role in promotion decisions, which may lead to stress. Police personnel may have to succumb to the pressures from politicians due to fear of losing their jobs or fear of being threatened by the bureaucrats. This may lead to distress as, following political pressures, they may be compelled to violate their own values and principles and follow unethical work practices. Further, political interference may contribute to delays in work, leaving the officers over-burdened with work. The finding of this study is echoed by research on police stress from other states in Indian research (see Bano, 2011).

Work overload has been stated as a source of stress irrespective of occupations (Johnson et al., 2005). In the present study, excessive workload may be attributed to manpower shortages in police stations (Kumar and Kamalanabhan, 2014). Police personnel housed in the police stations are required to perform varied roles which include investigation-related duties and jobs; crime prevention and preservation of peace and security; crime detection work; order maintenance and security jobs; enforcement of social legislation; minor, major and special acts; collection of intelligence; democratic and election related duties; natural calamities; disaster management and emergency duties; maintenance of Police Records; assistance to other departments; and other miscellaneous duties and functions. Juggling these tasks may lead to pressure of meeting deadlines which consequently leads to stress, especially when there is no clear division of work. This can be best explained by Yerkes-Dodson's (1908) law of an inverted U-shape relationship between different workloads and health outcomes which indicates that there is an optimal level of physical or psychological health at the mid-level of the workload distribution.

In the last few years, a small but growing literature has found associations between a lack of fairness at work and a decline in employee health indicated by lower self-rated health status, increased sick leave and more psychiatric disorders (Ndjaboué et al., 2015). The relationship between fairness and employee attitudes and behaviours has been well documented in meta-analyses and relevant literature (Colquitt, 2001). The current study also empirically demonstrated that perceived unfairness contributed to stress which is in line with an Australian study on police stress (see Noblet et al., 2009). The injustice-stress theory (Vermunt and Steensma, 2001) with respect to social-comparison has stated that when employees' objectives are unmet, they experience diminished satisfaction and heightened strain. Similarly, equity theory (Adams, 1965) explains the relationship between perceived justice/fairness and stress. This theory posited that individuals evaluate justice by comparing the ratio of inputs to outcomes. Further Walster et al. (1973) summarised that when individuals find themselves participating in inequitable relationships, they suffer from stress.

The present results demonstrate that work-family conflict is a significant source of stress for the police force. Several studies in the literature have found an association between work-family conflict and police stress (Bazana and Dodd, 2013; Lambert et al., 2017). The results show that when it is not possible to resolve the different demands of work and family, the employee is left stressed. The results suggest that the work environment of police personnel contributes to this work-family conflict as stressor. When individuals experience high levels of job demands, they tend to have less time with their family. This may perhaps be due to work overload, lack of time for family and work, strict deadlines and other police related activities, eventually leading to stress.

Finally, an inflexible work schedule was found to be a significant predictor of stress among the sample studied. This has been identified in numerous studies as a major stressor (see Abdollahi, 2002). Because policing is around-the-clock, many officers are forced to work early mornings, late evenings, sometimes even through nights. Having to work extensively long hours as enforced by the organisation may lead to stress (Ayres and Flanagan, 1994). The current situation is that Station House Officers (Inspector rank) are required to stay in the station 24×7 and monitor their respective jurisdictions. A lack of fixed working hours, work overload and manpower shortages perhaps could be the plausible reasons behind this factor as a source of significant stress (Kumar and Kamalanabhan, 2014).

The results of the present study highlight that EI, an internal protective factor and a personal resource, plays a key role in evaluating the stressors as threatening, eventually leading to a state of psychological stress. The findings of the study suggest that those who possess the qualities of an emotionally intelligent person will deal with the stressors in an appropriate way which may eventually prevent an individual from experiencing stress. Studies have indicated that those with high EI possess higher self-efficacy which aids in processing the stressor or stressful situation as less threatening and rather identifies such situations as challenging (Mikolajczak and Luminet, 2008). Mikolajczak et al. (2007) have also shown that high EI individuals secrete less cortisol in anticipation to a potentially stressful situation than their low trait EI peers. Under stress-inducing situations, EI skills save the individual from breaking under pressure or showing signs of helplessness and hopelessness (Mangal and Mangal, 2015). Mayer and

Salovey (1997) asserted that people with high levels of EI hold a greater ability to comprehend and analyse emotion, which leads to a positive effect. A critical characteristic of high EI people are positive affect and optimism (Salovey and Mayer, 1990). Such individuals may observe the procession of their thoughts and tend to ruminate productively on the antecedents and consequences of their problems. This, in turn, leads them to interpret stressful situations/conditions in a more benign and less stressful way, viewing them more as challenges than as threats. In the police force, a study by Bar-On and colleagues (2000) indicated that police officers who scored significantly higher on EI were less vulnerable to experience stress and coped with it better.

The findings presented in this chapter shed light on an important issue that directly affects police personnel and indirectly impacts the society. The outcomes of stress can be deleterious resulting in the development of burnout and lower the engagement levels of police personnel. This may further cause work impairment which may exact a heavy toll on the police organisation and the state and central government. This study has usefully generated knowledge on sources of stress (among Inspectors and Sub-Inspectors) prevalent in Delhi Police. These stressors warrant immediate attention and consideration to improve the well-being of the police, police organisation and the society at large. The current practices in Delhi Police must be revisited and modified. One of the core sources of stress is long working hours, which affects their family life. Thus we would recommend that the police administration introduces a shift system and develops incentives to expand manpower. To tackle perceived unfairness, awareness training among supervisors may help. Monitoring the political interference by senior government officials in the police department and where high police officials discourage political involvement may help reduce the impact of such intrusion on personnel. Finally, our results show the benefits of training police personnel to develop their EI to better handle and manage stress at an individual level. EI may also prove to be a useful tool for selection of police personnel, ensuring that they are protected and shielded from stressful work situations.

## References

Aaron, J. (2000). Stress & coping in police officers. *Police Quarterly*, 3, 428–450.

Abdollahi, K.M. (2002). Understanding police stress research. *Journal of Forensic Psychology Practice*, 2, 1–24.

Adams, J.S. (1965). Inequity in social exchange. In L. Berkowitz (Ed.), *Advances in experimental social psychology, 2*. New York: Academic Press.

Aiken, L.S., and West, S.G. (1991). *Multiple regression: Testing and interpreting interactions*. Newbury Park: Sage.

Anderson, G., Litzenberger, R., and Plecas, D. (2002). Physical evidence of police officer stress. *Policing: An International Journal of Police Strategies & Management*, 25, 399–420.

Anshel, M. H. (2000). A conceptual model and implications for coping with stressful events in police work. *Criminal Justice and Behavior*, 27, 375–400.

Aremu, O. (2009). The Inclusion of Emotional Intelligence in Nigerian Police Recruits Training Programme: Agenda for Police Personnel Prosocial Development and Effective Policing. *Journal of Research in Education and Society*, 2(1).

Austin, E.J., Dore, T.C. and O'Donovan, K.M. (2008). Associations of personality and emotional intelligence with display rule perceptions and emotional labour. *Personality and Individual Differences*, 44(3), 679–688.

Ayres, R.M., and Flanagan, G.S. (1992). *Preventing law enforcement stress: The organization's role*. Washington, DC: U.S. Department of Justice Bureau of Justice Assistance.

Bano, R. (2011). *Job Stress among Police Personnel*. Paper presented at International Conference on Economics and Finance Research, Singapore. Retrieved from http://www.ipedr.com/vol4/56-F10027.pdf.

Bar-On, R., Brown, J.M., Kirkcaldy B.D. and Thome, E.P. (2000). Emotional expression and implications for occupational stress; an application of the Emotional Quotient Inventory (EQ-i). *Personality and Individual Differences*, 28(6), 1107–1118.

Bazana, S. and Dodd, N. (2013). Conscientiousness, Work Family Conflict and Stress amongst Police Officers in Alice, South Africa. *Journal of Psychology*,4(1), 1–18.

Berg, A.M., Hem, E., Lau, B.H. and Ekeberg, O. (2005). Stress in the Norwegian police service. *Occupational Medicine*, 55, 113–20.

Bhaskar, S. (1986). Investigation into relation between job stress and personality factors among police. (Unpublished doctoral dissertation). University of Delhi, Delhi.

Bhowmick, S. and Mulla, Z. (2016). Emotional labour of policing: Does authenticity play a role? *International Journal of Police Science & Management*, 18(1), 47–60.

Biggam, F.H., Power, K.G. and MacDonald, R.R. (1997). Self-perceived occupational stress and distress in a Scottish police force. *Work and Stress*, 11, 118–133.

Blaug, R., Kenyon, A. and Lekhi, R. (2007). *Stress at Work: A report prepared for the Work Foundations principal partners*. Project Report. London: The Work Foundation.

Braun, V. and Clarke, V. (2006). Using thematic analysis in psychology. *Qualitative Research in Psychology*, 3(2), 77–101.

Brown, J., Cooper, C.L., and Kirkcaldy, B. (1996). Occupational stress among senior police officers. *British Journal of Psychology*, 87, 31–45.

Brown, J.M. and Campbell, E.A. (1994). *Stress and Policing: Sources and Strategies*. Chichester, John Wiley & Sons.

Buker, H. and Wiecko, F. (2007). Are causes of police stress global? Testing the effects of common police stressors on the Turkish National Police. *Policing: An International Journal of Police Strategies & Management*, 30(2), 291–309.

Burke, R.J. and Mikkelsen, A. (2005). Burnout, job stress and attitudes towards the use of force by Norwegian police officers. *Policing: An International Journal of Police Strategies & Management*, 28(2), 269–278.

Burke, R.J. and Mikkelsen, A. (2007). Suicide Ideation among police officers in Norway. *Policing: An International Journal of Police Strategies & Management*, 30(2), 228–236.

Chhabra, M. and Chhabra, B. (2009). Occupational Stress in BSF: Causes and Remedies. *The Indian Police Journal*, 56 (4), 85–94

Cohen, S., Karmarck, T. and Mermelstien, R. (1983). A Global Measure of Perceived Stress. *Journal of Health and Social Behaviour*, 24(4), 385–396.

Colquitt, J.A. (2001). On the dimensionality of organizational justice: A construct validation of a measure. *Journal of Applied Psychology*, 86(3), 386–400.

Ellison, K.W. and Genz, J. (1983). *Stress and the police officer*. Springfield, IL: Charles C Thomas.

Graf, F.A. (1986). The relationship between social support and occupational stress among police officers. *Journals of Police Science and Administration*, 14, 178–86.

Harpold, J., and Feenster, S.L. (2002). Negative influences of police stress. *FBI Law Enforcement Bulletin*, 71, 1–7.

Hart, P.M., Wearing, A.J. and Headey, B. (1995). Police stress and wellbeing: integrating personality, coping and daily work experiences. *Journal of Occupational and Organizational Psychology*, 68, 133–56.

He, N., Zhao, J., and Archbold, C.A. (2002). Gender and police stress: The convergent and divergent impact of work environment, work-family conflict, and stress coping mechanisms of female and male police officers. *Policing: An International Journal of Police Strategies and Management*, 25, 687–708.

Hourani, L.L., Williams, T.V. and Kress, A.M. (2006) Stress, mental health and job performance among active duty military personnel: Findings from the 2002 department of deference health-related behaviors survey, *Military Medicine*, 171(9), 849–856.

Johnson, S., Cooper, C., Cartwright, S. et al. (2005). The experience of work-related stress across occupations. *Journal of Managerial Psychology*, 20(2), 178–187.

Kirkcaldy, B., Cooper, C.L., and Ruffalo, P. (1995). Work stress and health in a sample of U.S. police. *Psychological Reports*, 76, 700–702.

Kop, N., Euwema, M. and Schaufeli, W. (1999). Burnout, job stress, and violent behaviour among Dutch police officers. *Work and Stress*, 13, 326–340.

Kumar, V. and Kamalanabhan, T.J. (2014). Sources of Stress among Police Officials: A Qualitative Investigation. *Indore Management Journal*. Retrieved from http://www.iimidr.ac.in/iimi/images/IMJ/Volume6/Sources.pdf

Lambert, E.G., Qureshi, H., Frank, J. et al. (2017). The relationship of work-family conflict with job stress among Indian police officers: a research note. *Police Practice and Research*, 18(1), 37–48.

Lazarus, R.S., and Folkman, S. (1984). *Psychological stress and the coping process*. New York, NY: Springer.

Liberman, A.M., Best, S.R., Metzler, T.J. (2002). Routine occupational stress and psychological distress in police. *Policing: An International Journal of Police Strategies & Management*, 25, 421–439.

Mangal, S.K. and Mangal S. (2015). *Emotional Intelligence: Managing Emotions to Win in Life*. PHI Learning Pvt. Ltd.

Maslach, C., Schaufeli, W.B. and Leiter, M.P. (2001). Job burnout. *Annual Review of Psychology*, 52(1), 397–422.

Martins, A., Ramalho, N. and Morin, E. (2010). A comprehensive meta-analysis of the relationship between emotional intelligence and health. *Personality and Individual Differences*, 49, 554–564.

Mathur, P. (1995). Perception of police stress: An empirical study of stressors and coping responses among police personnel in India. *Indian Journal of Criminology*, 23, 9–19.

Mayer, J.D. and Salovey, P. (1997). What is emotional intelligence? In P. Salovey & D.J. Sluyter (Eds.), *Emotional development and emotional intelligence: Educational implications*, New York: Harper Collins, pp 3-34.

Mayer, J.D., Salovey, P. and Caruso, D.R. (2000). Models of emotional intelligence. In R.J. Sternberg (Ed.), *Handbook of intelligence*, 396–420.

Mikolajczak, M., Luminet, O., and Menil, C. (2006). Predicting resistance to stress: Incremental validity of trait emotional intelligence over alexithymia and optimism. *Psicothema: Revista de Psicologia*, 18, 79–88.

Mikolajczak, M. and Luminet, O. (2008). Trait emotional intelligence and the cognitive appraisal of stressful events: An exploratory study. *Personality and individual differences*, 44(7), 1445–1453.

Mikolajczak, M., Menil, C. and Luminet, O. (2007). Explaining the protective effect of trait emotional intelligence regarding occupational stress: Exploration of emotional labour processes. *Journal of Research in Personality*, 41(5), 1107–1117.

Morash, M. and Haarr, R.N. (1995). Gender, workplace problems, and stress in policing. *Justice Quarterly*, 12(1), 113–140.

Morash, M., Haarr, R.N. and Kwak, D. (2006). Multilevel influences on police stress. *Journal of Contemporary Criminal Justice*, 22, 26–43.

National Crime Record Bureau (2015). *Crime in India.* Chapter 15. Police and Civilians Causualties. http://ncrb.nic.in/StatPublications/CII/CII2014/chapters/Chapter%2015.pdf. Accessed 2017.

National Crime Record Bureau (2016b). *Crime in India.* Chapter 16. Complaints against police personnel and Human rights violations by them. http://ncrb.nic.in/. Accessed 2017.

National Crime Record Bureau (2016a). *Crime in India.* Chapter 15. Police and Civilians Casualties. http://ncrb.nic.in/. Accessed 2017.

Ndjaboué, R., Brisson, C. and Vézina, M. (2015). Organisational justice and mental health: a systematic review of prospective studies. *Occupational and Environmental Medicine.* Online first: doi:10.1136/oemed-2011-100595.

Niederhoffer, A. (1967). *Behind the shield: The police in urban society.* New York: Anchor Books.

Noblet, A.J., Rodwell, J.J. and Allisey, A.F. (2009). Police stress: the role of the psychological contract and perceptions of fairness. *Policing: An International Journal of Police Strategies & Management*, 32(4), 613–630.

Norvell, N., Belles, D., and Hills, H. (1998). Perceived stress levels and physical symptoms in supervisory law enforcement personnel. *Journal of Police Science and Administration*, 16, 75–79.

Ransley, J. and Mazerolle, L. (2009). Policing in an era of uncertainty. *Police Practice and Research*, 10(4), 365–381.

Ranta, R.S. and Sud, A. (2008). Management of stress and burnout of police personnel. *Journal of the Indian Academy of Applied Psychology*, 34(1), 29–39.

Richmond, R.L., Wodak, A., Kehoe, L. and Heather, N. (1998). How healthy are the police? A survey of life-style factors. *Addiction*, 93, 1729–1737.

Salovey, P, and Mayer, J.D. (1990). Emotional intelligence. *Imagination, Cognition and Personality*, 9(3), 185–211.

Selokar, D., Nimbarte, S., Ahana, S. et al. (2011). Occupational stress among police personnel of Wardha City, India. *Australian Medical Journal*, 4(3), 114–7. doi: http//dx.doi.org/10.4066/AMJ.2011.562.

Singh, S. and Kar, S.K. (2015). Sources of occupational stress in the police personnel of North India: An exploratory study. *Indian Journal of Occupational and Environmental Medicine*, 19, 56–60

Slate, R.N., Johnson, W.W. and Colbert, S.S. (2007). Police Stress: A Structural Model. *Journal of Police and Criminal Psychology*, 22, 102–112.

Somodevilla, S.A. (1978). The psychologist's Role in the Police Department. *The Police Chief*, 45, 21–23.

Srinivasan, S. and Ilango, P. (2013). Stress Problems Faced by Police Constables in North Chennai. *Global Research Analysis*, 2(4). https://www.academia.edu/3313879/Stress_Problems_of_Police_Constables.

Subburaj, A., Shunmugasundaram, M., Sekar, M. and Sumathi, P. (2012). Big Five Personality Traits – A tool for Managing Stress. *Tactful Management Research Journal*, 1(2).

Suresh, R.S., Anantharaman, R.N., Angusamy, A. and Ganesan, J. (2013). Sources of Job Stress in Police Work in a Developing Country. *International Journal of Business and Management*, 8(13), 102–110.

Symonds, M. (1970). Emotional hazards of police work. *American Journal of Psychoanalysis*, 30(2), 155–160.

Toch, H. (2002). *Stress in policing*. Washington, DC: American Psychological Association.

Vadackumchery, J. (1998). *Indian Police: 2001 – What went wrong here?* Dehli: A.P.H. Publishing Corporation.

Valeria-Liliana-Amelia, P.N. (2013). An Analysis on Violence and Suicide among Police Officers. *Public Administration Research*, 2(1), 84.

Vermunt, R. and Steensma, H. (2001). Stress and Justice in Organisations. An Exploration into Justice processes with the aim to find mechanisms to reduce stress. In R. Cropanzano (Ed.), *From theory to practice: Vol. 2. Justice in the workplace*. NJ: Lawrence Erlbaum.

Violanti, J.M. (2004). Predictors of police suicide ideation. *Suicide and Life Threatening Behavior*, 34, 277–283.

Violanti, J.M. and Aron, F. (1993). Sources of police stressors, job attitudes, and psychological distress. *Psychological Reports*, 72, 899–904.

Walster, E., Berscheid, E., and Walster, G.W. (1973). New directions in equity research. *Journal of Personality and Social Psychology*, 25, 151–176.
Wright, K.N. and Saylor, W.G. (1991). Male and female employees' perceptions of prison work: Is there a difference? *Justice Quarterly*, 8, 508–524.

NINE

# Health status and lifestyle of the Oraon tea garden labourers of Jalpaiguri district, West Bengal

*Subrata K. Roy and Tanaya Kundu Chowdhury*

## Introduction

India is one of the leading countries in producing and exporting tea all over the world. According to the *61th Annual Report of Tea Board*, India produced 1.2 billion kilograms and exported 207 million kilograms of tea in 2014. This made it the second largest producer and exporter of tea after China (Tea Board of India, 2015). The tea industry is basically an agro-industry which depends largely on the work of manual labourers for its production. Given the heavily reliance on manual labour across the industry it is crucial to ensure that the workforce remains healthy. Poor health represents not only a threat to the person's well-being but to the economic fortunes of the companies involved. Studies have shown that healthy workers are more likely to be productive workers. Therefore, it is important to keep the tea garden labourers healthy. However, at present the health of tea garden labourers and the factors that affect it are not very well understood. On the basis of government regulation (Plantation Act, 1951), the tea garden authorities are required to provide medical facilities and other services such as subsidised food, free accommodation, piped running water and primary education for the children of labourers. It might well appear that access to these benefits should ensure that the workforce remains in good health. However, it is not clear whether this is the case as several studies have reported adverse health conditions among tea garden labourers (Biswas et al., 2002; Mittal and Srivastava, 2006; Medhi et al., 2006; Kundu et al., 2013). This presents an apparent paradox. Therefore, we hypothesised poor socioeconomic conditions may not the sole determinant of health but rather that the lifestyles and health behaviours of the labourers may play the key role in influencing their health.

The World Health Organization (WHO) has defined lifestyle as 'a way of living based on identifiable patterns of behaviour which are determined by the interplay between an individual's personal characteristics, social interactions, and socioeconomic and environmental living conditions' (WHO, 1998). To be more precise, the term lifestyle includes all human behaviours of day-to-day living. This is a complex and multidimensional concept. Hence, the lifestyle of a group of people is shaped by a range of factors like age, gender, level of education (Uitenbroek et al., 1996), economic conditions (Baker, 2006), social class (Blaxter, 1990), cultural values and norms (Cockerham, 2000), individual psychological condition (Cockerham et al., 2006), association with peer group and neighbour (Dressler, 1991), religious beliefs (Boswell et al., 2006) and ethnic identity (Sundquist, 1995). Furthermore, the media plays a crucial role in shaping lifestyles (Gough, 2007; Frosch et al., 2011). Mazengo et al. (1997) and Qu et al. (1997) have shown that urban lifestyles are different from rural lifestyles in activity patterns and food habits. Therefore, the lifestyle of a group of individuals is shaped through interaction of several circumstances and often varies between groups.

Lifestyles have been identified as a major factor in determining individual and group-level health (WHO, 2002). The key lifestyle components which determine health are physical activity, food habits and substance use (WHO, 2004). Studies have reported that optimal physical activity promotes good health (Frankish, 1998) while a lack of physical activity increases the risk of ill health and conditions such as obesity (Pietiläinen et al., 2008) and high blood pressure (Hu et al., 2004). Importantly though it is possible to do too much and studies have shown that excessive physical activity, such as hard manual labour, may cause musculoskeletal problems (Cole et al., 2001). Diets that contain a greater intake of fat, protein and sugar may also increase the chance of becoming obese (Singh and Kirchengast, 2011) and having high blood pressure and increased cholesterol (van Dam et al., 2003). Conversely a higher intake of fruits and vegetables decreases the chances of having metabolic disorders (Appel et al., 2006). Similarly, nutrient deficiency, especially micronutrients, leads to several other health problems (Tulchinsky, 2010). In the case of substance use, studies have shown that tobacco may cause several oral diseases (Johnson, 2001; Winn 2001), while alcohol consumption is associated with obesity, especially centroid obesity which is a particular risk factor for cardiovascular diseases (Brandhagen et al., 2012). Therefore, the effect of lifestyle on health varies across the population depending on the components of the lifestyle that one focuses on. Thus, the measured health condition of a group can be largely understood by observing/ measuring their lifestyles. However, studies on the lifestyles of the tea garden labourers are meagre or lacking. In view of this, we aim to understand the physical health status of Oraon tea garden labourers of Jalpaiguri district, West Bengal in the context of their working environment and way of living or lifestyle.

## Materials and methods

Our study was restricted to only one ethnic group, the Oraon, to eliminate possible ethnic and genetic variations between different communities in health-related traits. The Oraon are a Dravidian-speaking indigenous population who mainly inhabit the Chotonagpur regions and Santal Parganas of Bihar (Roy, 1915). Traditionally they were agriculturist but gradually shifted to other occupations. Around 150 years ago, the British tea garden authorities brought the Oraon in the tea gardens for work and from then they settled there and in several adjacent localities for generations (Choudhury, 1978). Data of the present study have been collected from Oraon tea garden labourers of Birpara tea garden, Jalpaiguri district (presently Alipurduar district since July 2014), West Bengal.

On sampling, it would have been ideal to generate a random sample, however, it was not possible to generate a completely random sample of the tea labourers. We felt that generating a random sample based on the employment registers might be seen as intrusive by the labourers and lead to suspicion and an unwillingness to participate. Thus we decided to invite people to volunteer for the study. This turned out to be a very successful approach and we were able to recruit a total of 500 adults for measurement of whom 286 were male and 214 were female tea garden labourers. Secondly, although there were people from other ethnic groups working at the plantation who could have provided general information regarding tea garden labourers and their health, it was not possible to include them in these analyses as the data form part of a larger biomedical project where controlling for potential ethnic and genetic effects was required. Hence the decision was to focus on just one ethnic group to do this.

We recorded data on a number of physical health traits which included anthropometric measures, blood pressure and haemoglobin levels. The anthropometric measures were height (cms), weight (kg), mid-upper arm circumference (cms), antero-posterior chest diameter (cms) and transverse chest diameter (cms). All the anthropometric measurements were taken by a single investigator (SKR) following the

International Biological Program's basic list of measurements, using standard techniques and instruments (Weiner and Lourie, 1981). Body mass index (BMI) was calculated using these measurements based on the formula: BMI = body weight (kg)/stature ($m^2$). Blood pressure data include systolic (SBP) and diastolic (DBP) blood pressure. They were measured using a mercury sphygmomanometer and a stethoscope. Pulse rate was also measured for 30 seconds using the radial artery on the left hand. The haemoglobin measures include packed cell volume (%) and haemoglobin level (g/dl). In the case of packed cell volume, blood samples were collected by finger pricking in standard heparinised microcapillary tubes (length 75mm, internal diameter 1mm). The microcapillaries were spun in the haematocrit centrifuge, shortly after collection (Dacie, 1958). Haemoglobin level was measured using oxyhaemoglobin method following standard techniques (Dacie, 1958). Besides these anthropometric data, additional lifestyle variables like food habits, sources of drinking water and hygienic practices were collected using a pretested questionnaire. Ideally we would have been able to collect other health data (such as lipid profile, body composition, stool examinations, lung function test) and lifestyle data (such as habitual physical activity, habitual food consumption, substance use, more data on hygienic practices) to provide greater insights into these issues as it was not possible due to financial and time constraints.

## Classification of data

Selected health traits, namely BMI, blood pressure, packed cell volume and haemoglobin level have been classified following standard cut off values. BMI values were classified as underweight (<18.50 kg/$m^2$), normal (18.50–24.99 kg/$m^2$), overweight (≥25.00–29.99 kg/$m^2$) and obese (≥30.00 kg/$m^2$) (WHO, 2004). Blood pressure data were classified as normal (SBP <120 and DBP >80 mm-Hg), pre-hypertensive (SBP 120–139 and DBP 80–89 mm-Hg), stage-1 hypertensive (SBP 140–159 and DBP 90–99 mm-Hg) and stage-II hypertensive (SBP ≥ 160 and DBP ≥100 mm-Hg) according to JNC-7 blood pressure classification (Chobanian et al., 2003). Data on packed cell volume were classified as normal and below normal (Dacie and Lewis, 1991). Haemoglobin level was classified as normal (male >13 g/dl, female >12 g/dl), mild anaemic (male 11.0–12.9 g/dl, female 11.0–11.9 g/dl), moderate anaemic (8.0–10.0 g/dl) and severe anaemic (<8.0 g/dl) according to WHO classification (WHO, 2011). Descriptive statistics in terms of means and standard deviations were calculated separately for men and women for all the selected health indicators: anthropometric measurements, blood pressure, pulse rate and haematological traits. Age and literacy level have been excluded from these analyses to aid the presentation and interpretation of the results. The collected data were analysed using SPSS version 16.0 (SPSS Inc., Chicago, IL, USA).

## Results

A brief socioeconomic background of the study population: both males and females worked as labourers (mainly as tea pickers) in the tea garden. They received weekly wages based on the total amount of tea leaves picked. In addition to their wages the labourers received food stuffs at subsidised rates, free housing and medical facilities and free primary education for their children. Three-quarters of the labourers› houses are brick walled with corrugated asbestos roofing and a quarter are mud walled with thatched roofs.

Table 9.1 shows the selected health practices of Oraon tea garden labourers. They reported taking their meals at regular times (76%), getting enough food to eat (94%) and consuming fish, meat and/or eggs at least once a week (74%). The Oraon in general are very fond of pork and tend to domesticate pigs in their houses, but for the Oraon families in our study, only 10% of families kept domesticated pigs or other animals inside the house. Most of the participants reported that

**Table 9.1: Selected health practices of Oraon tea garden labourers**

| | % |
|---|---|
| Do not keep regular meal times | 23.54 |
| Do not get enough food to eat | 6.28 |
| No consumption of fish/meat/egg in the last week | 26.23 |
| Keeps pig and other animals inside the house | 10.31 |
| Gets drinking water from: | |
| A tube well | 83.63 |
| Well or river | 1.12 |
| Piped water | 15.25 |
| Goes to the toilet: | |
| By the riverside | 61.43 |
| Inside the tea garden | 36.77 |
| By the railway line | 1.35 |
| In a toilet | 0.45 |

they drank water from a tube well[1] (83.63%) or from piped water (15.25%). However, a very small minority drank well/river water (1.12%) too. Very few have toilets (0.45%) in their home premises. Hence most people report that they go to the toilet by the riverside (61.44%) as well as inside the tea garden/open field (36.77%).

Table 9.2 shows the selected health traits of the Oraon tea garden labourers. The mean age of the male tea garden labourers is 28.47±7.91; for female tea garden labourers this is 31.43±9.90. Mean BMI values are 18.09±1.39 for men and 17.73±1.68 for women. In the case of blood pressure, the mean values of systolic blood pressure are 126.08 ±13.69 for men and 127.57±20.98 for women. For diastolic blood pressure the mean values are 75.66±9.76 for men and 80 ±13.83 for women. Lastly the mean values for haemoglobin levels are 11.53±1.75 for men and 10.0 7±2.09 for women.

Table 9.3 shows the classification based on standard cut off values of selected health traits of the Oraon tea garden labourers. The results for BMI show that most people irrespective of sex (male 59.44%, female 64.50%) are classified as underweight. Conversely, the majority of both men and women have normal blood pressure. However, there is

**Table 9.2: Selected health traits of Oraon tea garden labourers**

| | Male (n=286) | | Female (n=214) | |
|---|---|---|---|---|
| | Mean | SD | Mean | SD |
| Age | 28.47 | 7.91 | 31.43 | 9.90 |
| Height | 161.22 | 6.11 | 149.86 | 5.17 |
| Weight | 47.12 | 5.33 | 39.85 | 4.44 |
| BMI | 18.09 | 1.39 | 17.73 | 1.68 |
| Upper arm circumferences | 23.32 | 1.42 | 20.80 | 1.65 |
| Antero-posterior chest diameter | 16.85 | 0.98 | 15.92 | 1.10 |
| Transverse chest diameter | 24.27 | 1.50 | 21.94 | 1.11 |
| Systolic blood pressure | 126.08 | 13.69 | 127.57 | 20.98 |
| Diastolic blood pressure | 75.66 | 9.76 | 80.73 | 13.83 |
| Pulse rate | 76.75 | 13.24 | 87.61 | 12.06 |
| Packed cell volume | 39.03 | 6.87 | 32.80 | 6.22 |
| Haemoglobin* | 11.53 | 1.75 | 10.07 | 2.09 |

*Note:* *Male=109, female=100.

[1] A tube well is a type of water well in which a long, wide, stainless steel tube or pipe is bored into an underground aquifer. The lower end is fitted with a strainer, and a pump at the top lifts water for irrigation.

**Table 9.3: Classification based on standard cut off on selected health status of the Oraon tea garden labourers**

| | Male (n=286) | | Female (n=214) | |
|---|---|---|---|---|
| | N | % | N | % |
| **BMI category** | | | | |
| Underweight | 170 | *59.44* | 138 | 64.5 |
| Normal | 116 | *40.56* | 76 | 35.5 |
| **Blood pressure category** | | | | |
| Normal blood pressure | 196 | *68.53* | 117 | 54.67 |
| Pre-hypertension | 36 | *12.59* | 37 | 17.29 |
| Stage-1 hypertension | 46 | *16.08* | 35 | 16.36 |
| Stage-2 hypertension | 8 | *2.8* | 25 | 11.68 |
| **Packed cell volume** | | | | |
| Normal [M (≥40%) F (≥36%)] | 138 | *48.25* | 138 | 64.49 |
| Below normal [M (≥36%) F (<36%)] | 148 | *51.75* | 76 | 35.51 |
| **Haemoglobin level*** | | | | |
| Severe (<8.00) | 9 | *8.26* | 15 | 15.0 |
| Moderate (8.00–10.99) | 21 | *19.27* | 49 | 49.0 |
| Mild [M (11.00–12.99) F (11.00–11.99)] | 55 | *50.46* | 16 | 16.0 |
| Normal [M (≥13) F (≥12)] | 24 | *22.02* | 20 | 20.0 |

*Note:* *Male=109, female=100

a significant minority of around 16% in both sexes who have stage-1 hypertension. In the case of packed cell volume just over half of the men and around a third of the women in the study have a packed cell volume below normal level. The results for the analyses of the haemoglobin levels show that half of all men have mild anaemia and just under half of all women have moderate anaemia.

## Discussion

The present study aimed to investigate the physical health status of the tea garden labourers against the backdrop of their working environment and their way of living. The results for the analyses of the haemoglobin levels show that half of all men have mild anaemia and just under half of all women have moderate anaemia, and yet a number of people had hypertension. Also, almost half of the population have packed cell volume below normal level. These health statuses can be explained partially by the lifestyles of tea garden workers, which they have developed over generations for adapting to the particular work environment.

## Underweight

Around 60% of individuals irrespective of sex were underweight. Similar results from other studies (Biswas et al., 2002) on both tribal and non-tribal tea garden labourers have also been found, except one study (Mittal and Srivastava, 2006) which reported a comparatively lower percentage of underweight people over normal weight people. Underweight may have been caused due to undernutrition which has a relationship with low food intake, imbalance diet and high load of worm infestation (Ananthakrishnan et al., 1997). Additionally, people's attitudes, knowledge and food practices may have also played a role in the rates of undernutrition.

Most of the participants in the present study reported that they kept regular meal times (76.46%) and that they got enough food to eat (93.72%). They reported intake of fish/meat/eggs once a week (73.77%). However, when asked about what they eat for their meals the respondents said that during breakfast early in the morning (around 6.30 am) they have rice with boiled vegetables and any leftovers from breakfast are eaten for lunch at noon (around 1–1.30 pm). However, this appears to be an insufficient amount of food. It indicates that the labourers mostly consume cereals only with one portion of vegetables or with no vegetables. Mittal and Srivastava (2006) also reported insufficient intake of food grains, protein and vegetables among the Oraon tea garden labourers. Consumption of fats is also low as they mainly eat boiled or roasted foods. Thus, it seems that they do not get enough grain or sufficient protein and vegetables to eat, despite their beliefs to the contrary. One explanation for this is that the tea garden labourers often sell their food grains (which they purchase at subsidised rates from the tea garden) in the local market to buy locally brewed alcohol.

Tea garden labourers live in 'semi-katcha' or 'katcha'[2] houses with unhygienic conditions. They drink tube well water (83%) but the tube wells are 50 feet deep and thus they are really only able to lift surface water. Most of the people prefer to go to the river side (61.4%) to go to the toilet. This clearly results in greater risk of water contamination and worm infestation. Oraons generally prefer pork meat and domesticate pigs at houses. They do not wear shoes. All these habits make them vulnerable to worm infestation and waterborne diseases, which may further lead to undernutrition. Medhi and colleagues (2006) reported

[2] Houses made from mud, thatch or other low-quality materials are called katcha houses.

prevalence of worm infestation and undernutrition among tea garden labourers of Assam, and they argued that unhygienic living practices may be responsible for it.

Again, since all the adult members of a family, especially the females, work in the tea garden as labourers, the children at home are at risk of being neglected. As a result, undernourishment was a common phenomenon; ultimately the child grows up to be an underweight adult (Das and Banerjee,1964).

## Anaemia

The majority of male (77.98%) and female (80.0%) tea garden labourers were anaemic. This finding is similar to studies by Medhi and colleagues (2006) and Kundu and colleagues (2013). The high prevalence of anaemia may have been caused by food habits, hygiene practices, some beliefs and practices and available medical facilities. Bentley and Griffiths (2003) have argued that a lack of proper nutritional intake may be one of the reasons for anaemia. Previous studies on tea garden labourers have mentioned that worm infestation, especially tape worm infestation, is very common in this group (Mittal & Srivastava, 2006; Medhi et al., 2006). This is important as Farook et al. (2002) have shown that worm infestation may lead to anaemia.

The tea garden labourers enjoy free medical facilities. However, in most cases the hospitals operate with a shortage of health personnel, medicine and other facilities. Usually they only provide treatment for minor ailments or injuries. Again this observation is supported by evidence from elsewhere (Misra, 2003; Mittal & Srivastava, 2006). As a result, if a person suffers from anaemia or related ailments they do not get the proper treatment at the crucial time which means that the problem quickly develops to a state that is beyond control. Furthermore, as anaemia is not symptomatic, most people are not aware that they are anaemic and therefore are reluctant to go for treatment.

## High blood pressure

Although the majority of tea garden labourers of either sex of the present study had normal blood pressure, the prevalence of hypertension was also high. This trend is also evident in studies of Hazarika et.al. (2002) and Mahanta et al. (2008) who both reported a prevalence of hypertension. High blood pressure may be due to their food habits and/or substance use. The association between behavioural risk factors like excess salt and fat consumption, physical inactivity, tobacco use and alcohol consumption with increasing risk of hypertension is well documented (WHO, 2013). Participants in the present study also frequently consume pork as a delicacy. This high fat red meat may enhance the risk of high blood pressure. In the tea garden, all labourer families take tea with salt and consume locally brewed alcohol; smoking and chewing tobacco are also very common. This is supported by studies by Mahanta et al. (2008) and Hazarika et al. (2002).

## Conclusion and suggestions

The present study aimed to examine the health status of the tea garden labourers in the context of their working environment and lifestyles. This is a particularly important area of study given the size of the tea garden workforce throughout India. It is also a very interesting group to study given the apparent paradox between the availability of housing, subsidised food, medical care and schooling that the employer is obliged to provide and the well-documented levels of poorer health among this workforce. Indeed, our findings corroborate those from earlier studies and revealed quite high levels of poor health among the Oraon labourers irrespective of sex. Based on our findings it appears that one possible explanation for this paradox lies in the prevalence of poor health behaviours among the labourers that are having a detrimental impact on their health status. We were able to identify some of these factors that aggravated poor health among the labourers such as insufficient food consumption, low protein diet, consumption of locally brewed liquor, unhygienic living condition, drinking surface water, toilet habits, keeping domesticated animals inside the houses, consumption of excess salt, poor medical facilities. Actually, the tea garden labourers generally live in isolation (inside the garden), therefore, were largely isolated from local mainstream society. Modern media like television, mobile phone, video parlours were in theory available to them but have little access due to poor economic conditions. Therefore, exposure to mass media was relatively insufficient for the change in the cultural setup of the society itself. Substance use and gambling are the preferred pastimes after a long and monotonous day of work. Despite the importance of the present findings, there were some limitations in the study. We lacked a larger sample size and more objective ways to measure lifestyle. Therefore, future studies should be oriented with larger sample sizes, objective measures of lifestyle, and consider all the concomitants and rigorous study design, which may provide better insights into the problem. Our impressionistic view is that these tea garden labourers have a unique lifestyle which has been developed through its own cultural setup. Therefore, changing that cultural setup is difficult but not impossible. Moreover, it will take a long time to change, because people of the society have been brought up in that society. In view, it is suggested that (providing employers and policy makers wish to ensure the health of this crucial workforce) it would be beneficial to educate the labourers and let them know the basic health and hygienic practices that ensure better health. Regular health awareness campaigns and interventions are required to assess the progress of the interventions. The local Panchayat[3] should join together with the authority of the tea garden in such awareness programmes.

## References


Ananthakrishnan, S., Nalini, P. and Pani, S.P. (1997). Intestinal geohelminthiasis in the developing world. *The National Medical Journal of India*, 10, 67–71.

Appel, L.J., Brands, M.W., Daniels, S.R. et al. American Heart Association. (2006). Dietary approaches to prevent and treat hypertension: a scientific statement from the American Heart Association. *Hypertension*, 47, 296–308.

Baker, R.M. (2006). Economic rationality and health and lifestyle choices for people with diabetes. *Social Science & Medicine*, 63, 2341–2353.

Bentley, M.E., Griffiths, P.L. (2003). The burden of anemia among women in India. *European Journal of Clinical Nutrition*, 57, 52–60.

Biswas, D., Hazarika, N.C., Hazarika, D. et al. (2002). Study on nutritional status of tea garden workers of Assam with special emphasis to body mass index (BMI) and central obesity. *Journal of Human Ecology*, 13, 299–302.

Blaxter, M. (1990). *Health and Lifestyles*. London and New York: Routledge.

Boswell, G.H., Kahana, E., Dilworth-Anderson, P. (2006). Spirituality and health lifestyle. *Journal of Religion and Health*. 45, 587–602.

Brandhagen, M., Forslend, H.B., Lissner, L. et al. (2012). Alcohol and macronutrient intake patterns are related to general and central adiposity. *European Journal of Clinical Nutrition*, 66, 305–313.


[3] Panchayat is an elected body consisting of several members elected from each village. It is the smallest administrative unit in India and looks after the development of the village. The state government implements policies through the Panchayat.

Chobanian, A.V., Bakris, G.L., Black, H.R. et al. (2003). Seventh report of the joint national committee on prevention, detection, evaluation and treatment of high blood pressure, *Hypertension*. 42, 1206–1252.

Choudhury, M.R. (1978). *The tea industry in India: a diagnostic analysis of its geoeconomic studies.* Calcutta: Oxford Book and Stationary Co.

Cockerham, W.C. (2000). Health Lifestyles in Russia. *Social Science & Medicine*, 51, 1313–1324.

Cockerham, W.C., Hinote, B.P., Abbott, P. (2006). Psychological distress, gender and health lifestyle in Belarus, Kazakhstan and Ukraine. *Social Science & Medicine*, 63, 2381–2394.

Cole, D.C., Ibrahim, S.A., Shannon, H.S. et al. (2001). Work correlates of back problems and activity restriction due to musculoskeletal disorders in the Canadian national population health survey (NPHS) 1994–95 data. *Occupational and Environmental Medicine*, 58, 728–734.

Dacie, J.V. (1958). *Practical Haematology*. London: Churchill.

Dacie, S.J.V., Lewis, S.M. (1991). Reference ranges and normal values. In: *Practical Hematology*, S.J.V. Dacie and S.M. Lewis (Eds.), 8th edition, UK: Churchill Livingstone.

Das, A.K., Banerjee, A.K. (1964). *The impact of tea industry on the life of the tribals of West Bengal.* Cultural Research Institute. Kolkata.

Dressler, W.W. (1991). Social support, lifestyle incongruity, and arterial blood pressure in a Southern black community. *Psychosomatic Medicine*, 53, 608–620.

Farook, M.U., Sudharmini, S., Remadevi, S., Vijayakumar, K. (2002). Intestinal helminthic infestations among tribal populations of Kottoor and Achankovil areas in Kerala (India). *Journal of Communicable Diseases*, 34, 171–178.

Frankish, C.J., Milligan, C.D., Reid, C. (1998). A review of relationships between active living and determinants of health. *Social Science & Medicine*, 47, 287–301.

Frosch, D.L., May, S.G., Tietbohl, C. and Pagan, J.A. (2011). Living in the "land of no"? Consumer perception of healthy lifestyle portrayals in direct-to-consumer advertisements of prescription drugs. *Social Science & Medicine*, 73, 995–1002.

Gough, B. (2007). 'Real men don't diet': An analysis of contemporary newspaper representations of men, food and health. *Social Science & Medicine*, 64, 326–337.

Hazarika, N.C., Biswas. D., Narain, K. et al. (2002). Hypertension and its risk factors in tea garden workers of Assam. *The National Medical Journal of India*, 15, 63–68.

Hu, G., Barengo, N.C., Tuomilehto, J., et al. (2004). Relationship of Physical Activity and Body Mass Index to the Risk of Hypertension: A Prospective Study in Finland. *Hypertension*, 43, 25–30.

Johnson, N. (2001). Tobacco use and oral cancer: a global perspective. *Journal of Dental Education*, 65, 328–339.

Kundu, S., Prasad, S.K., Maji, B. et al. (2013). Nutritional status and productivity of female tea pluckers of a tea garden in Dooars, West Bengal. *International Journal of Biological and Medical Research*, 4, 3101–3106.

Mahanta, T.G., Ahmed, F.U., Mahanta, B.N. and Barua, A. (2008). Prevalence of hypertension and its risk factors in tea garden community of Dibrugarh district, Assam. *Indian Journal of Public Health*, 52, 45–47.

Mazengo, M.C., Simell, O., Lukmanji, Z. (1997). Food consumption in rural and urban Tanzania. *Acta Tropica*, 68, 313–326.

Medhi, G.K., Hazarika, N.C., Shah, B. and Mahanta, J. (2006). Study of health problems and nutritional status of tea garden population of Assam. *Indian Journal of Medical Sciences*, 60, 496–505.

Misra, U. (2003). Assam Tea: The Bitter Brew. *Economic and Political Weekly*, 19, 3029–3032.

Mittal, P.C., Srivastava, S. (2006). Diet, nutritional status and food related traditions of Oraon tribes of New Mal (West Bengal), India. *Rural Remote Health*. 6: Article no 385.

Pietilainen, K.H., Kaprio, J., Borg, P., et al. (2008). Physical inactivity and obesity: A vicious circle. *Obesity (Silver Spring)*, 16, 409–414.

Qu, J.B., Zhang, Z.W., Xu, G.F. et al. (1997). Urban-rural comparison of Nutrient intake by adult women in Shandong province, China. *The Tohoku Journal of Experimental Medicine*, 183, 21–36.

Roy, S.C. (1915). *The Oraons of Chotanagpur: Their history, economic life and social organization*. Ranchi: Crown Publications.

Singh, M., Kirchengast, S. (2011). Obesity prevalence and nutritional habits among Indian women: a comparison between Punjabi women living in India and Panjabi migrants in Viehna, Austria. *Anthropologischer Anzeiger*, 68, 239–251.

Sundquist, J. (1995). Ethnicity, social class and health. A population-based study on the influence of social factors on self-reported illness in 233 Latin American refugees, 33 Finnish and 126 South European labour migrants and 841 Swedish controls. *Social Science & Medicine*, 40, 777–787.

Tea Board of India, (2015). *61st Annual Report 2014–15*. Kolkata, India. http://www.teaboard.gov.in/pdf/bulletin/Consolidated_AR_2014_15.pdf Accessed on 22/3/2016.

The Plantation Labour Act. (1951). Government of India.

Tulchinsky, H. (2010). Micronutrient deficiency conditions: global health issues. *Public Health Reviews*, 32, 243–255.

Uitenbroek, D.G., Kerekovska, A., Festchieva, N. (1996). Health lifestyle behaviour and socio-demographic characteristics: A study of Varna, Glasgow and Edinburgh. *Social Science & Medicine*, 43, 367–377.

van Dam, R.M., Grievink, L., Ocke, M.C., Feskens, E.J.M. (2003). Patterns of food consumption and risk factors for cardiovascular disease in the general Dutch population. *The American Journal of Clinical Nutrition*, 77, 1156–1163.

Weiner, J.S., Lourie, J.A. (Eds.) (1981). *Practical Human Biology*. London: Academic Press.

Winn, D.M. (2001). Tobacco and oral disease. *Journal of Dental Education*, 65, 306–312.

WHO. (1998). *Health Promotion Glossary*. Geneva: WHO.

WHO. (2002). *The World Health Report 2002: Reducing risks, promoting healthy life*. Geneva: WHO.

WHO. (2004). *Global Strategy on Diet, Physical Activity and Health*. Geneva: WHO.

WHO. (2011). *Haemoglobin concentrations for the diagnosis of anaemia and assessment of severity*. Vitamin and Mineral Nutrition Information System, (WHO/NMH/NHD/MNM/11.1), World Health Organization, Geneva, Switzerland.

WHO. (2013). *A Global Brief on Hypertension*. Geneva, WHO.

TEN

# The role of work-family support factors in helping individuals achieve work-family balance in India

*Sarlaksha Ganesh and M.P. Ganesh*

## Introduction

Work and family are the two primary spheres in most people's lives, which makes it necessary to balance both. The two should complement each other in ways that help people to perform well in both. Due to recent developments in both spheres this has become an increasingly difficult task to achieve in India. This is evidenced by recent findings from the Randstad Workmonitor Survey (2015) which found that Indian employees had a poor work-family balance (WFB) as compared with countries in the Europe and the USA. Several reasons can be cited for this. On the family front, the rise of women in the workforce has certainly increased their expectations that domestic tasks should also be shared more equally (Russel et al., 1988; Aryee et al., 1999). Though women still appear to bear the brunt of the unpaid household work (see Chapter 5), the pattern is slowly changing with men also starting to contribute their share over the past few years. This said there is still considerable room for improvement in India to make it a more female-friendly culture (Dreze and Sen, 2014). Alongside increased rates of female labour market participation, the continued rise in the cost of living has made it imperative for both partners to earn money which can have a negative impact on WFB.[1] There has also been a rapid rise in the number of nuclear families which has tended to have a negative impact on the availability of crucial family support in India, making it more difficult to balance work and family life. Finally, the growth in both internal and external migration means that families are increasingly dispersed

[1] Many of these factors have been outlined in Chapter 4, 'Employment trends in India: Some issues for investigation', by Prof A.V. Jose in the current volume.

across wide geographical locations (Banerjee, 1981; Singh, 1984; Desai and Banerji, 2008). On the work side factors such as the increase in labour market participation among older members of society, the increasing number and types of jobs, an increase in the salary being offered, emergence of more and more team-based work (including virtual teams), a trend towards globalisation resulting in more global competition, staffing reductions, travelling on work duties and so on have all contributed to making WFB an increasingly challenging task to achieve (Nasscom, 2003; Taylor and Bain, 2005; Taylor and Bain, 2006; Som, 2007) (see Chapter 4).

Hence balancing work and family demands has become an important topic of research for organisations, researchers and practitioners alike (Guest, 2002). In fact, as noted in the introductory chapter to this book, the European Union has identified the lack of work-life balance (WLB) – often due to long or unconventional work hours – as one of the four important stressors at work (see Chapter 4). The health consequences of high levels of stress due to work are well known (see Chapter 2 for an overview). However, it is also important to know that the positive consequences of achieving such a balance are immense, not only for the employee, but for the organisation and their family. Many Western countries have realised the importance of striking this balance, and have addressed the issue not only from a research or theoretical perspective, but have implemented WFB programmes in their organisations to help their employees achieve it (Fagan et al., 2012). In fact, several companies in such countries are even giving perks to their employees for striking a healthy balance between their personal and professional lives. Forbes for example, encourages employees to take leave and time off from work so that they can attend to any personal needs or even take a break from the humdrum of their regular jobs (Forbes India, 2015). This is seen as a strategy to retain talented employees in the organisation as well as motivating them to work at their best. Such practices also help to attract talent to the company. PricewaterhouseCoopers, in Europe, also found that implementing the right WLB initiatives improved the WLB of their employees by about 30% and led to increased productivity, while the Inland Revenue in the UK also found similar benefits from offering a good WLB for their employees (European Agency for Safety and Health at work, 2005; 2016). Similarly, Oriflame, a cosmetics company, is using its worker-friendly policies and work environment as a marketing tool to attract more talented employees to the organisation (European Agency for Safety and Health at Work, 2016). All these initiatives in different countries show that there is an increasing need for WLB that is being recognised at the organisational level. Also, implementing policies that can help improve the WFB of the employees has only had fruitful benefits for the company and the employee, making it a win-win situation (Smeaton et al., 2014). While WLB is being recognised as a national as well as corporate-level issue worldwide, in the case of India, both research and practice of WLB is yet to gain momentum. Hence it is important to first understand WLB in the Indian context.

## Work-family balance in India

There are two important dimensions to the scenario of WLB in India – the national debate on WLB/WFB on the one side, and researchers' and practitioners' views of WLB/WFB on the other.

It makes sense to first understand the timeline of WFB and WLB developments in the country. In a detailed study of the profile of WLB in India, Rajadhyaksha (2012) notes that the 1970s saw the first report on the status of women in India. Working women, in the formal economy, were a completely new phenomenon in India at this time and the decade saw a dramatic increase in both the numbers of women pursuing higher studies as well as those taking up jobs. Before that, Indian women were generally considered to be content being homemakers and living on the income of their father or husband. Between the 1980s and 1990s there was enough data to reveal gender differences in WLB. Hence, there were signs of change in the previously dominant patriarchal structures in society as people started to accept women going to work and/or further studies. By the mid-1990s, systematic research to highlight the norms of patriarchy and the structural constraints it posed had begun. Slowly but surely, both men and women realised that it was essential for both partners to earn to make ends meet. The expected standard of living had increased and money was required to maintain that standard. Women had started to strongly resist the oppressive family life they were leading, and were no longer content to remain at home. From the late 1990s onwards, the information technology (IT) and IT enabled services (ITeS) companies boomed and many practices were adopted from the West, making the WLB/WFB scene better for many employees, especially in the IT/ITeS industries (Chawla and Sondhi, 2011). This situation continues to hold today as well.

In a cross-national study on different aspects of WFB, it was noted that while 57% of employees on a global scale stated that employers expect them to be available outside regular office hours, in the case of

Indian employees this increased to 75%. Also, 78% of Indian employees felt that they were expected to be available on phone or over email, as opposed to the global average of 47%. It has almost become the norm to handle work matters during private time, either because the employee wants to feel involved or they feel pressured to take these calls and respond to emails as soon as possible so that they are considered good employees. The study also points out that Indians are most active in looking for new jobs with new employers as this gives them better options to balance work and personal lives (Randstad Workmonitor, 2015). Overall, the figures suggest that in India employees are far more pressured than employees in other countries.

The social structure and norms in the country provide the platform to gain an understanding of the dynamics of WLB for people in the country. With respect to the overall culture, India is a largely patriarchal society, although there is a slow but constant shift to create a more gender-equal culture (Ganesh and Ganesh, 2014). The increase of women in the workforce has not been accompanied by a corresponding increase in the sharing of household work by men. This makes it a double shift for working women – they work at home and now also outside home. They seem to be stressed both before and after work hours. Very few women, including those in relatively good jobs, seem to have enough time for their hobbies, friendships and other social relationships, even though time for these could actually help them perform better at home and at work (Ranjan and Prasad, 2013).

If this is the case for women in relatively good jobs, the case is worse for both men and women working in daily wage jobs in the country. About 7 million children accompany their parents to building sites, where the parents work as construction labourers (Evans, 2000). These sites are both unhealthy and dangerous for the children, but the parents have no other choice as they have to work to make a living and cannot afford day care for their children. WLB is a dream and will continue to remain a dream for such workers. Even in the lower socioeconomic classes, though the woman may earn as much or more than the men in the household, women continue to shoulder an unfairly large share of the household responsibilities (see Chapter 5), making WLB very difficult to achieve. Even men who take up mundane jobs requiring less education but more time and energy consuming (such as railway drivers, bus drivers, construction workers, call centre workers) find it difficult to balance work and family needs (Ranjan and Prasad, 2013). Such jobs are, however, abundant in India and provide few benefits to these workers. They have fewer holidays, fewer social interactions, long and atypical hours, low pay and so on.

The other socially significant aspect of Indian culture is its collectivistic nature (Hofstede, 1980; 2001). The existence of many joint or extended families is very common throughout the country (though as noted earlier there has been a consistent rise in the number of nuclear families as well). The joint family system is extremely useful when the extended family is able to provide support for childcare or older people care, both physically and emotionally. However, in cases where older relatives stay at home but are unable to provide physical support, the duty of taking care of them largely falls on the woman. This means that she will have the double responsibility of caring for the children as well as for older people. While there are many day care centres available for the children, there are not as many older people care facilities (Rajadhyaksha, 2012). This makes it difficult for working women to balance the needs at home and those at work. Many women are known to neglect their health to ensure the health of their family members (Sudha and Karthikeyan, 2014).

Though the situation today is better than it was a few decades ago, the proportion of women in the formal workforce is minimal (Rajadhyaksha, 2012). There are certain laws in the country that relate to women in the workforce, and which help them to have a better WLB. There are acts that relate to maternity leaves (12 weeks paid leave for child birth – Maternity Act, 1961), childcare facilities where there are more than 30 women employees with children below 6 years (the Factories Act, 1948). However, although the number of childcare facilities has increased in recent years, there are no laws governing them. Different states have different guidelines to regulate creches, but monitoring for quality is rarely done. Those that do comply with the rules are unaffordable for most couples. Yet a handful of companies have begun on-campus creches for their employees in the past two to three years. These include Indian brand Godrej, retail giant Hindustan Unilever and cosmetics firm L'Oréal (Limaye, 2016). There are also policies aimed to ensure equal pay to both men and women for equal work and to prevent harassment (physically or mentally of women in the workplace, elimination of gender discrimination of any form and so on) (Desai, 2006). However, whether these policies have really been implemented stringently in India is a serious question even now. Companies often try to dodge the responsibilities which arise from legislation (McDonnell, 2011). For example, between 2008 and 2012 the labour courts in India received more than 900 complaints of denial of maternity benefits by employers. It is not surprising then that only 18–34% of married women In Delhi continued working after having a child. As Anu Aga, MP and leading businesswoman, stated in an interview with the BBC India (Arya, 2015):

> 'there is a tendency to give greater importance to a man's job than a woman's job in India. So companies are not willing to make special allowances to integrate women after they take a break for becoming mothers.'

Apart from the laws for women, there are also laws that apply to both men and women. Regarding the maximum working hours per day, the Factories Act states that employees should be made to work for a maximum of 8 hours per day with the exception of two hours overtime on some days, to not exceed 48 hours per week. There are also policies around casual leave, sick leave and festival holidays apart from providing at least one day of holiday per week. Notwithstanding the laws pertaining to work hours and leave in India, it is not uncommon to see men and women alike made to work for longer than the stipulated hours, or working even after coming home (Subramaniam, 2008). Many employees today are forced to work for longer hours for fear of losing their job or not getting their due promotion if they work only 8 or 9 hours a day. Indeed, many of the employees work over time without even getting paid for the extra hours they have put in (Kumar, 2011). This is the scenario of workers in the Indian context.

The second dimension of WLB in India is the researchers' and practitioners' views on the situation. Though many studies abroad have focused on the positive effects of WLB, theoretical, empirical or experimental studies in India are still in the nascent stage. However, popular magazine and newspaper articles have emphasised the need for more research in this area. One such article states that 'Indians care about work-life balance more than money' (Sharma, 2008). Another author cries out against the 'Outrageous hours that corporate India seems to demand' in the open page of *The Hindu*, a very popular Indian newspaper (Subramaniam, 2008). The author clearly points out that the corporate Indian economy strives to meet the needs of customers in other parts of the world in a way that compromises both the health and family life of employees in India. A relatively crude piece of research on employees' take on WFB found that in seven major cities in India, around 750 employees had quit because of WLB issues. The top management have realised that it is crucial to provide their employees with ample opportunities for WFB to retain top talent as well as keep their employees motivated (Deodhar, 2016). Though such articles have gained importance at the level of the print media, systematic research on WLB (much needed in our country, given her steady progress towards greater socioeconomic development) still has a long way to go.

All the same, there has been some empirical research that has given the area of WLB in India much needed attention. One study examined the antecedents and consequences of work-family enrichment in the manufacturing and IT sectors (Baral, 2009). Another study looked at WLB and burnout as predictors of job satisfaction in the IT and ITeS industries (Kanwar et al., 2009). Rajadhyaksha (2012) provided an in-depth analysis of the WLB scenario in India. There has also been a clear rise in studies focusing on the issue of WLB among Indian female professionals (Chawla and Sondhi, 2011; Valk and Srinivasan, 2011; Delina and Raya, 2013; Sudha and Karthikeyan, 2014; Raajarajeswari and Saravanan, 2015). Such studies relating to WLB issues in India have gained momentum and a respectable place in systematic research work over the last few years only. Hence many workers in India, especially women workers, struggle to achieve a good WLB. Not only does this have a detrimental effect on the health and well-being of the person but these negative effects can spillover into the family, community and workplace. Hence it is crucial for us to consider the evidence for the factors that can improve WLB and see how they can be improved in India. In the next section, we will turn our attention to key modifiable factors that have been identified in the literature and look at how they might be improved in the Indian context to promote good WLB for all.

## Social support factors

In India social support factors play an extremely crucial role, considering the collectivistic nature of the country (Hofstede, 1980, 2001). Hence, it becomes vital to understand the role of such factors in influencing the WLB for employees. These factors are, however, not only vital for Indian employees but employees all over the world who wish to achieve a good balance between their professional and personal lives. Support for WLB can come from four main external sources: 1) family, 2) co-workers, 3) supervisors and 4) the organisation. These four sources each function in different ways to help the employee to realise a good WLB. Here are a few things that each of these sources can do to help the employee improve their family and work lives.

## Support from the family

Firstly, the family of a person consists of his/her well-wishers (parents, relatives, siblings, and so on). In India, support from the extended family is usually very high. Help is usually received from the extended family members in one's own family and that of the family that one marries into. These people mainly help by providing emotional support when he/she needs it and also by providing instrumental support for the family-level activities and personal responsibilities. Family members can be an important source of informal or emotional support. Many studies have shown that this sort of support is crucial for alleviating work stress (Cohen, and Wills, 1985; Thoits, 1995). From the family member's side, it can help to just listen to the employee when he or she is back, if the employee wishes to share what went wrong. Sometimes, it may be that the employee wants to be left alone to just unwind, in which case it would be better to stay away. Families can also provide instrumental support by taking care of some of the domestic responsibilities such as caring for the children or older relatives at home, shopping for groceries, helping with household work and making repairs. Such support is expected by most people (whether they are single or married). Hence it is important to recognise that there are two components to WLB and it is important to create supportive environments at work and outside work.

For married people, though there are additional responsibilities associated with married life and family life, extra support comes in the form of a spouse and their children. One can normally expect a good level of emotional and instrumental support from one's spouse and children. When and where possible, it would be beneficial if family members try and develop some routines such as eating together, sharing the day with others, playing games at the end of the day, or even watching a movie/series together, going to the restaurant or malls on Friday evenings to provide opportunities to bond as a family and to get away from the rigours of work. Another way to promote good WLB would be if the whole family could go on a vacation (even a short one is helpful). Such small getaways from the regular day-to-day work can go a long way in making life outside work exciting for all the family members. It is up to the family members to be as imaginative as possible and see how to break the monotony of the everyday humdrum.

This source of support is very important for most professionals, since it has an impact on many aspects of a person's work such as mood at work, efficiency in achieving tasks, social relationships at work, professional growth, work ethics, values and so on. While developed countries have a lot of community support systems such as day care centres, older people care options and registered offices for nannies the situation in India is still somewhat behind. Certainly, there has been a growth in the number of day care centres in the metropolitan cities. However, in smaller cities the family is still largely the main source of support. This makes it crucial for the employee to strike a good WLB (Chawla and Sondhi, 2011).

## Support from co-workers

Secondly, a person's co-workers (either their own team members or others working in the same company) play a crucial supportive role. Having understanding and cheerful team members not only boosts team morale but also provides mutual support to each team member. Studies on team cohesion have shown that it can lead to work-family enrichment (Hunter et al., 2010), while co-worker support has been a key player in improving job satisfaction (Ducharme and Martin, 2000) and performance (Babin and Boles, 1996). It would certainly bring out the best in everyone if they work in a team that both understands one's professional strengths and complements them. Co-workers can bring a lot of energy into the team and contribute to each other's professional successes. One Indian study showed that co-worker support improves the quality of work life for frontline employees in the banking industry (Ganesh and Ganesh, 2014). The potential of co-worker support for improving the WLB of the employee is an area that needs much attention in India.

Team members can also provide emotional assistance and instrumental support on the job (by helping a colleague do part of their work when they are stressed out). In many industries today, team work has become integral. This can be seen as a boon such that team members can help colleagues to leave early when necessary, share the burden of the team member or even help the team member to learn new skills. Also, since team members are on the same hierarchical level as the employee, the question of power distance does not come into the picture. This would help the employee to discuss topics ranging from work to movies to sports to personal events, which can help build their social capital. Colleagues can also break the routine and go out for activities such as team lunches, movies or play cricket/baseball together while discussing work. Such small efforts not only help team cohesion but also create synergy in the team. Hence, this also becomes an important form of support in boosting WLB. It makes sense for Indian organisations to invest in building cohesive teams, as the benefits of such an investment for the employee are clear from studies that have been conducted abroad. Not only would such initiatives help the employee, but would also impact the bottom line of the company through increased productivity, higher retention of talent, lower stress levels and burnout for employees and more.

## Support from supervisors and managers

Thirdly, supervisors and managers are key players in making the employee feel supported (Griffin et al., 2001; Baral, 2009). Supervisors act as a link between the employee and the larger organisation. Since many supervisors and managers are directly involved in the design and implementation of organisation-related policies (including WLB policies), they also become vital in helping or hindering the employee in using these policies. Supervisors who help the employee to become aware of these policies and use the policies themselves help alleviate stress levels among the workforce.

Due to the relatively strict hierarchy in India (Hofstede, 2001), subordinates seldom approach their managers for WLB support. A manager who understands these dynamics could overcome them by taking the initiative to voluntarily provide support for their workers. They would act as a catalyst in improving the employee's performance levels by encouraging the employee whenever possible thereby giving the employee a lot of confidence. It is important for a supervisor to encourage the team to speak up, to understand the needs of the team and the team dynamics. In so doing, they would help to develop a good team culture which allows the team more control over their work and encourages team members to hone their skills and perform at their best. Being more experienced than the subordinate, the supervisor can also provide some level of instrumental support when the employee encounters problems with work-related issues, in addition to providing him/her with emotional support. All these initiatives would certainly help the employee on the work front. It might also be beneficial to take some interest in the personal life of the employee, as this would help build a great rapport and help the employee be open about why he/she is not performing at best when personal limitations are the reason. Above all, it is essential for a supervisor to understand that he/she should act as a mentor for a team or the subordinate, rather than be a ringmaster whom the subordinates are frightened of. These characteristics of the supervisor would help the employee feel more comfortable in maintaining a good WLB. Especially in India, where very few supervisors act as mentors to their subordinates, such characteristics of the supervisor would definitely help the employee and the team. Vineet Nayar (2010) celebrated CEO of HCL Technologies has written a book titled *Employees First Customers Second – Turning Conventional Management Upside Down*, emphasising the role of management in enabling employees to be their own masters and making the management accountable to the value delivered to employees. This book was one of its kind, and the implementation of this philosophy has made it one of the fastest growing firms in the IT field. Such paradigm shifts only go to show that Indian companies are also realising the value of providing a good WLB to the employee. So what is it that the management can do?

## Support from the organisation

An organisation that understands the WLB needs of its employees is likely to design customised policies that would truly contribute to the WLB of its employees. Rather than having many policies that are useful to only few of the employees, a supportive organisation would make sure that the few policies it designs are useful to as many employees as possible. More importantly, the work-culture in an organisation can be developed to be worker friendly and supportive, so that a mutually beneficial relationship can be realised between the worker and the organisation (in addition to improving the image of the organisation in the eyes of potential employees and competing companies). This is more relevant for Indian companies, which have just begun to establish their presence in the global market. Especially in the service industries where employees provide support or services directly to customers (such as the airline industry, hospitality, tourism and banking) it is essential for employees to be helped to be as happy as possible, since most industries in this category will have long and sometimes unconventional working hours.

Some of the best practices that have been implemented by companies in India to help employees achieve a good WLB are giving a paid vacation/holiday hours to the employee, allowing the employee to leave work when needed, offering the employee the option of telecommuting (this is especially relevant for those who do not need to be physically present at the office to do their work or those who live far away from their workplaces), a compressed workweek, flexible scheduling of work, offering sabbaticals after working for a certain number of years and job sharing. Apart from these, a lot of companies with good human resources (HR) practices also offer other perks for employees such as childcare at the workplace at subsidised rates and offering subsidised or free meals for employees at work so that they can save time on cooking. We suggest that even small changes such as taking the employees off-site or simply holding meetings in a different place could all go a long way. However, the extent to which these policies or initiatives will be successful in India depends on the top management in the organisation and how creative they are at devising new and novel means to attract new talent into the organisation and retain existing talent. These moves by companies provide evidence that the Indian work environment is slowly and steadily making the way for employees to balance out their work and personal lives.

Organisations that wish to provide a better working environment for their employees should bear in mind that if they wish their business to flourish, it is important that they have a satisfied, happy and motivated workforce. This is especially the case for industries such as hospitality and banking, as service quality is the key to profit. Even in this age of mechanisation, the service industry relies extensively on the quality of service provided by frontline employees for attracting new customers and also maintaining the existing customer base. Therefore, it becomes crucial to have happy employees who perform well, as their service becomes the main competitive edge for the organisation. Therefore, the organisation must communicate through various means to the employees that they encourage them to maintain a reasonable balance between their personal and professional lives.

## Incorporating work-life balance policies as part of organisational strategy

Having discussed the positive effects of employees experiencing a good WLB, it is important that service organisations incorporate related policies adequately. In the Indian context, most organisations do not look at provision of WLB as a strategic advantage. However, the situation is changing in light of the growing body of evidence that shows that the effective implementation of such policies can have very positive outcomes for the employees and the organisation. As already noted these include increased job satisfaction of employees, greater involvement in organisational citizenship behaviours, improved organisational commitment, better job performance, reduced attrition rate in the organisation and specifically with respect to service organisations, happier and more satisfied customers (Guest, 2002; White et al., 2003; Beauregard and Henry, 2009; Lazar et al., 2010;

Odle-Dusseau et al., 2012; Cegarra-Leiva et al., 2012; Butts et al., 2013). While some of the policies such as maternity and paternity leave, and provision of health insurance for the employees' family members are common, organisations should look to incorporate policies beyond these, so that they attract more talent to their organisation and do not lose their existing talent. Particularly in the service industry where most frontline employees lack a good WLB, organisations should view provision of usable policies as a strategic advantage. Marriot hotels for example realised that they were making better profits overall and that both the top-line and bottom line were impacted significantly when they changed the culture of facetime (Munck, 2001). This suggests that such practices can be a strategic advantage for other such companies as well.

## Making organisation and employee specific work-life balance policies

While there are certain WLB policies that are useful for most employees, it is important for organisations to realise that just as their services are customised, their policies should also be tailor-made taking into account the needs of the organisation and the employees. For example, hotel employees do a lot of night shift work, while bank employees do not. Moreover, the nature of the job for a HR manager in a hotel would be very different from that of a frontline worker or an event manager. Such differences call for designing unique WLB policies that help these employees to actually reduce any conflicts between their working life and their personal life and improve their overall WLB. Moreover, policies should cater to the needs of both single and married employees, so that single employees do not feel left out. Having recreational activities for single employees such as a party evening once a month or paid vacations for them as well, would help make single employees feel that that the organisation is also supporting them. The organisation can also help single employees spend their leisure time productively by providing them with opportunities to go to the gym, learn yoga and meditation, engage in sports, learn fine arts and more. Involving employees in designing the policies by having frequent open houses where employees are able to contribute to the designing of policies and using suggestions and complaint boxes to help address employee concerns can go a long way in customising WLB policies and also helping the HR department to understand how useful the policies are for their employees.

## Increasing family-related policies and support

Organisations should look at increasing family-related support to their employees, not only to show that they care for them, but also so that the employees are able to focus and perform well on the job. In a collectivistic country like India, it is understandable that employees might give more preference for their families over work. Apart from providing monetary support such as paid maternity leave and medical insurance for the employees and their dependents, other initiatives should also be undertaken. For example, providing childcare facilities, older people care facilities and having company outings with the family members can go a long way in making the employees' families feel supported (Redmund et al., 2006). A good example of this are Marriot Hotels India, who allow their employees paid vacation for a few days close to their birthday. Also, a meal for six on their birthday is free of cost, which can help the employee's family feel included. This is one of the most appreciated HR policies that has helped the hotel chain retain its talent (by making the employee feel valued and giving them something back). Such initiatives show that if necessary and when and where possible the employees' family members should be included in major decisions for the employee's job such as transfers. Moreover, family-related support/policies should be useful for both married and single employees. Since single employees do not always stay with their families, organisations can look at options such as sponsoring a family holiday for the best employee of the year. Such initiatives would also motivate employees to give their best for the organisation, which is what the organisation ultimately needs.

## Effective communication of work-life balance policies

While having WLB policies is important, what matters more is to effectively communicate these policies to the employees. Organisations should look at developing good communication channels for the WLB policies available in the organisation. During employee induction, a list of policies available should be provided and the employee should be encouraged to get additional details from the HR manager, supervisor or co-workers. It is equally important to make it clear to the employees that they will not be penalised in any manner for using the policies to have a better WLB. It is also important to show through the culture of the organisation that people who work long hours are not going to be the only ones who are promoted or rewarded. If an employee can work smartly and achieve their goals within the expected time, such employees should also be recognised. Supervisors should be instructed clearly by the top management that the organisation favours and encourages employees to use the policies as and when possible, and that it believes in a culture that supports a good WLB for their employees, irrespective of whether they are single or married. Supervisors must understand that even subtle signals such as looking up at an employee who is leaving early from work or hanging around in the office when really not necessary could send strong signals about the culture of the organisation to the employee. While it takes time to build such a culture in Indian companies due to hierarchical structures and power imbalances, once such a culture is ingrained, the benefits it reaps are sustained and considerable.

## Using positivity to counter negativity of work-life balance

Previous research suggests that employees can be made to understand that a lot of the experiences and resources gained at work can help in achieving a good WLB (Beauregard and Henry, 2009; Butts et al., 2013). Organisations can look at organising participative workshops or training programmes on how positive experiences at work can help employees to overcome unpleasant experiences at work or home. Supervisors can also be encouraged to participate in these workshops so that they understand the importance of their employees' work-family enrichment (how work can have a positive influence on family and vice-versa) for their motivated performance in the organisation. Additionally, HR practices should look to cover and address all aspects of the quality of life at work. While most organisations address the physical and safety needs of the employees at work, higher order needs such as employees' needs for creativity, expressing their complete potential at work, good social relationships and so on are usually not addressed sufficiently. Satisfaction of these needs is vital for employees to experience a good quality of life at work overall, which could become the key competitive edge for the organisation.

## Using work social support effectively

Both supervisor support and co-worker support have positive consequences for the WLB of the employee, while reducing their work-family conflict (Carlson and Perrewé, 1999). Hence, social support at work is an important resource for improving the work experience of an employee. Supervisors can support the employees by providing details of the available policies, the kind of work that is expected from them, encouraging the employee when he/she performs well or even providing emotional support to the employee when he/she is feeling low. They must be approachable and someone who employees want to take tips from for working well, and feel comfortable discussing reasons for ineffective performance at work. Co-workers on the other hand can provide instrumental support to the employee by taking on a part of the employee's work, exchanging shifts to suit the convenience of another employee or helping their colleagues when they have a new job to do. Additionally, they can also provide emotional support to their colleagues by encouraging them during tough times or providing a lending ear after the employee has gone through an unpleasant experience. Such support will be effective in helping employees to perform well even under stressful conditions and help them to overcome the day-to-day stresses which they face on the job. Hence, both the top management and HR managers should help supervisors and co-workers know and understand their roles in creating a work-life friendly environment.

## Training for helping employees achieve a good work-life balance

While it may not be possible to entirely change the personality of employees, training programs or workshops on positive traits such as emotional intelligence, coping and techniques for stress management, time management and so on can act as an opportunity for employees to learn how to manage the resources they have – both tangible and intangible – such that they can balance their personal and professional lives well. Moreover, such initiatives should focus on helping employees to understand how they can use their psychological resources to combat work-family conflicts and achieve a better WLB. Apart from this, organisations should also look at other training options that can relieve employee stress such as yoga activities, stress management programs, laughing clubs, gym exercises to release stress, using stress journals to help employees introspect and so on. Not only do these help in reducing the stress levels of the employee, but they also convey to the employees that the organisation cares for their personal well-being. This could be looked at as another strategy to attract and retain the human capital in the organisation, while helping the employee achieve a good WLB. This initiative would be a clear signal to the employee that the company cares for their personal needs as much as it cares for the business.

## Responsibility for work-life balance and quality of life of employees at work

Organisations should look at the WLB and work-life quality of their employees as a part of responsible management practices of the company. There should be ownership of both these aspects, and this can only be achieved when there is adequate support from the top management. In most cases, the HR department or the training department generally design the policies but do not often have the time or resources to ensure that the policies are being implemented and used adequately. Companies that provide services should realise that happy employees can create happy and satisfied customers, which is the bottom line for the profit of the organisation. Therefore, the top management should provide enough support and encouragement to the HR and training departments so that they are able to improve the WLB and work-life quality of the employees. Furthermore, the top management should emphasise to the HR and training departments that they should take ownership for the WLB and work-life quality of their employees. Regularly surveying the employees anonymously to understand their WLB and work-life issues can provide a wealth of information to the HR and the company about what they can do. Even small steps such as putting up posters on maintaining a good WLB and enjoying one's work can be considered. Finally, employees should be informed and encouraged to discuss WLB related problems with their supervisors and the HR department, and assured that their problems would be addressed in as best a way as possible.

## Conclusion

On the whole, it can be said that the family, co-workers, supervisors and organisations can play a major role in improving the WLB of their employees. Currently it is a concern that WLB issues do not appear to be high on the agenda for many Indian organisations. However, there are some encouraging signs that some companies, such as Marriot Hotels, are taking the lead to implement positive WLB policies. As yet the research in this field in India is still in its infancy so it will take time to properly assess the impact that these developments might have. However, by looking at the evidence from abroad, which we have sought to present in this chapter, we feel confident that such initiatives will deliver pay-offs for both the employer and the employee. By building such an evidence base we hope to be able to show that both employers and employees can take action to improve their WLB and that there are many sources and opportunities for them to do so. Given India's collectivistic nature, support from these sources would be completely expected by the employees and useful for the company as a whole. Each one has a significant role to play in helping the employee to achieve a good WLB. More than any of these support factors however, is the fact that the employee must want to experience the positive aspects of both their personal and professional lives rather than just wish for these. At the end of the day, it is the employee who is capable of using these resources, and making it a win-win situation for their personal and professional lives.

## References

Arya, D. (2015). Why motherhood makes Indian women quit their jobs. BBC Hindi. 23/4/2015. http://www.bbc.co.uk/news/world-asia-india-32377275

Aryee, S., Luk, V., Leung, A. and Lo, S. (1999). Role stressors, interrole conflict, and well-being. *Journal of Vocational Behavior*, 54, 259–278.

Babin, B.J., and Boles, J.S. (1996). The Effects of Perceived Co-Worker Involvement and Supervisor Support on Service Provider Role Stress, Performance and Job Satisfaction. *Journal of Retailing*, 72(1), 57–75.

Banerjee, B. (1981). Rural-urban migration and family ties: an analysis of family considerations in migration behaviour in India. *Oxford Bulletin of Economics and Statistics*, 43(4), 321–355.

Baral, R. (2009) Examining Antecedents of Work-Family Enrichment and its Effects on Individual, Family and Organizational Outcomes. Unpublished Doctoral Dissertation, Indian Institute of Technology, Bombay, India.

Baral, R. and Bhargava, S. (2005). *Work Family Issues: A Review of Recent Literature and Agenda for Future Research*. Paper presented at Consortium of Management Research, Indian Institute of Science, Bangalore, India.

Beauregard, T.A. and Henry, L.C. (2009). Making the link between work-life balance practices and organizational performance. *Human Resource Management Review*, 19(1), 9–22.

Butts, M.M., Casper, W.J. and Yang, T.S. (2013). How important are work–family support policies? A meta-analytic investigation of their effects on employee outcomes. *Journal of Applied Psychology*, 98(1), 1.

Carlson, D.S. and Perrewé, P.L. (1999). The role of social support in the stressor-strain relationship: An examination of work-family conflict. *Journal of Management*, 25(4), 513–540.

Cegarra-Leiva, D., Sánchez-Vidal, M.E. and Cegarra-Navarro, J.G. (2012). Work-life balance and the retention of managers in Spanish SMEs. *The International Journal of Human Resource Management*, 23(1), 91–108.

Chawla, D. and Sondhi, N. (2011). Work-Life Balance Among Indian Women Professionals. *Indian Journal of Industrial Relations*, 47(2), 341–352.

Cohen, S. and Wills, T.A. (1985). Stress, social support, and the buffering hypothesis. *Psychological Bulletin*, 98(2), 310.

Delina, G. and Prabhakar Raya, R. (2013). A study on Work-Life Balance in Working Women. *International Journal of Commerce, Business and Management*, 2(5), 274–282.

Deodhar, S. (2016). Definitive steps to maintain work-life balance for employees. *Forbes India*. 03, Mar 2016. http://www.forbesindia.com/blog/the-good-company/definitive-steps-to-maintain-work-life-balance-for-employees/

Desai, S. and Banerji, M. (2008). Negotiated identities: male migration and left-behind wives in India. *Journal of Population Research*, 25(3), 337–355.

Desai, T.P. (2006). *Managing work and family conflict in contemporary India: Luxury and necessity for the urban workforce – A macroperspective*, Presented at 'Why Workplace Flexibility Matters – A Global Perspective' International Conference, 16–18 May, Chicago, Illinois.

Dreze, J. and Sen, A. (2014). *An Uncertain Glory: India and its Contradictions*. London: Penguin.

Ducharme, L.J. and Martin, J.K. (2000). Unrewarding work, co-worker support and job satisfaction. *Work and Occupations*, 27(2), 223–243.

European Agency for Safety and Health at Work (2005). *Family Issues and Work-Life Balance*. https://osha.europa.eu/en/tools-and-publications/publications/e-facts/e-fact-57-family-issues-work-life-balance. Accessed 2/4/2016.

European Agency for Safety and Health at Work. (2016) *'Ourtime' – A Work-Life Balance Project*. https://osha.europa.eu/en/tools-and-publications/publications/2018our-time2019-2013-a-work-life-balance-project-inland-revenue. Accessed 2/4/2016.

European Agency for Safety and Health at Work. (2016) *Work-Life Balance and Employees Participation Programme*. https://osha.europa.eu/en/tools-and-publications/publications/work-family-balance-and-employees-participation-programme. Accessed 2/4/2016.

Evans, R. (2000). Uncertain future for mobile creches. BBC News, 26 May, cited in C. Hein (2005). *Reconciling work and family responsibilities: Practical ideas from global experience.* International Labour Organization: Geneva, 17.

Fagan, C., Lyonette, C., Smith, M. and Saldana-Tejeda, A. (2012). *The Influence of Working Time Arrangements on Work–Life Integration or 'Balance': A Review of the International Evidence.* Geneva: ILO. http://www.ilo.org/travail/whatwedo/publications/WCMS_187306/lang--en/index.htm.

Forbes India (2015). *Forget Work-Life Balance, Strive for work-life harmony.* http://forbesindia.com/blog/business-strategy/forget-work-life-balance-strive-for-work-life-harmony/#ixzz42UVtDBpL. Accessed 2/4/2016.

Ganesh, S. and Ganesh, M.P. (2014). Effects of Masculinity-Femininity on Quality of Work-Life: Understanding the moderating roles of gender and social support. *Gender in Management: An International Journal*, 29(4), 229–253.

Guest, D.E. (2002). Perspectives on the study of work-life balance. *Social Science Information*, 41(2), 255–279.

Hofstede, G. (1980). *Culture's Consequences: International Differences in Work-Related Values.* Beverly Hills, CA: Sage Publications.

Hofstede, G. (2001). *Culture's Consequences: Comparing Values, Behaviors, Institutions and Organisations across Nations.* Thousand Oaks, CA: Sage Publications.

Hunter, E.M., Perry, S.J., Carlson D.S. and Smith, S.A. (2010). Linking team resources to work-family enrichment and satisfaction. *Journal of Vocational Behaviour.* 77, 304–312.

Kanwar, Y.P.S., Singh A.K. and Kodwani, A.D. (2009). Work-Life Balance and Burnout as predictors of Job Satisfaction in the IT-ITES industry. *The Journal of Business Perspective.* 13(2), 1–12.

Kumar, M. (2011). Work-Life Balance in India – An Innovative Approach. *Social Science Research Network* [online] Available from doi: http://dx.doi.org/10.2139/ssrn.1803884 Accessed 2/4/2016.

Lazar, I., Osoian, C. and Ratiu, P. (2010). The role of work-life balance practices in order to improve organizational performance. *European Research Studies*, 13(1), 201.

Limaye, Y. (2016). Will new maternity law help keep Indian women in work? BBC News. http://www.bbc.co.uk/news/world-asia-india-35371454. Accessed 25/1/2016.

McDonnell, A. (2011). *It is Your Responsibility to make Work-Life Balance for Your Employees*. http://thehiringsite.careerbuilder.com/2011/02/11/is-it-your-responsibility-to-make-worklife-balance-work-for-your-employees. [Accessed 8/2/2016].

Munck, B. (2001). Changing a Culture of Facetime. *Harvard Business Review*, 125–131.

Nasscom. (2003). *Strategic Review: The IT Industry in India*. New Delhi: Nasscom.

Nayar V. (2010). *Employees First, Customers Second: Turning Conventional Management Upside Down*. Harvard Business Review Press. Boston.

Odle-Dusseau, H.N., Britt, T.W. and Greene-Shortridge, T.M. (2012). Organizational work–family resources as predictors of job performance and attitudes: The process of work–family conflict and enrichment. *Journal of Occupational Health Psychology*, 17(1), 28.

Raajarajeswari, M.A. and Saravanan, R. (2015). Work-Life Balance of Women Employee: A Literature Review. *Paripex – Indian Journal of Research*. 4(10), 80–82.

Rajadhyaksha, U. (2012). Work-Life Balance in South East Asia: The Indian Experience. *South Asian Journal of Global Business Research*. 1(1), 108–127.

Randstad Workmonitor. (2015). *Working Hours Vs Private Time: Blurred Lines*. Group Communications Randstad Holdings: Amsterdam, Netherlands.

Ranjan, R. and Prasad, T. (2013). Literature Review Report on Work-Life Balance of Loco Pilots (Railway Drivers) in India. *European Journal of Business and Management*, 5(19), 17–28.

Redmond, J., Valiulis, M. and Drew, E. (2006). *Literature Review of Issues Related to Work Life Balance and Workplace Culture*, Crisis Pregnancy Agency, Dublin, Ireland.

Russel, G., James, D. and Watson, J. (1988). Work/family policies: the changing role of fathers and the presumption of shared responsibility for family. *Australian Journal of Social Issues*, 23, 249–267.

Sharma, R. (2008). Indians care about work-life balance more than money, Livemint.com (*The Wall Street Journal*), 27/7/2008.

Singh, J. P. (1984). The changing household size in India. *Journal of Asian and African Studies*, 19(1–2), 86–95.

Smeaton, D., Ray, K. and Knight, G. (2014). Costs and Benefits to Business of Adopting Work Life Balance Working Practices: A Literature Review. Department for Business Innovation & Skills, available at: www.gov.uk/bis

Som, A. (2007) What drives adoption of innovative SHRM practices in Indian organizations? *International Journal of Human Resource Management*, 18(5), 808-828

Sudha, J. and Karthikeyan, P. (2014) Work Life Balance of Women Employee: A Literature Review. *International Journal of Management Research & Review*, 4(8), 797–804.

Taylor, P. & Bain, P. (2005). India calling to the far away towns: the call centre labour process and globalization. *Work, Employment and Society*, 19(2), 261–282.

Taylor, P. and Bain, P. (2006). Work organisation and employee relations in Indian call centres, in J. Burgess and J. Connell (eds) *Developments in the Call Centre Industry*, London: Routledge, 36–57.

Thoits, P.A. (1995). Stress, Coping and Social Support Processes: Where are we? What Next? *Journal of Health and Social Behaviour*, Extra Issue: Forty Years of Medical Sociology: The State of the Art and Directions for the Future, 53–79.

Valk, R. and Srinivasan, V. (2011). Work-family balance of Indian women software professionals: A qualitative study. *IIMB Management Review*, 23(1), 39–50.

White, M., Hill, S., McGovern, P., Mills, C. and Smeaton, D. (2003). 'High Performance' Management Practices, Working Hours and Work-Life Balance. *British Journal of Industrial Relations*, 41(2), 175–195.

ELEVEN

# Working conditions, health and well-being among the scavenger community

*Vimal Kumar*

## Introduction

India has the second largest scavenging population in the world after China. Although the exact number of manual scavengers remains disputed, the 2011 census showed that between 800,000 to 1,000,000 people are engaged in manual scavenging in India (The New Indian Express, 2013). Scavenger communities are known by the different names in the India: Bhangi, Hadi, Thotti, Mehter, Dhanuk, Valmiki, Chuhra[1] and Balmiki (Haryana). Whatever they are called, they are placed in the lowest rung of the Hindu caste hierarchy (Freed, 1970) and are trapped into performing 'unclean' occupations through the generations. The overarching conceptual identification of these occupations intersecting with communities is explored here through a focus on manual scavengers. Manual scavenging refers to the removal of human waste/excreta using brooms, tin plates and baskets from the dry latrine for disposal and the people engaged doing it are referred to as manual scavengers. Contemporary debates around the exact name of these communities is disputed and remains contested. This chapter uses the neutral English term 'scavenger'. This may to refer to 'Chuhra' 'Balmiki' 'Bhangi' 'Mehtar' 'Hadi' 'Dom' and so on. The Government of India also uses the term 'Safai Karamchari' in Hindi language which in English translates as manual scavenger. As a continuation of this

[1] List of scheduled castes according to 'Welfare of Scheduled Caste & Backward Classes Department', Government of Haryana.

a National Commission for Safai Karamcharis was formed by the government to look into issues of the scavenger community.[2]

In Indian caste-based society, identity, social status and respect of communities/people are directly related to the occupation they are ascribed to perform. Work and occupation such as manual scavenging is given the lowest status in the society. India is also known as 'Hindustan' and this is the most common word in Indian society. The meaning of 'Hindustan' is the country of Hindus. Therefore, large populations of India are influenced by the Hindu religion and beliefs, following the Hindu code and ideas which have been set out by the controversial Hindu law giver Manu and is commonly known as 'Manusmriti'. These ideas, as described by Blunt (1981), hold that a particular caste group will be engaged in a particular type of work or profession based on their birth and descent. This theory is still widely accepted by a very large orthodox section of Hindu society.

## Caste and occupation of the scavenger community

The low status and lack of respect accorded to the manual scavenging community is directly related to their occupation which is identified as disgraceful work. This has led to the perception and practice of 'untouchability' against the community. As already argued, the scavengers are traditionally confined to the least desirable forms of work such as the removal of human excreta and dead animals, leather work, working as messengers to deliver news of deaths and butcher work. Ghurye (1961) has shown that those who belong to the scavenger community are required to clean night soil and have been performing this occupation throughout history in India. Within the caste hierarchy, it is well documented by Hutton (1946) that the scavenger caste is positioned at the lowest grade in the Hindu social structure. This is the case despite government policies that outlaw such discrimination. According to The Protection of Civil Rights Act, 1955 (Act No. 22 of 1955) 7(A): 'unlawful compulsory labour, when to be deemed to be a practice of "untouchability".[3] Whoever compels any person, on the ground of "untouchability", to do any scavenging or sweeping or to remove any carcass, or to flay any animal, or to remove

[2] The National Commission for Safai Karamcharis is formed by the Indian government for the welfare of various communities including scavengers and manual scavengers. http://ncsk.nic.in/index.asp

[3] See The Protection of Civil Rights Act, 1955 (Act No. 22 of 1955) 7(A) http://scstwelfare.delhigovt.nic.in/act%20no22.html

the umbilical cord or to do any other job of a similar nature shall be deemed to have enforced a disability arising out of "untouchability".[4]

Caste position is not limited to lower castes, but is deeply rooted in Indian sociocultural hierarchy. Within the lower castes (now identified as scheduled caste by the Indian Government) community, sub-castes and hierarchies are even more pronounced and significant. Dumont (1980) points out that of the total 25 untouchable castes, there are 12 castes which will not touch the scavenger caste. For instance, the sub-caste known as 'Balmikis' is considered the lowest among scheduled castes, while 'Jatavs' are higher in status. The former are engaged in manual scavenging jobs, while the latter are engaged in leather crafts, indicating that status within the caste. These practices among communities are closely linked to Brahmanical notions of purity and pollution which run across all caste groups. Therefore, even though the Indian Constitution bans the practice of untouchability and has identified the scavenger community as scheduled caste, they face discrimination from other upper castes and even within those who are also identified as scheduled castes.

Occupations performed by the scavenger community are highly stressful and unhygienic and due to the stigma of being lower caste, further stress is added to an already hash and disagreeable situation. Having been treated as the most polluted and socially disgraced group within the Hindu society, as well as among Dalits (scheduled caste), scavengers are struggling to change their plight in the fight for their rights within the existing system.

Interestingly even today, after the 70th year of India's independence, most of the people belong to the sweepers community, working in the Municipal Corporation,[5] Nagar Nigam[6] and Gram Panchayat level belong to the scavenger community. They work as manual scavengers sweeping roads and streets, cleaning sewage and sanitation and dumping dead animals from the residential areas.

---

[4] See Protection of Civil Rights Act, 1955 (Act No 22 of 1955) 7(A). http://scstwelfare.delhigovt.nic.in/act%20no22.html

[5] In India state governments formed departments to support the development of metropolitan cities, i.e. those with a population of more than 1 million. The growing population and urbanization in various cities of India were in need of a local governing body that can work for providing necessary community services like health centers, educational institutes, housing, property tax, and cleaning work in the city.

[6] A Nagar Palika or Municipality or is an urban local body that administers a city of population 100,000 but less than 1,000,000 along with sanitation work.

> 'Castes other than Balmiki (Scavenger) are not willing to take up this polluting work. In the case of sweepers, the caste and its occupational association have not broken down. In Balmiki (Scavenger) community, many youths after working as semi-skilled labour, have taken up sweeping, a highly stigmatized job.' (Aggarwal and Ashraf, 1976)

As they belong to this particular caste, society and the state have allocated them to the scavenging occupation while other communities are prevented from doing this work. In direct and indirect ways such occupations are imposed on this particular caste. Therefore, there are fewer chances to move away from these inhuman occupations and their concomitant stigma.

Many members of the scavenger communities have been observed to be converting or are being converted to other religions with a hope that they would receive an improved social status as well as a more dignified life. The main religions that they have converted to in order to escape untouchability and discrimination are Sikhism, Christianity, Arya Samaj and Islam. On this count, M.N. Srinivas, a sociologist, noted that 'conversion to Christianity only changed the faith but not the customs, the general culture, or the standing of the converts in society' (Srinivas, 1995). In the states of Haryana and Punjab in India, some people of the Chuhra (scavenger) community converted to Sikhism and are known as 'Mazhbi' or 'Rangreta' in the Sikh religion. The status of Rangreta (scavengers) still remains the lowest in the Sikh religion and they are still engaged in scavenging work, facing daily discrimination and untouchability. In the book 'Punjab caste' Ibbetson and Denzil (1974) argued that 'the Ramdasi is still a "Chamar" and the Rangreta still a "Chuhra". The change has been recent and is still in progress'. After converting to different religions, the manual scavengers remain excluded, living as a community outside the confines of the city, performing unclean jobs with their old brooms. So it could be argued that religious conversion among the scavenger community has not really altered their social status. On the contrary, religious conversions have broken their community unity and fragmented them as a group.

In Indian society, it is very complicated to split caste hierarchy as power structures are formulated on caste lines and there are vested interests that benefit from its persistent perpetuation. M.K. Gandhi was a freedom fighter during the British rule in India and is commonly known as 'Bapu Gandhi' and sometimes 'The Father of the Nation'. Dominant castes among Indian society revere Gandhi. However, on the issue of scavengers, while trying to reverse the caste hierarchy Gandhi ended up describing and eulogising 'The Ideal Bhangi' in the *Harijan* on 28 November 1936. His message romanticised the issue of manual scavenging, writing in 1936 that 'a Bhangi (scavenger) does for society what a mother does for her baby. A mother washes her baby of the dirt and ensures his health. Even so the Bhangi protects and safeguards the health of the entire community by maintaining sanitation for it' (Gandhi, 1936). Still, after nearly 70 years of independence the Prime Minister Mr Narender Modi, then the minister of the state of Gujarat, repeated Gandhi's argument and tried to romanticise the issue of manual scavenging. In his book *Karmayog* Modi (2007) wrote: 'Scavenging is a 'Spiritual Experience' (IBNLive, 2013). These two statements from two political leaders of India confirms the prevalence of a casteist mindset in society which perpetuates a romantic notion of the scavenger community. Unfortunately, most of Indian society accepts these ideas, put forward as they are by such esteemed political leaders. With political forces working against scavengers the processes of discrimination and exclusion are further reinforced and policy makers give little attention to the issues among the scavenger community.

While scavenging is considered an indispensable occupation, scavengers are neglected by the government, solid waste management experts, international development agencies and even by many of the non-governmental organisations (NGOs) that operate in India (Medina, 2007). They remain as deprived as ever and face political discrimination at every step. A report by N.R. Malkani, (1994) published by the Planning Commission of India, highlighted the plight and extreme working conditions of scavengers in India. The report observed that 'such atmosphere charged with filth and squalor cannot but have depressive effects not only on the human dignity and personality of these workers but also on their mental make-up and their whole attitude of life. The nature of their work has made them most despised section of the working class'.

The Indian government formed national commissions called the 'National Commission for Safai Karamcharis' and the 'National Safai Karamcharis Finance & Development Corporation'.[7] These two organisations are national-level government bodies meant for the welfare and rehabilitation of scavengers and their dependants. Mostly, executive members of the commissions are recommended by the

[7] The National Safai Karamcharis Finance & Development Corporation is formed to implement the rehabilitation schemes for the scavengers in India. http://nskfdc.nic.in/

ruling political party in the central government. Thus they are under various political and local pressures which can limit their effectiveness. The recommendations made by these commissions are neither taken up nor implemented by the concerned parties; some reports[8] have revealed the dependency and helplessness of these commissions. In short, the commissions have not been able to play the important and powerful role envisaged for them. The national commissions which have been set up to safeguard the rights of the marginalised in our society have failed in performing their responsibilities. More recently in 2014 the government launched Swachh Bharat Abhiyan (Clean India Campaign). In so doing Prime Minister Modi stated that; 'A clean India would be the best tribute India could pay to Mahatma Gandhi on his 150th anniversary of his birth in 2019' (2014). The Government of India has invested significant funds in this campaign and the media regularly carry inspirational pictures of political leaders holding brooms to signify their support. The campaign has attracted significant support from the public with many posting pictures on social media using #MyCleanIndia. The programme itself boasts some significant successes, notably in reducing open defecation through a programme of toilet building in some areas of the country. However, while this appears at first sight to be a positive development concerns have been raised. Firstly, there are many signs that despite a promising start the campaign has failed to meet many of its targets. As Shalini Nair (2015), writing for the *Indian Express*, notes:

> 'Only 20–25% of the target in terms of toilet construction has been achieved while on the garbage management front, the results are even more abysmal. Rankings released earlier show several major cities such as Mumbai, Delhi, Hyderabad, Patna, Lucknow, Jaipur among others fare poorly on the cleanliness scale.'

Secondly it is possible that this increased public awareness of issues around public hygiene might add another burden on sweepers. Representatives from the community have been overlooked as central partners in the development. Yet members of the public are now looking to them to increase their workload to meet the centrally planned targets. Without additional funding and support this would likely increase the stress on the already overworked scavengers and

[8] See the annual reports of 'National Commission for Safai Karamcharis' http://www.ncsk.nic.in/main11.asp

potentially lead to more work-related accidents and health problems. While it is too soon to be able to properly evaluate the impact of this campaign, it will be important to monitor developments.

The hazardous work environment of scavengers is stated to be dangerous for health and to greatly enhance the chance of death. Due to the practice of this unclean work, there is a high prevalence of alcohol consumption and smoking among scavengers as a coping mechanism to avoid the smell. The principal reason for this high level of addiction is the filth and unpleasant nature of work and most of those who use alcohol and tobacco only began to do so after they started working. According to a report by *Tehelka* magazine 'at least 22,327 workers from the scavenger community die every year' (Anand, 2007). This translates to more than 61 scavenger deaths every day. However, the story of discrimination does not end with the death of scavengers. After the death of a scavenger, their family has to fight with the system to get compensation and justice (The Hindi, 2014).

The degree and frequency of discrimination against the scavenging community clearly identifies them as the most discriminated group in Indian society. In this context it is imperative that every aspect related to the scavenger community is understood. Yet there are hardly any studies on the issues of the scavenger community. With these realities in mind, it is essential to explore in more depth the current working conditions of the most excluded group and to know how they are living with this unclean occupation in modern India.

This study of the realities of the scavenger community has been conducted to explore the problem of the work environment, stress and health of scavengers due to scavenging work and presents recommendations to protect the rights of scavengers. This research also explores the connection between caste and occupation in Indian society. There are very few studies related to the health and work environment issues of scavengers in India. This research therefore will be very helpful for researchers, academics and policy makers and will hopefully influence them to work with and think more seriously about the issues of scavenger community.

## Material and methods

The fieldwork for this study took place in Ladwa in November 2013. Ladwa is a town in Kurukshetra district in the Indian state of Haryana situated in the north-western region surrounded by Himachal Pradesh from the north, Uttarakhand from the north-east, Rajasthan from the south, Uttar Pradesh and Delhi from the east and Punjab from the north-west (see Figure 11.1). During the period of data collection, there were 50 sweepers on the payroll of the Ladwa Municipal Committee in November 2013. After random sampling 25 sweepers (20 male and 5 female), which is 50% of total respondent population, were selected for the survey. Data were collected through home visits, workplace visits and by an interviewer-administered questionnaire. The questionnaire was divided into seven parts aimed at collecting different types of information on stress in the work environment, caste-based taunts during work, relationships with supervisors, substance use, unpaid jobs, accessibility of safety equipment, physical injury, anxiety and so on. Some open-ended questions were also asked to explore the perceptions of scavengers themselves of their work, working conditions and the reasons behind the problems of work stress.

**Figure 11.1: The location of Ladwa, Haryana province**

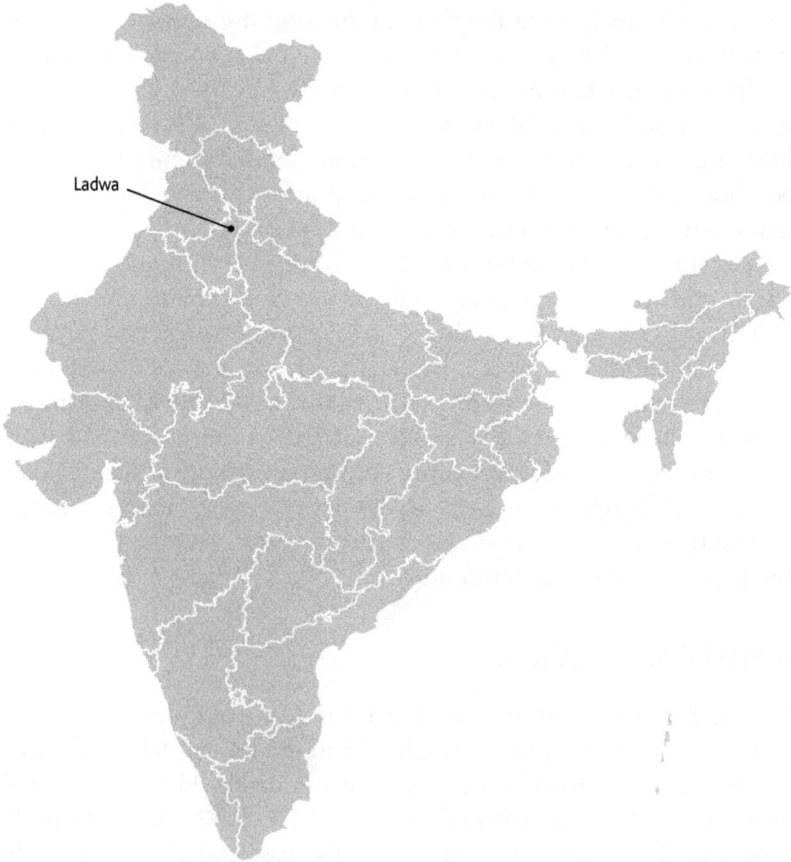

## Health status

The current health and working conditions of scavengers was a major focus of the study. The data show the prevalence of health-related problems among scavengers in Ladwa city of Haryana state, India. Figure 11.2 shows that scavengers face a considerable burden of poor health. The list of problems they suffer from is extensive: headaches, anxiety, chest pains, sleeplessness, back ache, neck ache, stomach disorders and physical injury are common complaints among the participants. These health complaints are symptomatic of the types of problems associated with poor working conditions. According to Baker (1985) the 'working environment plays a very crucial role in making a stressful or a comfortable work environment for the workers. Due to the uncomfortable and harmful workplace or work environment scavengers are facing different types of stresses'. The impact of work and the work environment for the health of Indians has also been highlighted in many of the previous chapters in this book.

Just over half of the respondents experienced persistent headaches and around a quarter report that they suffer from these sometimes. Given the exposure to toxic fumes, working in noisy, dangerous and unsanitary conditions this finding is to be expected. Nonetheless it is extremely worrying as persistent headaches have been associated with a marked negative influence on people's lives, compromising

**Figure 11.2: The prevalence of health problems among scavengers in Ladwa**

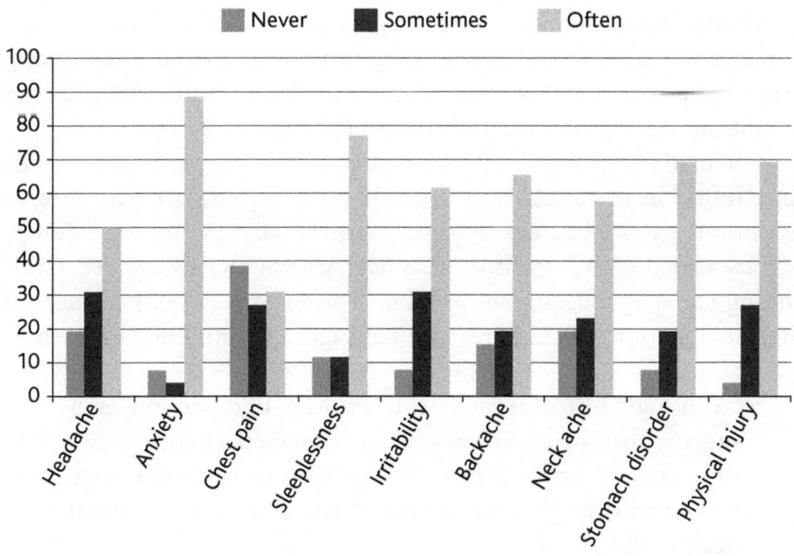

their sense of well-being and their ability to function in different roles (D'Amico et al., 2003). Equally concerning are the extremely high rates of problem sleep in this group. Eight of ten of those asked reported that they experienced sleeplessness. Numerous studies have shown that ensuring good sleep is essential for maintaining good health (Gottlieb et al., 2006; Patel and Hu, 2008; Gallicchio and Kalesan, 2009; Cappuccio et al., 2010). There are also high levels of musculoskeletal complaints among this group. More than 60% of the respondents said that they often suffered from backache, with a further 20% reporting that they sometimes had backache. Roughly similar figures are reported for neck ache. This is in line with findings from studies in the USA and Egypt which have shown higher levels of musculoskeletal problems, notably in the neck, hip and lower back, among municipal waste collectors (An et al, 1999; Englehardt et al., 2003; Abou-ElWafa et al., 2012). This suggests that this group spend long periods of time crouching or in twisted body positions as they pick up refuse and clean the streets which leads to pain and tension in the back and neck.

Gastrointestinal problems are also high and around 80% of respondents said they often suffered from stomach disorders. Again these figures are similar to those found in research with municipal waste or garbage collectors in other countries. In their study of Danish rubbish collectors Sigsgaard and colleagues (1994) found that they were exposed to high levels of dust and microorganisms. Consequently, this group suffered from a range of problems including chest tightness, flu-like symptoms, itching eyes, itching nose, nausea, vomiting and diarrhoea. These findings were supported by another Danish study which not only found high rates of gastrointestinal symptoms among waste collectors but that these were exacerbated by working in hot conditions during the summer (Ivens et al., 1997). This latter finding is particularly relevant for the current study as scavengers often work in extreme heat. Similarly, a Turkish study found that exposure to poisonous gases and microorganisms in the air near garbage dumps was associated with respiratory disorders, gastroenteritis and dermatitis among garbage collectors in Istanbul (Issever et al., 2002). Hence, in their review of the field Perez and colleagues (2006) concluded that:

> 'Although not extensive, the existing body of research suggests that there is an association between the performance of job tasks involving the handling of municipal solid waste and various respiratory, dermatologic and gastrointestinal health effects.'

Finally, an alarmingly high proportion of the respondents (68%) reported that they often had a physical injury during work. Again these figures highlight the extremely hazardous and stressful nature of the work that scavengers do across India. Leigh and colleagues (1999) have shown that there are around 1 billion global occupational injuries worldwide each year, of which India accounts for 17 million non-fatal injuries and 45,000 fatal injuries. More recently epidemiologists have estimated that every year there are 36,700 occupational fatalities observed in India, as well as 1,830,000 cases of occupational injury and 1,850,000 cases of occupation-related diseases (Brecker, 2010).

## Hazardous working conditions and health

As is to be expected given the nature of their work and position in society scavengers face harsh working conditions. They are exposed to extreme temperatures, environmental hazards, toxic substances, discrimination and even physical abuse. Figure 11.3 shows the extremely hazardous and stressful work environment that respondents in this study experienced. More than 95% of survey respondents reported being exposed to noise, dust or fumes, overcrowding, excessive heat in the

**Figure 11.3: Prevalence of work environment complaints among scavengers in Ladwa**

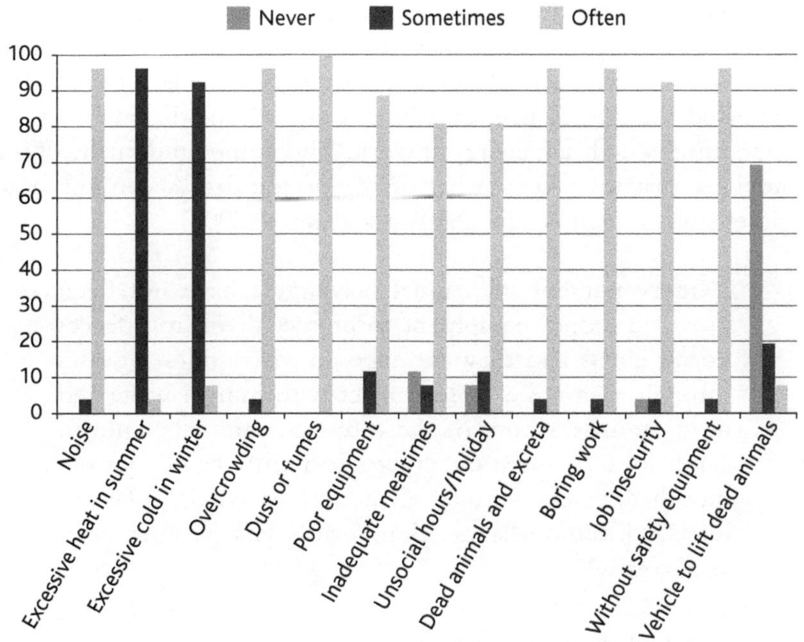

summer and excessive cold in the winter. Sometimes the temperature in summer reaches between 45°C and 47°C. Many scavengers report feeling faint or light-headed during work due to working throughout the day in these intolerable temperatures. In contrast, in the winter they generally work in temperatures as low as 1°C without sufficient warm clothing or protection from the cold. Both of these weather conditions are extremely challenging for scavengers as they have to perform their work in open environments like roads. This fits with the evidence presented by Sahoo in Chapter 6 of this book which showed that casual workers are more prone to respiratory disease, joint pain and so on, showing that this group is at high risk for these types of diseases.

Scavengers have to reach the municipal office to report for work by 6.30 am. Often this means rising very early as many of them have to make their way on foot to the office. To ensure that the scavengers are punctual and regularly turn up for work there are strict provisions and laws. For instance, The Haryana Municipal Act, 1994 under section 303(1) states that: 'if any sweepers will found absent without permission or leave, then he/she will be punished by the imprisonment which may extend to one month or Rs.1000/– or both'.[9] This law shows the domineering attitude of the government towards scavengers. Therefore, they have to reach their place of work at any cost and usually work under pressure. These early starts mean that many of them do not have breakfast. In the present survey 80% of scavengers reported that they regularly start their work without breakfast and have to work on empty stomach. The lack of breakfast increased the risk of malnourishment and means that workers are often hungry and lack energy at work. This compounds many of the problems that they face during their working day. According to an earlier study conducted by Darokar and Beck (2006):

> 'Ninety percent of manual scavengers have not been provided proper equipment to protect them from faeces borne illness and they are exposed to countless diseases through their daily, close contact with human waste and dead animals. Some of these diseases are tuberculosis, campylobacter infection, cryptosporidiosis, hand, foot and mouth diseases, hepatitis a, meningitis (viral), rotavirus infection, salmonella infection, thrush, viral gastroenteritis and worms.'

[9] See the Haryana Municipal Act, 1994.

The lack of proper protection is therefore a serious issue for scavengers. In light of the health hazards that result from the lack of proper health and safety equipment and clothing it is a great concern that all of the respondents in the current study reported that they worked without even basic safety equipment like gloves, masks or boots. Figure 11.4 shows a scavenger cleaning debris from a gutter without any protective clothing. All the respondents regularly work in dusty environments among crowds and traffic without facemasks to filter out pollutants and particles. Sweepers are at most risk of constant exposure to hazardous levels of dust raised during scavenging work (Smilee et al., 2013). People working in this field are at higher risk of countless diseases because they are coming into direct contact with human and animal waste (Kumar, 2014). According to the International Labour Organization (2007) the continued inhalation of dust during

**Figure 11.4: A scavenger cleaning gutters without any protective clothing**

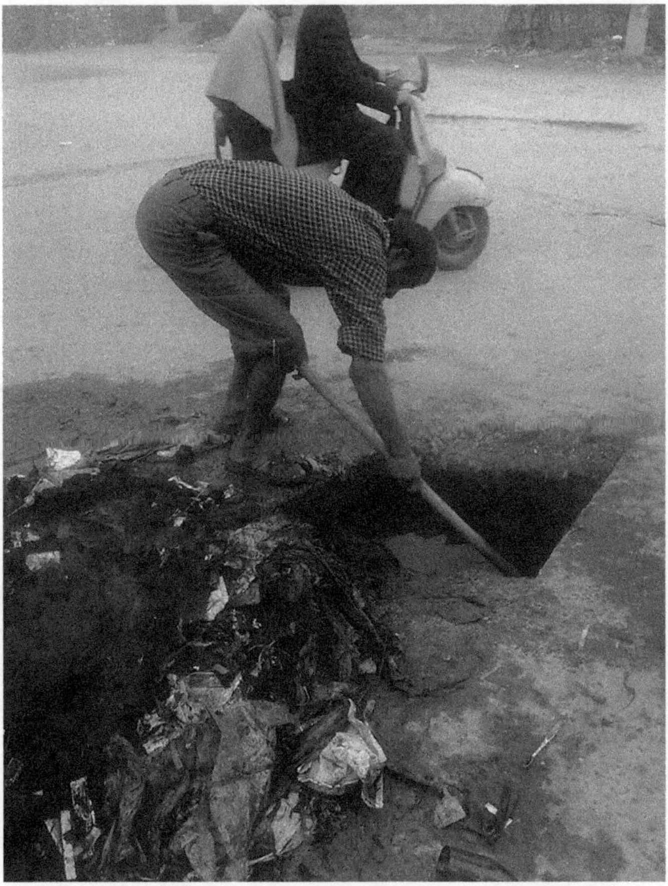

street sweeping can lead to impaired lung function and may cause acute and chronic respiratory health diseases. Therefore, the dusty work environment is a major cause of the poor health conditions of scavengers.

However, dust is not the only problem faced by these workers. More than 60% of respondents do not have hand carts to lift the dead animals that they must clear from the streets and roads. Therefore, they must physically drag or lift the often-rotting corpses of dead animals with their bare hands which exposes them to the risk of numerous infections along with unpleasant odours. As one of the interviewees explains:

> 'People put pressure on us to lift the dead animal when it produces smells and worms and then we have to clean it after drinking alcohol. That day we are not in any condition to eat.' (Niranjan)

It should be noted that being forced to clean human excreta and dead animals is a crime and a punishable offence and was banned by the government of India under the act of 'Prohibition of Employment as Manual Scavengers and Their Rehabilitation Act, 2013'.[10] However, despite this legal protection, the practice of manual scavenging continues. The reason for this paradox becomes apparent when we consider that 84% of respondents said that they felt insecure about their job. This lack of job security meant that they often felt obliged to do such debasing and dangerous work even though they did not want to do so. The finding strongly suggests that scavengers are still forced to carry out these disgusting and dangerous tasks by unscrupulous local government officials or members of the upper castes. Indeed, all of the respondents in the survey reported that they had been forced by the municipality to remove dead animals and clean human excreta using their bare hands. While this work is inhuman and banned under The Employment of Manual Scavengers and Construction of Dry Latrines (Prohibition) Act, 1993, in the 19 years it has been in force there has not been a single conviction. Given the government's record in enforcing the law against manual scavenging, one wonders whether another law would make any difference. On this count the government has set numerous deadlines by which it hoped to eradicate this practice and has never been able to meet them.

[10] See Prohibition of Employment as Manual Scavengers and Their Rehabilitation Act, 2013.

## Impact of scavengers' occupation on their children

There is now a substantial body of work which shows that the experience of adversity in childhood can have long-lasting detrimental effects on development that can be felt across the life course and even into late old age (Holland et al., 2000; Poulton et al., 2002; Graham and Power, 2004). Therefore, the poor living environment and status of the scavenger community in society also affects the lives of their children. Education is one of the major indicators of social and individual progress and key for the development of any country. In recognition of this the Indian government has invested substantial efforts into improving the level of education throughout the country and has instituted compulsory and free education for all children until the age of 14 under the Right to Education Act, 2009.[11] However, the occupation of the scavenger community has a negative impact on the educational status of their children. In the morning scavengers do not have time to prepare their children for school and they cannot supervise their attendance at school. Therefore, the very early timing of work is a major factor in the very high school dropout rates for the children from the scavenger community (Government of India, 2001). Scavenging work is the major cause of educational backwardness of the scavenger community (Mohanty, 2014). The children of the scavenger community have the lowest education status in society and also among scheduled castes. Table 11.1 shows the lowest educational status and high dropout of students after primary school education among the scheduled castes of Haryana.

**Table 11.1: Educational status of scheduled castes of Haryana**

| Category | Literate without educational level | Below primary | Primary | Middle | Metric/ secondary/ higher secondary | Technical/ non-technical diploma and so on | Graduate and above |
|---|---|---|---|---|---|---|---|
| All scheduled castes | 1.8 | 32.1 | 33.6 | 14.9 | 15.2 | 0.6 | 1.9 |
| Chamar | 1.4 | 28.7 | 32.8 | 16.1 | 17.7 | 0.7 | 2.4 |
| Dhanuk | 2.1 | 37.0 | 33.8 | 12.8 | 12.5 | 0.5 | 1.3 |
| Balmiki (Scavengers) | 2.2 | 37.4 | 35.8 | 13.0 | 10.4 | 0.2 | 1.0 |

*Source:* Census of India, 2001

[11] See The Right of Children to Free and Compulsory Education Act, 2009.

## Work, stress and substance use

The link between work-related stress and excessive use of alcohol and other substances has been demonstrated in earlier research (Cooper et al., 1990; Carney et al., 2000; Wiesner, 2005; Frone, 2008; Marchand, 2008). In his seminal study on this link Frone (1999) identified some common work stressors such as dangerous working conditions, noxious physical work environments and unfair treatment of workers and job insecurity. When they reached chronic levels, these led workers to turn to alcohol as part of a set of coping mechanisms. Although most of this research has been undertaken in the USA, which has a different drinking culture to India, it is probable that the high rates of stress faced by scavengers as a result of the demanding and dangerous work that they do would also be a major risk factor for substance use and addiction. Indeed, the results of the current study show that scavengers often rely on alcohol, tobacco chewing and smoking to relieve the stress of their work. However, the results also reveal a very interesting, highly gendered pattern of substance use among this group.

Looking first at tobacco use the analyses show that 65% of male respondents are chain smokers and 20% are habitual tobacco chewers (see Figure 11.5). The health risks of smoking are well documented. However, chewing tobacco, a less common practice in the West, is also associated with a number of serious health conditions (Benowitz et al., 1988). In fact, Boffetta and colleagues (2008) estimate that

**Figure 11.5: Prevalence of alcohol and tobacco use among scavengers in Ladwa**

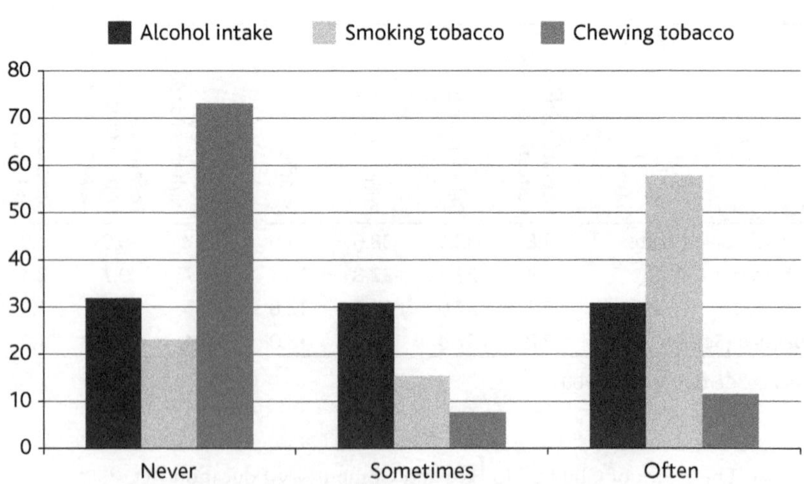

more than half of all oral cancers are attributable to smokeless tobacco products in India. Alongside this 35% of the men in the study reported that they regularly drank alcohol. Conversely, none of the female scavengers reported any levels of substance use. This gender difference raises the question of why we only see these behaviours in men. The results of the observations carried out in the research provide a possible answer. It quickly became evident that the removal of dead animals was exclusively performed by male scavengers. Indeed, if an animal died in the working area of a female scavenger than she normally asked a male scavenger to attend to the task of removing it. The fact that it is only the men who do this unhygienic job – remember gloves and handcarts are not available – and it is only men who drink and smoke clearly points to the role that substance use plays as a coping mechanism in this group. A number of men in the study reported that they usually have to have a drink or smoke to prepare themselves for when they have to remove dead animals or human corpses from public places. Indeed, most scavengers say that they only started to drink and smoke after they started working.

## Discrimination and abuse during work

As the previous sections have shown the workplace and the wider environment are very unpleasant and hazardous for scavengers. On top of this caste-based or racial taunts during work are a common stressor for the workers (von Onciul, 1996). According to data analysis in this study 92% of respondents reported that they have experienced caste-based taunts during work. The scavengers have to perform their job mostly in public places among crowds, such as roads, parks, public toilets, market and fairs. Therefore, they are constantly surrounded by people in public places. This means that there is a high chance that they or their broom might accidentally brush against someone which would result in verbal and sometimes even physical abuse. This is a clear example of the persistent ideas of untouchability and it generates high levels of stress and anxiety among scavengers as they constantly fear being abused or insulted in public as they go about their work.

To ask for water from strangers for human beings is a normal practice all over the world. But in India for a member of a scheduled caste to ask for water from a member of an upper caste is strange and uncomfortable. The sharing of food and water between the upper castes and scheduled caste does happen, but often those in the upper caste refuse to share water and food with scheduled castes (Jodhka, 2002). Scavengers usually perform their work on the streets.

During their working day scavengers also suffer from the stigma of untouchability. For an instance, scavengers often have to work without any water and shelter. Whenever they feel thirsty they are generally obliged to ask members of the public for water as their employers do not provide it for them. However, when they ask for water they often face discrimination and people are reluctant to give them any due to this notion of being untouchable. As one of the female respondents, Sheela, recounts:

> 'One day I was very thirsty when I was working in the summer and I knocked on a door to ask for drinking water, then a woman came out and shouts at me and warned me that "do not touch the door again because we have to purify our door after you touch it, if you want water than just call from outside the house."'

This is one of the normal incidents of untouchability faced by the scavengers. Due to excessive heat many scavengers regularly feel weak and light-headed. Hence it is common for scavengers to be thirsty and not receive sufficient hydration during their working day.

Scavengers are also bound to do unpaid jobs for those in the upper castes and the local authorities. All the respondents reported that they regularly do unpaid jobs apart as well as the work they are required to do by the government. Scavengers are usually called on by those in the upper castes and those in the municipal authorities to do jobs such as renovating houses and shops, working as labourers, doing farm work, removing dead animals, unblocking toilets and cleaning septic tanks. As one of the make respondent Mohinder notes:

> 'we have to do all these unpaid work for the officers of the municipality and for the relatives of the officers. Otherwise, they will put more workload on us and they will discriminate against us as a punishment for not doing these unpaid jobs. We are destined for this work; it is the fate of our caste.'

Mohinder's statement shows the helplessness and feeling of slavery as a scavenger. There are many people like Mohinder who do not want to do these unpaid and demeaning jobs but who feel that they must because of their social position and lack of security and legal protection. Figure 11.6 shows that all of the respondents in Ladwa municipality frequently do unpaid jobs for the political leaders, officers and relatives of the officers. If someone is not available or unfit to do these unpaid jobs, then they must send their children or any family member to perform this unpaid work as a substitute. The data show that more than 40% have had to send their children, wife, husband or family members to do this work in their stead.

One of the 14-year-old boys in the study is used to doing scavenging work as a substitute for his father. During his work he was cutting grass with an electric lawnmower when he lost control of the machine and fell down. As he fell the blades of that machine injured him and he suffered a serious cut to his left hand. However, perhaps the saddest part of this story is that after the accident the scavenger's son was crying and his hand was bleeding but nobody from the staff of the municipality took him to hospital. Eventually they called a cycle rickshaw puller to go with the boy to hospital for the treatment. Until the family members reached the hospital, the boy was alone in the hospital for treatment. This story is repeated up and down the country and shows that although this substitute work is illegal many municipal officers feel they can ignore the laws because these issues are related to the most deprived and weakest section of the society.

Despite the countless services that scavengers perform for society they remain undervalued by government officials and the public. More than 80% of the scavengers in the study report that they never feel appreciated for their work (Figure 11.6). Instead they continually face discrimination, taunts and complaints during work. The public also behaves like an authority over the scavenger community and humiliates them continuously based on caste. Many problems came

**Figure 11.6: Proportion of scavengers who report discrimination and abuse during work**

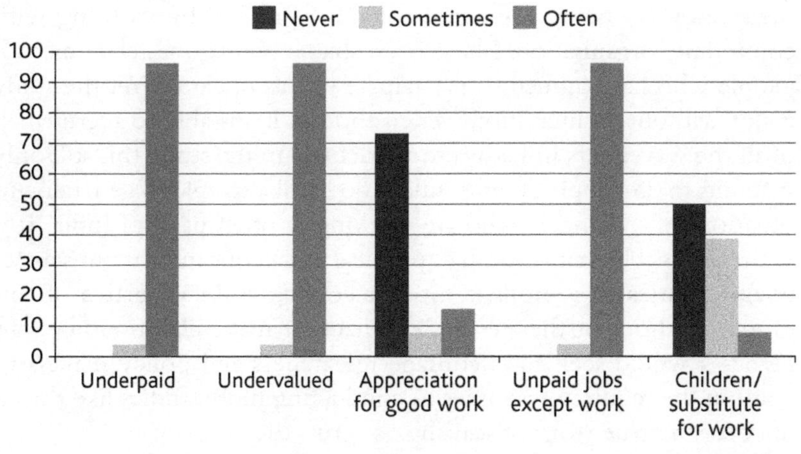

to light during this small study of the scavenger community related to health, work environment, caste and administration. The study also indicates that the state itself plays a crucial role in the rights of the scavenger community and is also partly responsible for their stressful lives.

## Conclusion

India is a developing country and is investing in areas such as the arts, sciences, technology and economy. However, despite strong constitutional provisions and judicial interventions, government agencies have been negligent in engaging with the most excluded and poorest groups in society. Even to this day, successive generations of one particular caste group are being forced, through the legitimacy provided by the caste structure, to perform some of the most distasteful and dangerous occupations, defying the logic of human worth and dignity. Given the evidence uncovered in this study and elsewhere it is hardly surprising that members of the scavenging community are extremely depressed about their situation and want better conditions for themselves and their children. However, most are trapped in this situation because of a lack of alternative livelihoods.

This study was carried out to present the working conditions and health problems of scavengers working in India. This is a hugely important study as, even though there are estimated to be around 1 million people employed in this occupation, very little is known about their working conditions and their health. Furthermore, this is a difficult area to access for research. Given their social situation and experience of contact with government officials members of the scavenger caste can be wary about talking to researchers from outside their caste. By being a member of this caste and by working with community organisations I have been able to build good relations with people who have agreed to participate in this research. Yet the study is not without its limitations. Even though I was able to recruit half of all the scavengers in Ladwa to participate in the study this still only amounts to 25 people. This is much too small a sample to generalise to situations of scavengers who are working in other parts of India. It is entirely possible that the social, political and economic circumstances in other cities or regions is more accepting and supportive of this group. Without further research we cannot make claims either way. Hence I would seek to encourage researchers and policy makers to commit the required resources to conducting more studies like this to uncover the true story of scavengers across the country.

Nonetheless, by combining quantitative and qualitative methods the current study has revealed the horrific working conditions of the scavengers and the intransigent and careless attitude of the government and society at large. With the exception of a few advocacy groups, even solid waste management experts, international development agencies and NGOs in India are non-responsive to the realities of scavengers. The municipality which is responsible for looking into the quality of work and life of its employees was not conscious of the health hazards of the occupation and the continuous violation of the rights of the scavengers. They are publicly humiliated by the municipal officers daily. Proper working tools and safety equipment are not provided for them and, due to the lack of this equipment, they are often forced into manual scavenging, falling prey to occupational hazards like exposure to harmful gases, skin infections and respiratory disorders.

Finally, it is important to note that while some government policies, schemes and reservation facilities[12] are available for the scheduled castes of India, comparatively, the scavenger community does not receive equal benefits of reservation and schemes as the scheduled castes do due to their most excluded status in the caste hierarchy. There is feeling of hopelessness among the scavenger community. This is a crucial issue and immediate attention needs to be paid to the development and rights of this community via special quotas and policies. In this context there is a need to focus seriously on the various aspects of the life of this community especially on their socioeconomic status, caste discrimination, working conditions, health, education of their children, vocational trainings and implementation of law and policies.

## References

Abou-ElWafa, H.S., El-Bestar, S.F., El-Gilany, et al. (2012). Musculoskeletal disorders among municipal solid waste collectors in Mansoura, Egypt: a cross-sectional study. *BMJ Open*, 2(5), p.e001338.

An, H., Englehardt, J., Fleming, L. and Bean, J. (1999). Occupational health and safety amongst municipal solid waste workers in Florida. *Waste Management and Research*, 17(5), 369–377.

[12] The Government of India in recognition to the peripheral status of the marginalised social communities has consistently promulgated various legislations and statutes, which are influenced by two main considerations, first, to overcome the multiple deprivations of the marginalised social groups inherited from exclusion in the past, and to the extent possible bring them at par with the others; second, to provide protection against exclusion and discrimination in the present by encouraging their effective participation in the general economic, social and political processes of the country.

Anand, S. (2007). Dying In The Gutters. *Tehelka magazine*, 4(47).

Baker, D.B. (1985). The study of stress at work. *Annual review of public health*, 6(1), 367–381.

Benowitz, N.L., Porchet, H., Sheiner, L. and Jacob, P. (1988). Nicotine absorption and cardiovascular effects with smokeless tobacco use: comparison with cigarettes and nicotine gum. *Clinical Pharmacology & Therapeutics*, 44(1), 23–28.

Blunt, E.A.H. (1981). *The Caste System of Northern India*. Ann Arbor, MI: University Microfilms International.

Brecker, N. (2010). Occupational health in India. *Occupational Medicine*, 60(7), 577.

Boffetta, P., Hecht, S., Gray, N. et al. (2008). Smokeless tobacco and cancer. *The Lancet Oncology*, 9(7), 667–675.

Cappuccio, F.P., D'Elia, L., Strazzullo, P. and Miller, M.A. (2010). Quantity and Quality of Sleep and Incidence of Type 2 Diabetes A systematic review and meta-analysis. *Diabetes Care*, 33(2), 414–420.

Carney, M.A., Armeli, S., Tennen, H. et al. (2000). Positive and negative daily events, perceived stress, and alcohol use: a diary study. *Journal of Consulting and Clinical Psychology*, 68(5), 788.

Cooper, M.L., Russell, M. and Frone, M.R. (1990). Work stress and alcohol effects: A test of stress-induced drinking. *Journal of Health and Social Behavior*, 260–276.

D'amico, D., Usai, S., Grazzi, L., Rigamonti, A., Solari, A., Leone, M. and Bussone, G. (2003). Quality of life and disability in primary chronic daily headaches. *Neurological Sciences*, 24(2), s97–s100.

Darokar, S. and Beck, H. (2006). *Study on Practice of Manual Scavenging in the State of Gujarat*. Mumbai: Tata Institute of Social Sciences.

Dumont, L. (1980). *Homo hierarchicus: The caste system and its implications*. University of Chicago Press.

Aggarwal, P.C. and Ashraf, M.S. (1976). *Equality through Privilege: A Study of Special Privileges of Scheduled Castes in Haryana*. New Delhi: Shri Ram Centre for Industrial Relations and Human Resources.

Englehardt, J.D., Fleming, L.E. and Bean, J.A. (2003). Analytical predictive Bayesian assessment of occupational injury risk: municipal solid waste collectors. *Risk Analysis*, 23(5), 917–927.

Freed, S.A. (1970). Caste ranking and the exchange of food and water in a north Indian village. *Anthropological Quarterly*, 1–13.

Frone, M.R. (1999). Work stress and alcohol use. *Alcohol Research and Health*, 23.4, 284–291.

Frone, M.R. (2008). Are work stressors related to employee substance use? The importance of temporal context assessments of alcohol and illicit drug use. *Journal of Applied Psychology*, 93(1), 199.

Gallicchio, L. and Kalesan, B. (2009). Sleep duration and mortality: a systematic review and meta-analysis. *Journal of Sleep Research*, 18(2), 148–158.

Gandhi, M.K. (1936). The Ideal Bhangi: Harijan. In *Collected work of Mahatma Gandhi*, LXIV.

Ghurye, G.S. (1961). *Caste, class and occupation*. Bombay: Popular Book Depot.

Gottlieb, D.J., Redline, S., Nieto, F.J. et al. (2006). Association of usual sleep duration with hypertension: the Sleep Heart Health Study. *Sleep*, 29(8), 1009–1014.

Government of India. (2001). *Census 2001*, Data Highlight, table number 2. Educational levels attend by major SC groups in Haryana.

Graham, H. and Power, C. (2004). Childhood disadvantage and health inequalities: a framework for policy based on lifecourse research. *Child Care, Health and Development*, 30(6), 671–678.

Holland, P., Berney, L., Blane, D. (2000). Life course accumulation of disadvantage: childhood health and hazard exposure during adulthood. *Social Science & Medicine*, 50(9), 1285–1295.

Hutton, J.H. (1946). *Caste in India: Its nature, function and origins*. Cambridge: Cambridge University Press.

Ibbetson, D. (1974). *Punjab Castes*. Lahore: Sh. Mubarak Ali.

IBNLive. (2013). *Modi's Book 'Karmayog' Offends Dalits*. 1/6/2013.

International Labour Organization. (2007). *The Baseline Survey of the Occupational Safety and Health Conditions of Solid Waste Primary Collectors and Street Sweepers in Addis Ababa*.

Issever, H., Gul, H., Erelel, M. (2002). Health problems of garbage collectors in Istanbul. *Indoor and Built Environment*, 11(5), 293–301.

Ivens, U.I., Ebbehøj, N., Poulsen, O.M. and Skov, T. (1997). Season, equipment, and job function related to gastrointestinal problems in waste collectors. *Occupational and Environmental Medicine*, 54(12), 861–867.

Jodhka, S.S. (2002). Caste and Untouchability in Rural Punjab. *Economic and Political Weekly*, 37(19), 1813–1823.

Leigh, J., Macaskill, P., Kuosma, E. and Mandryk, J. (1999). Global burden of disease and injury due to occupational factors. *Epidemiology-Baltimore*, 10(5), 626–631.

Kumar, V. (2014). Scavenger Community at the Crossroads: Reflection on State Intervention, Welfare and Abstruse Welfarism. *Indian Journal of Dalit and Tribal Social Work*, 2(1), 1.

Malkani, N.R. (1994). *Report of the committee on Customary Rights to Scavenging*. Delhi: Ministry of Home Affairs.

Marchand, A. (2008). Alcohol use and misuse: What are the contributions of occupation and work organization conditions? *BMC Public Health*, 8(1), 1.

Medina, M. (2007). *The world's scavengers: salvaging for sustainable consumption and production*. Rowman AltaMira.

Modi, N. (2007). *Karmayog*, Government of Gujarat. Unreleased publication.

Mohanty, P. (2014). Non-enrollment and Dropout in Elementary Education: A Study of Scavenger's Children Living in Urban Slums of Lucknow and Kanpur. *European Academic Research*, 1(12), 5664–5677.

Nair, S. (2015). *A year of Swachh Bharat and it's been no clean sweep. Here is why*. http://indianexpress.com/article/explained/one-year-of-swachh-bharat-and-its-been-no-clean-sweep/. Accessed 4/4/2017.

National Commission for Safai Karamcharis. http://www.ncsk.nic.in/main11.asp

Patel, S.R. and Hu, F.B. (2008). Short sleep duration and weight gain: a systematic review. *Obesity*, 16(3), 643–653.

Perez, H.R., Frank, A.L. and Zimmerman, N.J. (2006). Health effects associated with organic dust exposure during the handling of municipal solid waste. *Indoor and Built Environment*, 15(3), 207–212.

Poulton, R., Caspi, A., Milne, B.J. (2002). Association between children's experience of socioeconomic disadvantage and adult health: a life-course study. *The Lancet*, 360(9346), 1640–1645.

Prime Minister of India. (2014). *Towards a Swachh Bharat*. http://www.pmindia.gov.in/en/government_tr_rec/swachh-bharat-abhiyan-2/. Accessed 6/4/2017.

Sigsgaard, T., Malmros, P., Nersting, L. and Petersen, C. (1994). Respiratory disorders and atopy in Danish refuse workers. *American Journal of Respiratory and Critical Care Medicine*, 149(6), 1407–1412.

Smilee, J.S., Dhanyakumar, G., Vivian S.T. et al. (2013). Acute lung function response to dust in street sweepers. *Journal of Clinical and Diagnostic Research*, 7(10), 2126.

Srinivas, M.N. (1995). *Social change in modern India*. Orient Blackswan.

The New Indian Express (2013). *13 lakh Dalits still engaged in manual scavenging*.

Von Onciul, J. (1996). ABC of work related disorders. Stress at work. *BMJ*, 313(7059), 745.

Wiesner, M., Windle, M. and Freeman, A. (2005). Work stress, substance use, and depression among young adult workers: an examination of main and moderator effect model. *Journal of Occupational Health Psychology*, 10(2), 83.

TWELVE

# Lessons and future research directions from work environment research in India

*Martin Hyde, Holendro Singh Chungkham and Laishram Ladusingh*

## Introduction

The chapters in this book represent state-of-the-art research on work and health in India. They cover a wide range of topics across a variety of different socioeconomic groups and locations. Yet the task of providing an overview of the issues raised is challenging. Indeed, the overriding impression one gets from the evidence presented throughout the book is that India is a country of contradictions. This is perhaps hardly surprising given its sheer diversity. India is a country of some 1.2 billion people covering an area of 3.3 million km$^2$. In comparison the European Union is home to 508 million people over 4.3 million km$^2$ and few people would treat this as a culturally, politically or even economically homogenous entity. Indeed, the degree of regional diversity is probably greater in India than most other comparable regions of the world. As Dreze and Sen (2014) wryly observe India is part California and part sub-Saharan Africa. It has some of the most dynamic, fastest-growing, modernising cities in the world. Visitors to Mumbai, Delhi or Kolkata will be struck by the sheer scale of the cities, the pace of economic activity and the number of easily recognisable global corporate logos dotted around the city. Yet these economic successes coexist alongside extreme poverty. As Dreze and Sen argue (2014, 47):

> 'Contrary to the increasingly used rhetoric which suggests that India is well on its way to becoming an economic 'superpower', this is far from the real picture, even in terms of per capita income. In fact, despite rapid economic

> expansion in recent years, India remains one of the poorest countries in the world.'

Evidence of this persistent poverty can be seen not only in the mega-slums that have grown up around these global cities but in the countryside too where famines and droughts continue to plague the lives of millions. Recently severe water shortages have taken a terrible toll on the lives and livelihoods of many famers in the country (Akhef and Joshi, 2015).

This level of diversity is reflected in the findings presented in the book. On the one hand there are some very clear indicators of modernisation and rapid development in the country, as noted in several chapters. If one looks at GDP, India has experienced relatively high and sustained economic growth over the past few decades. As is shown in Chapter 4, this has in turn been accompanied by dramatic changes in the sectoral composition of the workforce as India moves away from being a predominantly agricultural economy. The statistics show the rapid rate of industrialisation and the tremendous growth of the service sector, both in terms of employment and economic outputs. Drawing on a wealth of historical data A.V. Jose shows that India is undergoing the same sort of economic transformation that Western economies, such as the UK and Sweden, experienced in the previous century. The speed and extent of these changes have also caught the public imagination through news stories of the growth of Indian manufacturing giants such as Tata Motors and media images of Indian call centre workers providing IT support for western multinational corporations. As more and more workers are pulled into the growing manufacturing and service sectors it is likely that they are now subject to the same sorts of workplace stressors as their European and American counterparts. There has also been a rapid expansion of the middle classes in India (Murphy, 2011). This is expected to grow from 5% of the population to 40% over the next few years (Ablett et al., 2007). These workers face many of the same 'post-industrial' issues, such as flexiwork, ICT use and organisational change, as workers in the West. Alongside these economic changes we have also witnessed a no-less-dramatic change in the patterns of morbidity and mortality in India. As Chapters 6 and 7 show, India is passing through a period of epidemiological transition as the main causes of poor health and death shift from communicable diseases such as tuberculosis to non-communicable diseases such as cardiovascular disease. As with the economic changes, these epidemiological changes are reminiscent of those that characterised the development of the western industrial economies throughout the 19th and 20th centuries (Omran, 1971). It is these twin trends that prompted us to write this book. As Magnusson-Hansson et al. observe in Chapter 2 there is now a well-established body of research that links stressful psychosocial working conditions to an increased risk of many chronic diseases, most notably cardiovascular disease. Hence we were interested to see whether these economic developments were leading to the creation of the same sorts of psychosocial working conditions that employees experience in the advanced industrialised economies and, if so, whether these could be linked to the rise in non-communicable diseases.

## Work and health in India

As has been noted in several chapters we are not alone in this endeavour. There is a growing body of research on the effects that industrialisation and globalisation are having on the health and well-being of workers in India (Agnihotram, 2005). However, the vast majority of this work focuses on the impact of the physical work environment, such as exposure to dust (Chaudhury et al., 2010; Ahmad, 2017), extreme heat (Sett and Sahu, 2014) and heavy lifting (Yasobant and Rajkumar, 2014). As was noted in Chapter 3, to date there is relatively little work that has explicitly looked at the role that the psychosocial work environment might have on health in India. Yet, the existing studies find similar relationships between poor psychosocial working conditions and a range of health and health behaviour outcomes among Indian workers (Mohan et al., 2008; Peters et al., 2010; Basnet et al., 2010; Rameshbabu et al., 2013; Roy and Chowdhury, 2013). Indeed, when we look at the findings from the relevant chapters in this book we are also confronted with all-too-familiar work environment issues. In their study of stressors among Inspectors and Sub-Inspectors in the Delhi police Kumar and Kamalanabhan (Chapter 8) found that work overload, lack of perceived fairness, family to work conflict, work-family conflict and inflexible work schedules were significant predictors of psychological stress. Not only are these findings in line with previous research on police stress, both in India and in other countries, but they resonate with the broader literature on the impact of stressful working conditions on health and well-being (see Chapter 2). Their findings on the negative impact of a poor work-life balance provide a clear empirical example of the wider issues raised by Ganesh and Ganesh in Chapter 10. The study showed that the 24×7 nature of policing means that many officers are forced to work early mornings, late evenings and sometimes also through the night to monitor their respective jurisdictions. However, as Ganesh and Ganesh show, this is not unusual and many workers in India have a poor balance between the demands of work and family life. Drawing on international data they show that over three-quarters of Indian workers feel that they are expected to be contactable outside of office hours. This compares unfavourably to a 'global' average of around 47% of workers. Indeed, throughout their chapter they paint a rather bleak picture of the current state of work-life balance in the country and have a fairly pessimistic prognosis for its future improvement. Yet, although the specific manifestations of these issues are played out somewhat differently in the Indian context, for the most part the drivers of these changes are the same in India as are they are throughout the West. These are the increased economic necessity of dual-earner families, increased pressure to work longer, increased time spent commuting to and from work, lack of good childcare or older people care support and more. In a very extreme case we can see the impact this can have on children when we look at the findings from Kumar's work with the scavenger community in Ladwa (Chapter 11). In his study Kumar shows how the long, unsociable working hours and always being 'on call' for any odd jobs for local government officials means that scavengers have little time to spend with their children. This in turn impacts on the lives of their children through lower school attendance and lower educational achievement, creating a viscous circle of intergenerational and life course disadvantage. The study also details the intolerable working conditions that scavengers must endure and the detrimental impact that these have on their well-being. Here again, although the specific conditions are far removed from anything that workers in the West might encounter, we still see evidence of universal associations between stressful work, poor health and health behaviours. Similar evidence comes from the study of tea pickers by Roy and Chowdhury (Chapter 9). The story of strained financial circumstances, lack of proper provision of necessary facilities and resources leading to poor health and poor diet is one that many workers from around the world could easily identify with.

However, alongside these more familiar, universal findings it is important not to lose sight of the specific national and local contexts in which these studies were conducted. As Dreze and Sen (2014: 65) point out there are still very stark differences between India and not just the Western economies but even other developing countries. For example, literacy rates are still relatively low in India compared with other countries with a fifth of all Indian men in the age group of 15–24 years, and one quarter of all women in the same age group, reportedly unable to read and write. India also has a very poor international record in terms of rates of child immunisation and the extent of undernourishment among children. While many other developing economies, such as China and Brazil, have managed to eradicate malnourishment more than 40% of all children below the age of five in India are underweight. To some extent, these issues reflects the fact that India is still much poorer than other developing countries. Thus, despite the aforementioned rate of economic growth, GDP per capita in India is less than half of that in China, one third of Brazil, and a quarter of that in Russia. The impact of these wider socioeconomic differences were evident in some of the findings from the chapters which differed markedly from what we would expect to find in studies from Europe or North America. The vast body of work on socioeconomic inequalities in health in the West shows that there is a social gradient in health with those in the poorest positions suffering the worst health (Marmot and Wilkinson, 2005; Mackenbach et al., 2008). Yet the findings from Chapters 6 and 7 on the relationships between activity status and occupational social class and chronic diseases appear to contradict this. In contrast to findings from studies in Europe and North America, Sahoo's analysis of the risk of reporting a chronic condition or being hospitalised show that it is those who are in the most advantageous socioeconomic positions, notably employers, who suffer the greatest burden of ill health. Similarly, Mohanty and Kastor in Chapter 7 of this book show that the rates of non-communicable diseases are higher among those in the higher socioeconomic classes. These findings are in contrast to findings from developed countries but in line with other studies in India. Although the authors of both chapters point to some possible methodological reasons for these findings (which are discussed in greater detail below) they also reflect the fact that India is at a different stage of economic development than countries in the West. In epidemiological terms India could be seen to be transitioning between Omran's (1971) 3rd and 4th phases and as such is facing a double-burden of disease as both communicable and non-communicable diseases co-exist. However, very much like Europe in the late 19th and early 20th centuries, many non-communicable diseases such as cardiovascular disease have become the 'diseases of affluence'. Hence these findings suggest that access to more privileged socioeconomic positions has allowed certain groups in India to escape the scourge of communicable diseases, such as tuberculosis, but in so doing they have become exposed to the risk factors for chronic diseases.

## Unequal India

However, although the chapters in this book make a valuable contribution to the growing evidence base for the relationship between work and health in India it is clear that they go beyond this and raise a number of broader issues about wider inequalities in India, notably those of gender, class, caste and the intersections between them.

As Dreze and Sen (2014, 224) note gender inequality is exceptionally high in India, particularly in large parts of the northern and western regions. This is supported by more recent research by the McKinsey Global Institute who found the states of Bihar, Uttar Pradesh, Assam, Madhya Pradesh and Jharkhand had levels of gender inequality that were similar to impoverished Chad and war-torn Yemen. This has tremendous ramifications not only for women themselves, but also men and children who would benefit from a more active, informed and equal participation of women in social and public life. As the report's authors go on to note in India women contribute a mere 17% of India's GDP through paid work which is very low compared with China where women account for 41% of GDP, or even sub-Saharan Africa where it is 39% (Woetzel et al., 2015). These findings correspond strongly to those presented in Chapter 5 by Ladusingh which show that women in India are largely excluded from the formal labour market. The results of India's only Time Use Survey to date clearly show that traditional gender roles prevail with women spending more time per week than men doing unpaid household work. Moreover, this holds even when women are engaged in paid market work which leads to a double-burden of doing both paid work and unpaid household work. This in turn connects with the issues raised by Ganesh and Ganesh in Chapter 10, that it is most often women who suffer from having a poor work-life balance as they continue to bear the responsibility of caring for the family as well as going out to work in the 'New India'. However, there does appear to be some evidence of change and positive developments.

Social class is another key dimension of social inequalities that runs through many of the chapters. This fits with wider concerns about the growing levels of economic inequality in the country. As Dreze and Sen (2014) observe the social reach of economic progress in India has been remarkably limited. Income inequalities have grown over the past few years due to the relatively stagnant real wages among the working classes and unskilled or causal labour in particular. As noted earlier, however, the evidence presented in this book and elsewhere shows that socioeconomic patterning of chronic diseases in India follows a somewhat different pattern. As Sahoo shows the principle distinction appears to be between those who are in the formal labour market and those who are out of the formal labour market. Still even among those who are working for pay there are notable socioeconomic differences between the different groups. This accords with the findings in Montany and Kastor's chapter (Chapter 7), which show that the prevalence of chronic diseases is significantly higher among professional/technical workers followed by managerial/administrative and clerical workers. As they note this is in line with other research and is not surprising in the Indian context as working in the private sector, in which there are a large proportion of managerial and administrative jobs, often involves working long hours in stressful conditions.

While the relationship between social class and chronic illness might be different in India to Europe, class itself is a familiar concept. However, Kumar's study in Chapter 11 on the plight of scavengers draws attention to the role that caste continues to play in India. This is an alien concept in the West. Yet, as Dreze and Sen (2014, 219) note, India seems to be quite unique in terms of the centrality of caste hierarchies and their continuing hold in modern society. They go on to note that in previous times Dalits were not allowed to wear sandals, ride bicycles, enter temples, or sit on a chair in the presence of higher castes. However, despite legislation that outlaws caste-based discrimination, the respondents in Kumar's study reported that these and similar forms of discrimination persist today. His study offers an almost unique insight into the terrible social and occupational conditions experienced by this most marginalised group. His findings reveal the horrific working conditions of the scavengers and the intransigent and careless attitude of the government and society at large. Proper working tools and safety equipment are not provided for them and accordingly they are often forced into manual scavenging, falling prey to occupational hazards like exposure to harmful gases, skin infections and respiratory disorders. Depressing as this is it becomes even more so when one understands the structural constraints that this system places on members of this group which mean that, through the legitimacy provided by the caste structure, successive generations are often forced to follow their parents into this most distasteful and dangerous of occupations. As Dreze and Sen (2014) note class and caste intersect making it more difficult for the economically underprivileged to organise and bargain for a better deal. They go on to cite B.R. Ambedkar, the famous social reformer who fought for rights for Dalits, that 'the Caste System is not merely a division of labour. It is a division of labourers.'

## Methodological challenges and recommendations

Throughout the book methodological challenges are, explicitly and implicitly, raised. Some of these are specific to the Indian context while others are shared by all research on the relationship between work and health. In his review of the state of occupational health research in India, Agnihotram (2005) identified a number of key research issues that required attention. He noted that most of the studies that have been conducted are very small-scale, community-based studies often with sample sizes between 200–300 subjects. Moreover, the variety of different study designs, control groups, interview procedures, self-reporting biases and statistical techniques used in these studies make the interpretations very complex making it difficult, if not impossible, to generalise the findings to the wider population. In many respects several of the studies that have been included in this book are subject to these limitations. They are based on small samples with particular groups, such as police inspectors, tea pickers and scavengers, in particular areas. The authors of those chapters recognise these limitations and acknowledge that larger sample sizes and the use of more standardised or even objective measures, notably for health, should be used to generalise their findings beyond these particular locations. To redress these limitations Agnihotram (2005) recommends some possible solutions. Firstly, he suggests that researchers explore the possibilities of using administrative sources which hold information about occupation, such as ration cards, driving license and death certificates, to examine occupational patterns of disease and illness. As these are already routinely collected data this is a potentially ingenious and low-cost solution to this issue and reflects what is already being done in European countries, mainly the Nordic countries, where linked register data on health and occupation are available. However, in the Indian context this approach is likely to be severely limited by gaps in the coverage of certain groups in the population. For example, if only those from the more economically well-off sections of Indian society hold a driver's license then these data would be useless for looking at the health of those in the lower social classes. Another alternative he proposed would be to conduct geographical (ecological) correlation studies to generate hypotheses about occupational risks in various parts of India. Again this possible solution has the advantage of being relatively easy to perform as data are collected at the state level on the main forms of industry as are key vital statistics for the area. These can be accessed via the Indian Statistical Office. This approach is similar to that taken by a number of health geographers in the UK and Europe who have looked at the impact of area level disadvantage and health (see Dorling and Thomas, 2016). However, many of the states in India have populations that are larger than many European countries. For example, Uttar Pradesh, the largest state in the country, has a population of just under 200 million people. This is almost as large as the combined populations of the UK, France and Germany. Hence the danger of committing an ecological fallacy, where inferences about the nature of individuals are deduced from inferences about the state in which they live, would be very high with such a study design. Ultimately then he argues that large-scale nationally representative studies using standardised measures would be required to generate reliable and representative data on occupational health in India. However, this requires the political will and resources to fund large-scale studies on work environment issues which at present do not seem to be forthcoming.

Moreover, as both Chapters 6 and 7 in this book show, even when large-scale surveys are used they do not completely resolve these problems. As Sahoo notes there may be serious flaws in the healthcare surveys, which are primarily dependent on self-reported illnesses by the respondents. There are many reasons why a respondent may not report ill health. Some respondents might be reluctant to admit that they are suffering from an illness for personal or cultural reasons, respondents might lack the information to be able to report that they have an illness or, alternatively, the survey might not ask about the illness that the respondent has. This fits with the findings from Chapter 7 that there is a lower incidence of non-communicable diseases among farming and related workers. This could be because many of the diseases go undiagnosed among these groups. This is supported by recent studies that have shown that poorer and less well-educated groups are more likely to remain undiagnosed for chronic diseases (Aroikasamy et al. 2012). These arguments warrant an immediate attention of the survey designers to adopt more appropriate methodologies to address these issues. Finally, future surveys should also aim to collect prospective longitudinal data to be able to properly track intra-individual changes and therefore be better placed to look at how the relationships between work and health develop over time.

Ultimately the data derived from these studies would help researchers and occupational health professionals to design intervention studies to reduce or eliminate the impact of work-related stress on health. In our review of the current literature we only discovered one intervention study in India designed to reduce work-related stress. This study looked at the potential for a yoga-based intervention to reduce job anxiety and perceived stress among 96 IT workers in Bengaluru. Importantly the study found that after an 8-week course participants reported a significant reduction in their levels of anxiety and stress (Srinivas et al., 2015). Although this was a small-scale study in only one location the results are promising and suggest that it is possible to design effective interventions to combat the negative effects of work-related stress on health.

## Policy challenges and recommendations

Alongside these methodological issues some challenges and recommendations for policy makers are raised by the foregoing chapters. First and foremost is that the government should take measures to ensure that improving health for all is central to plans for economic growth. The data presented throughout the book show that in contrast to India's economic development many Indians still suffer from poor health and poor health behaviours. However, according to a 2012 survey of 260 stakeholders of the World Bank in India, health was considered to be a very low priority when asked about economic growth (World Bank, 2012). This is creating a gap between economic growth and healthcare provision in the country. To redress this the government and other key stakeholders, such as companies, trade unions and non-governmental organisations, should prioritise the following: 1) invest in healthcare, 2) create healthy working environments and 3) reduce inequalities.

In 2011 *The Lancet* ran a special issue which focused on the state of healthcare in India. In the opening article for the issue Hortona and Dasa (2011) summed up what they saw as the cause and consequence of underfunding of public healthcare in the country:

> 'India suffers deep inequities, mainly because of insufficient government funding for health… Put simply, too many politicians in India do not take the health of those they claim to represent seriously enough.'

The lack of reinvestment of the public revenues generated from India's tremendous economic growth can be seen in the low levels of spending on healthcare. Government spending on healthcare in India represents 1.2% of GDP which compares poorly with China which spends 2.7% of GDP on healthcare (Dreze and Sen, 2014). This lack of public spending means that India has one of the most fragmented and commercialised healthcare systems in the world. This in turn has an impact on the ability of ordinary Indians to access suitable healthcare. Because public spending on health has remained low, private out-of-pocket expenditures on health are among the highest in the world (Dreze and Sen, 2014; Patel et al., 2011). Thus, as Montany and Kastor note in Chapter 7 instead of helping people get better and enabling them to return to work healthcare become an important cause of household impoverishment and debt in India. Hortona and Dasa (2011) concluded their article with a 'call to action for universal healthcare in India' which would require increased public spending on health, the creation of an Indian national health service, better health information, stronger regulation of the private sector, and the improvement of preventive and curative health services. However, in a follow-up issue in 2015 the journal found that despite a 2014 agenda developed by the government to improve healthcare investment, there was still a substantial 'unmet need for public-provided health care and the unmet need for any type of biomedical health care' which was perpetuating social inequalities in health in India (The Lancet, 2015). As Gupta and Muraleedharan (2014) observe the objective of universal health coverage, set out in India's 12th Five Year Plan, will be difficult to realise because of a lack of adequate health infrastructure and a shortage of trained medical professionals.

However, although it is crucial to ensure that once people become ill they have access to proper and affordable healthcare it is equally important to work towards eliminating those conditions that create poor health in the first place. If all are to benefit equally in this 'New India' then development needs to be thought of in broader terms and not simply measured by GDP growth. As Dreze and Sen (2014: x) argue 'development is best seen in terms of an expansion of people's basic freedoms, or human capabilities. In this perspective, we have to recognise the importance of the two-way relationship between economic growth and the expansion of human capability'. For us this means that the Indian government and businesses should not just be looking at the creation of jobs but should strive to ensure that economic growth creates quality jobs with a good working environment. The balance between health and economic growth should not be seen as a zero-sum relationship, such that investment in healthy jobs will act as a break on economic growth, but as a virtuous circle. There is a wealth of evidence that shows that a healthy workforce is a more productive workforce (Karasek and Theorell, 1992). One key area in which this can be achieved is in ensuring a good work-life balance for all employees. As Kumar and Kamalanabhan's study of Delhi police inspectors shows a poor work-life balance leads to stress which in turn can lead to a range of deleterious outcomes both for the officer and the public alike. To counter this, in Chapter 10 Ganesh and Ganesh offer a range of practical policies that organisations can offer to support their employees. These include providing recreational activities for staff, supporting staff to take parental leave, providing childcare and older people care facilities for staff and organising company outings for staff and family members. However, the government has a role to play here too by ensuring that companies fulfil their obligations under the current laws to provide statutory parental leave and not to infringe on the working time legislation. As Ganesh and Ganesh note many companies do not abide by these laws thus forcing staff to work longer or to come back to work too soon after giving birth.

Kumar and Kamalanabhan present other practical recommendations for the police to tackle stress in the workforce. They suggest that the police administration introduce a shift system and develop incentives to expand manpower. Training supervisors may help to tackle perceived unfairness awareness. Monitoring the political interference by senior government officials in the police department and where high police officials discourage political involvement may help reduce the impact of such intrusion on personnel. Finally, they propose training police personnel to develop their emotional intelligence to be able to deal with stress. This fits closely with the recommendation by Roy and Chowdury, referring to the poor health of tea pickers, that employers should provide heath and diet information courses and resources to educate the employees about the negative impacts of poor health behaviours.

However, as Agnihotram (2005) argues, although these individual-focused programmes are useful they need to be supported by better occupational health and safety legislation with adequate enforcement machinery and the creation of centres of excellence in occupational medicine throughout the country. He notes that Indian doctors and nurses are very poorly trained to deal with occupation health-related morbidity and that there are too few medical schools that offer this sort of specialised training. He also laments the small number of factory inspectors in India, a mere 300, who are responsible for checking industrial safety in companies throughout the country. He compares this with the 3,000 factory inspectors in a small country like Japan as evidence of the low level of concern in the government for industrial safety and occupational health. To address this, he suggests that the government should engage with key stakeholders such as industrialists, medical professionals and researchers and trade unions to develop suitable policies and practices to ensure healthy and safe workplaces.

Alongside this we would argue that psychosocial working conditions need to be included in occupational health assessments. India has a well-established National Institute of Occupational Health which operates under the aegis of the Department of Health Research within the Ministry of Health and Family Welfare. However, its work is almost exclusively focused on the impact of the physical work environment, such as exposure to dust, or occupational injuries. While these are clearly still important issues that need to be addressed the Institute needs to update its profile of occupational risks to include emerging factors such as work-related stress, burnout and isostrain, to meet the challenges of an increasingly modernised workforce.

Finally, all of this needs to be integrated into a broader political commitment to reduce inequalities between socioeconomic groups to ensure that all can equally benefit from the general improvements in health that are being seen across the country. As previously noted inequalities in India are widening across a range of socioeconomic dimensions. These need to be addressed to ensure that marginalised groups are not left behind and trapped in a cycle of poverty and poor health. This appeal comes across most clearly in the work by Kumar on the situation of those working as scavengers. He argues forcefully that there is a need to focus seriously on the various aspects of the life of this community especially on their socioeconomic status, caste discrimination, working conditions, health, education of their children, vocational trainings and implementation of law and policies. However, as Dreze and Sen note (2014: vii) this will be difficult to achieve as there is little public discussion about the state of inequalities in the country. Instead media and political discourses are dominated by the rich and powerful groups while the 'issues that affect the lives, and even survival, of those who have been comprehensively left behind tend to receive remarkably little attention'.

## Future research directions

The chapters in this book represent some of the state-of-the-art research on the relationship between work and health in India. We feel that both individually and collectively they have made some significant contributions to our understanding of these issues. However, as India continues to go through economic and epidemiological changes we should expect to see a rapid growth in the number of studies in this area. As such it is important to identify areas that should be the focus of future research: 1) occupational or industry-specific studies to capture new forms of working; 2) the development of nationally representative prospective cohort studies of the work environment and health; and 3) greater multidisciplinary dialogue.

As was noted in a number of chapters in the book, the Indian economy is becoming more diversified as new industries and forms of working emerge. It is crucial therefore that researchers examine what the working conditions are for these new groups of workers, most notably those engaged in the ICT and IT enabled services sectors which are growing rapidly throughout India. Hence, even though we aimed to get a good breadth of coverage of topics in the book there are also noticeable absences. Despite our best efforts we were unable to find an author to contribute a chapter on working conditions and health for call centre workers in India. Given the prominence of this group of workers in the popular and academic discourses, it deserves serious attention. However, it is not just these hi-tech jobs that need to be studied. Although much of the research on export-processing zones has been on their growth in other Asian countries such as China, Malaysia and Bangladesh there has been a rapid growth of these new forms of industrial agglomerations in India over the past decade or so (Aggarwal, 2004). The relative lack of research on export-processing zones in India is potentially worrisome as research by the International Labour Organization has shown that workers in these zones often lack proper protection under labour laws, have poorer working conditions, have restrictions on forming labour unions or other forms of association and tend to work very long hours, often in violation of national laws on working time (Milberg and Amengual, 2008).

Also we are sensitive to the arguments made by Dreze and Sen (2014) that concerns about psychosocial stress at work may appear to reflect the needs of the more affluent and overlook the real hardships faced by millions of ordinary Indians. We certainly do not want to diminish the hardship experienced by those who toil on the land or in the informal economy. Indeed, we hope that we have shown, through including the studies on tea pickers and scavengers, that we are very much aware of these issues. However, again there was a group of workers that was largely absent from our analyses. With the exception of the chapter by Ladusingh there was little mention of child labourers here. Yet there are an estimated 70–115 million children in the Indian workforce. These are very much concentrated in the agricultural sector which accounts for 80% of child labourers in India. In his review of the state of occupational health Agnihotram (2005) found evidence from a number of studies that child labourers were at an increased risk of acute musculoskeletal pain, serious injury, disease and even death when compared with children of the same age who were not working.

This is a group that requires further research to ensure that they are protected from adverse working conditions.

It is important to continue to build our knowledge about the nature of working conditions for different types of workers through these industry or occupationally specific studies. Yet our ultimate aim has to be the creation of a nationally representative prospective cohort study to be able to properly explore the prevalence of adverse physical and psychosocial working environments and their impact on health. As already noted much of the work in this area is so far limited to small-scale studies. This means that even when we find clear evidence of an effect of working conditions on health we cannot be sure that these findings would be generalisable to other groups in India or even people in the same occupation working in different parts of the country. The lack of a set of harmonised measures of both working conditions and health further compounds this problem. Hence we cannot be sure that we are even comparing like with like across different studies. The cross-sectional nature of the current state of the research in this field also means that we cannot be confident of the direction of causal relationships between working conditions and health. At best we can say that these are associated. However, it is likely that poor health might cause people to have poor working conditions, what is called the 'social selection effect' or 'reverse causation'. The development of a truly nationally representative longitudinal cohort study would solve these problems and give us the high-quality evidence that we need to be able to convince policy makers to act to create healthy working conditions for all. Following on from this it would be good to see the development of more intervention studies to explore what factors could help to reduce the levels of work-related stress and/or the negative consequences of such stress.

Finally, there needs to be greater dialogue between work environment researchers, social scientists, epidemiologists, occupational health and safety planners and developmental economists to ensure that economic growth is accompanied by the growth of sustainable work environments. As has been shown throughout the book issues of work and health cannot be considered in isolation from wider social, political, economic and cultural contexts. To understand the complex interconnections between these factors will require a collective effort among experts from a variety of fields. However, the rewards for doing so will be immense if we are able to improve the working conditions and health for many millions of people.

## References

Ablett, J., Baijal, A., Beinhocker, E. et al. (2007). *The 'bird of gold': The rise of India's consumer market.* Washington: McKinsey Global Institute.

Aggarwal, A. (2004). *Export processing zones in India: analysis of the export performance.* Indian Council for Research on International Economic Relations. Working Paper no 148. http://icrier.org/pdf/wp148.pdf. Accessed 25/03/2016.

Agnihotram, R.V. (2005). An overview of occupational health research in India. *Indian Journal of Occupational and Environmental Medicine*, 9, 10–14.

Ahmad, A. (2017). Socio-economic and health status of sandstone miners: a case study of Sorya village, Karauli, Rajasthan. *International Journal of Research in Medical Sciences*, 3(5), 1159–1164.

Akhef, M. and Joshi, P. (2015). *300 farmer suicides in Marathwada since January.* http://timesofindia.indiatimes.com/india/300-farmer-suicides-in-Marathwada-since-January/articleshow/47240967.cms Accessed: 12/04/2016.

Basnet, P., Gurung, S., Pal, R. et al. (2010). Occupational stress among tunnel workers in Sikkim. *Industrial Psychiatry Journal*, 19(1), 13–19. http://doi.org/10.4103/0972-6748.77626.

Chaudhury, N., Phatak, A., Paliwal, R. and Raichaudhari, C. (2010). Silicosis among agate workers at Shakarpur: An analysis of clinic-based data. *Lung India*, 27(4), 221–224

Dorling, D. and Thomas, B. (2016). *People and Places: A 21st-century atlas of the UK.* Bristol: Policy Press.

Dreze, J. and Sen, A. (2014). *An Uncertain Glory: India and its Contradictions.* London: Penguin.

Gupta, M.D. and Muraleedharan, V. (2014). Universal health coverage. *Economic & Political Weekly*, 49(35), 29–32.

Hortona, R. and Dasa, P. (2011). Indian health: the path from crisis to progress. *The Lancet.* 377 (9761), 181–183.

Karasek, R. and Theorell, T. (1992). *Healthy work: stress, productivity, and the reconstruction of working life.* New York: Basic Books.

Mackenbach, J.P., Stirbu, I., Roskam, A. (2008). Socioeconomic inequalities in health in 22 European Countries. *The New England Journal of Medicine*, 358(23), 2468–2481.

Marmot, M. and Wilkinson, R.G. (2005). *Social Determinants of Health.* 2nd edition. Oxford: Oxford University Press.

Milberg, W. and Amengual, M. (2008). *Economic development and working conditions in export processing zones: A survey of trends.* Geneva: International Labour Organization.

Mohan, G.M., Elangovan, S., Prasad, P.S.S. et al. (2008). Prevalence of job strain among Indian foundry shop floor workers. *Work*, 30, 353–357.

Murphy, J. (2011). Indian call centre workers: vanguard of a global middle class? *Work Employment and Society*, 25(3), 417–433.

Omran, A. (1971). The epidemiologic transition: A theory of the epidemiology of population change. *The Milbank Memorial Fund Quarterly*, 49(4), 509–538.

Patel, V., Kumarc, A.K.S., Paul, V.K. et al. (2011). Universal health care in India: the time is right. *The Lancet*, 377 (9764), 448–449

Peters, D.H., Chakraborty, S., Mahapatra, P. and Steinhardt, L. (2010) Job satisfaction and motivation of health workers in public and private sectors: cross-sectional analysis from two Indian states. *Human Resources for Health*, 8, 27. doi: 10.1186/1478-4491-8-27.

Rameshbabu, A., Reddy, D.M. and Fleming, R. (2013). Correlates of negative physical health in call center shift workers. *Applied Ergonomics*, 44(3), 350–354. doi:10.1016/j.apergo.2012.09.002.

Roy, S.K. and Chowdhury, T.K. (2013). Differences in Selected Health Traits between Occupational Groups among Oraons of Jalpaiguri District, West Bengal. *Journal of Anthropology*. doi:10.1155/2013/582036.

Sett, M., and Sahu, S. (2014). Effects of occupational heat exposure on female brick workers in West Bengal, India. *Global Health Action*, 7, 10.3402/gha.v7.21923. http://doi.org/10.3402/gha.v7.21923

Srinivas, P.S., Kumari, S., Akhilesh, K.B., Nagendra, H.R. (2015) Is job anxiety and perceived stress modifiable in Indian IT professionals? An experimental study using yoga-based intervention. *Journal of Health Research Review*, 2, 81–5.

The Lancet, (2015). Editorial. India—small progress in health care, decline in rural services. *The Lancet*, 386(9996), 830.

Woetzel, J., Madgavkar, A., Gupta, R. et al. (2015). *The power of parity: Advancing women's equality in India.* London: McKinsey Global Institute.

World Bank. (2012). India: The World Bank Country Survey 2012. Report of Findings. http://microdata.worldbank.org/index.php/catalog/1842/data_dictionary. Accessed 3/5/2016

Yasobant, S. and Rajkumar, P. (2014). Work-related musculoskeletal disorders among health care professionals: A cross-sectional assessment of risk factors in a tertiary hospital, India. *Indian Journal of Occupational and Environmental Medicine*, 18(2), 75–81.

# Index

NOTE: page numbers in italic type refer to figures and tables.


## A

absenteeism 109
abuse, of scavengers 229–32
active work 30
activity status see economic activity status; employment status
Aga, A. 196
age
  and cause of death 140, *141*
  and hospitalisation *125*
  and illness 118, *120*, 130
  of labour force 70, 81, 82
  and occupational class 140–1
  and time use 10, 96–100
Aggarwal, P.C. 216
Agnihotram, R.V. 244, 248, 250
agricultural sector 8, 80, 82, 147
  *see also* rural/urban locations
ailments see morbidity/ill health
alcohol use 219, 228, 229
An, X. 88
anaemia 183, 185
animal carcases 226, 229
Argentina 52
Ashraf, M.S. 216
asthma 143, 144, 145, 146
authoritarian leadership 54

## B

Bano, R. 158
Bar-On, R. 159, 169
Bartley, M. 28
Basnet, P. 53
Beck, H. 224
Bhojani, U. 109
birth rates 11, 107, 108
Black Report 136–7
blood pressure 144, 145, 182, 185–6
BMI (body mass index) 182
*see also* weight
Brazil 58
BRIC nations 6–7, 58–60
Bridgman, B. 88
Buker, H. 157
burnout 33
Buse, K. 60

## C

career growth 164
caring activities 91
  age comparisons 99, 100
  employment 87–8
  gender comparisons *94*, 95, 99, *100*
  residence comparisons *94*, 95, 99, *100*
  women's *94*, 95, 96, 99, *100*, 102, 195
caste 213, 214–17, 229–32, 243
  *see also* scavenger community
CATS (cognitive activation theory of stress) 34
causality 251
Chhabra, B. 159
Chhabra, M. 159
Child Development Services scheme 102
childcare 100–1, 102, 195
  *see also* caring activities
children
  in labour force 82, 231, 250–1
  in parents' workplace 194
  of scavenger community 227, 231
  undernourished 185
Chile 52
China 52
Chowdhury, T.K. 16, 53, 177, 240
chronic disease
  and occupational class 133, 142–8
  *see also* communicable diseases; non-communicable diseases
Chungkham, H.S. 25, 237
Clark, C. 88
class see occupational classes; social class
Clean India Campaign 218–19
co-workers 199–200
cognitive activation theory of stress (CATS) 34
Colombia 52
Commission on Social Determinants of Health (CSDH) 6
commissionerate system of policing 156
communicable diseases 241

decrease in 107, 108, 109, 134
and hospitalisation 124, *126*
and mortality *141*
prevalence of 113, *115*, 121–3
communication, of work-life balance policies 204–5
complaints, against police 156
Concha-Barrientos, M. 17–18
construction sector 194
control 29–30
*see also* demand-control model
cooking 100–1
*see also* unpaid household work
Copenhagen Psychosocial Questionnaire (COPSOQ) 35
correlation studies 244–5
Cox, T. 3
creative work 54, 56, 59

## D

Darokar, S. 224
Darshan, M.S. 53
Dasa, P. 246
data analysis 92, 161–4
data classification 180–1
data sources 244
death rates see mortality rates
decision authority 29
decision latitude 29
demand-control model 5, 15, 29–30, 32, 51, 58
demand-control-support model 30, 32, 35, 36
Demand-Control Questionnaire (DCQ) 35
demands, in effort-reward imbalance model 31
demographic change 1–2, 11, 107, 108, 134
developing countries
health inequalities research in 135–6, 138–9
variation between 240–1
work and health in 5–7, 26, 46–8, 51–60
development 247
diabetes 143, 144, 145, 146
diagnosis 111, 147, 245
diet/nutrition 2, 178, 184–5, 224
disabilities 107, 116, 119, 124, 127
discrimination, against scavengers 214–15, 217, 219, 229–32
disease see communicable diseases; morbidity/ill health; non-communicable diseases
distributive justice 32
diversity in India 237–8
Dollard, M.F. 53
domestic work see caring activities; unpaid household work
Dong, X.-Y 88
Dreze, J. 237–8, 242, 243, 249
Duraisingam, V. 53

## E

economic activity status 11–13, 241
and hospitalisation 124–8
measurement of 111–12
prevalence of ailments by 113–20, 129
relationship with health status 13, 110–11, 129
types of disease by 120–3
*see also* employment status; occupational classes
economic globalisation 5–6, 54
economic growth
in India 1, 7, 67, 238
and labour market *see* labour market changes
relationship with health 246, 247
relationship with healthcare 246
economic inequality 237–8
*see also* socioeconomic inequality
economic sectors 8
*see also* employment sectors
economic value of unpaid work 87, 88–9, 100, 102–3
educational level
and gender 83
of labour force 71–3, 81–2, 83
and occupational class 142
of scavengers 227
effort-reward imbalance model 5, 30–1, 35, 36, 51, 52
emotional dissonance 159
emotional intelligence (EI) 158–60, 164, 168–9
emotional labour 159
employee training 206
employees
WLB policies customised for 203
*see also* labour force
employment population ratios 71–3
employment sectors
changing patterns 1, 8, 69, 70, 76, 80–2, 238
future research on 250
and work-life balance 193, 194, 201, 202, 203
*see also* primary production activities; secondary production activities
employment status
of labour force 70, 78–80
*see also* economic activity status; occupational classes

epidemiological transition 11–14, 107–8, 134, 238, 241
equity 32
equity theory 167–8
European social model 71–4
export-processing zones 250
extended families 195, 198

## F

fairness 32, 167–8
family
  extended 195, 198
  role in work-life balance 198–9
  in WLB policies 204
  work-family conflict 168
Ferrant, G. 88
fertility rate 11
fight-or-flight response 50
financial costs of ill health 109–10, 135, 147, 247
flexibility/inflexibility 32–3, 168
Folkman, S. 159
Forbes India 192
Frone, M.R. 228

## G

Gandhi, M.K. 216–17
Ganesh, M.P. 16, 191, 240, 242, 248
Ganesh, S. 16, 191, 240, 242, 248
gastrointestinal problems 222
GDP (gross domestic product) 68, 87, 88
gender comparisons
  alcohol use 229
  informal sector 100–1
  literacy and education 83
  occupational class and NCDs 144
  part-time employment 73–4
  time use 94–9, *100*
  unpaid household work 10–11, 87–8, *94*, *95*, *99*, *100*, 101, 194, 242
  vulnerable employment 47–9
  work-life balance 193, 194–6, 242
gender composition, of labour force 9–10, 70, 76–9, 242
gender inequality 242
generalisability 244, 251
Global Burden of Disease project 45
globalisation 5–6, 54
Goldschmidt-Clermont, L. 88
Gómez Ortiz, V. 52
government policy
  challenges and recommendations 246–7, 248–9
  European social model 74
  relating to scavengers 217–19, 226
  relating to women workers 102–3
  *see also* legislation
gross domestic product (GDP) 68, 87, 88
Gupte, M.D. 14

## H

Harr, R.N. 157
Hawkes, S. 60
headaches 221–2
health
  determinants of 110
  impact of lifestyle on 138, 178–9, 183–7
  impact of police stress on 154–5
  improvements in 1–2
  relationship with activity status *see* economic activity status
  relationship with economic growth 246, 247
  relationship with work 28–9, 35–6
    future research 249–51
    *see also* psychosocial work environment
  socioeconomic differences in 109, 242–3
  of tea garden labourers *see* tea garden labourers
  *see also* morbidity/ill health
health awareness campaigns 187
health behaviours 138
  *see also* lifestyle; tea garden labourers
health data, in tea garden labourers study 179–80
health hazards, for scavengers 223–6
health inequalities research 136–9
health insurance 147
health and safety equipment 224–5
health and safety policies 248
healthcare, and economic growth 246
healthcare costs 109–10, 135, 147, 247
healthcare spending 246–7
heart disease 143, 144–6
hierarchies
  of police personnel 156, 158
  and stress 50
high blood pressure 144, 145, 185
high strain 30
Hindu society 214
Hirway, I. 89
Hortona, R. 246
hospitalisation 124–8
household work see unpaid household work
Hyde, M. 6, 25, 45, 237
hygiene 184
  *see also* scavenger community
hypertension 143, 144, 183, 185–6
hypothalamic-pituitary-adrenal (HPA) axis 50

hypothalamic-pituitary-gonadal (HPG) axis 50

## I

Ilango, P. 158
ill health see morbidity/ill health
ILO (International Labour Organisation) 2–3, 47
income inequality 142, 242
independence at work 54, 57, 60
India Human Development Survey-II 139
inequalities
in India 1, 237–8, 242–3, 249
*see also* economic inequality; gender inequality; health inequalities research; income inequality; socioeconomic inequality
infant mortality 1–2
inflexible work schedules 168
informal sector 58, 78–9, 100–1
information technology sector 193, 201, 250
informational justice 32
injuries 116, 124, 127, 223
injustice-stress theory 167
Inland Revenue 192
insecure work see job insecurity
intellectual work 54, 55, 58, 59
interactional justice 32
International Labour Organisation (ILO) 2–3, 47
interpersonal trust 164
intervention studies 245–6
interviews 34
iso-strain 30, 36
Issever, H. 222
IT sector 193, 201, 250
Ivens, U.I. 222

## J

Job Content Questionnaire (JCQ) 35
job demands-resources (JD-R) model 33–4
job exposure matrices 34
job insecurity 37, 46, 226
job strain 30, 36
Jose, A.V. 9, 67
Juárez-García, A. 52
justice 32, 37

## K

Kamalanabhan, T.J. 15, 153, 239, 247–8
Kar, S.K. 158
Karasek, R. 29
Kastor, A. 133, 241, 243
Korean Working Conditions Surveys 52
Kumar, Vaijayanthee 15, 153, 239, 247–8
Kumar, Vimal 17, 213, 240, 243, 249
Kuznets, S. 69, 88

## L

labour force
age composition 70, 81, 82
children in 82, 231, 250–1
educational composition 71–3, 81–2, 83
employment sectors 1, 8, 69, 70, 76, 80–2, 238
employment status 70, 78–80
gender composition 9–10, 70, 76–9, 242
increase in India 1, 75–6
rural/urban 69–70, 76–83
*see also* economic activity status; police personnel; scavenger community; tea garden labourers; work-life balance
labour market changes 9
developments in India 74–83
historical context 67–70
recent European developments 71–4
labour market protection 74
Ladusingh, L. 9, 87, 242
Lazarus, R.S. 159
leadership styles 54
legislation 195–6, 214–15, 224, 226
Leigh, J. 223
Li, J. 52
life expectancy 1, 11, 12, 47–9, 107, 134
lifestyle
definition and components of 178
impact on health 138, 178–9, 183–7
of scavengers 219
lifestyle data 180
literacy levels 82–3, 240–1
living standards 68, 193
Longitudinal Aging Study in India (LASI) 147
low and middle income countries (LMICs)
health inequalities research in 135–6, 138–9
variation between 240–1
work and health in 5–7, 26, 46–8, 51–60
low strain 30

## M


Maddison, A. 68
Magnusson-Hansson, L.L. 3, 25
Malkani, N.R. 217
malnourishment 184–5, 224
managers 200–1, 206, 207
manual scavenging 213
  *see also* scavenger community
manual work 54, 55, 58, 59
manufacturing sector 8
marital status 203, 204
Marmot, M. 50
Marriot Hotels 203, 204
Maternal and Child Health Program 102
maternity leave 195
Mayer, J.D. 168–9
MDGs (Millennium Development Goals) 6, 45
medical expenses 109–10, 135, 147, 247
medical facilities 185
medical poverty trap 135
men see gender comparisons
mentors 200–1
methodology
  challenges 34–5, 129–30, 147, 148, 186–7, 232, 244–6
  study of morbidity and activity status 111–12
  study of occupational health inequalities 139–40, 147, 148
  study of police and stress 160–1
  study of scavengers 219–20, 232
  study of tea garden labourers 179–80, 186–7
  study of unpaid household work 89–90
middle class 8
middle income countries see low and middle income countries
migration of workforce 69–70, 81–2, 96
Millennium Development Goals (MDGs) 6, 45
Modi, N. 217
Mohan, G.M. 53
Mohanty, S.K. 13, 133, 241, 243
Morash, M. 157
morbidity/ill health
  activity status differences 13, 113–23, 129
  activity status and types of 120–3
  age differences 118, *120*, 130
  causes of 14–15
  changing patterns of 2, 11–14, 107–9, 134, 238, 241
  communicable *see* communicable diseases
  hospitalisation 124–8
  and job insecurity 46
  and lifestyle *see* lifestyle
  measurement of 111, 245
  NCDs *see* non-communicable diseases
  occupational class differences 13–14, 133, 142–8
  and psychosocial work environment 35–7
  regional differences 109, 111, 112–13, *114–16*, 128–9
  of scavengers 219, 221–6
  socioeconomic differences 109, 129–30
  of tea garden labourers 182–6
mortality
  and cause of death 11, *12*, 140, *141*, 238
  and scavengers 219, 223
mortality rates 1–2, 11, 107, 108, 134
motivation 31
multidisciplinarity 251
musculoskeletal problems 222


## N


Nair, S. 218
National Commission for Safai Karamcharis 217–18
National Institute of Occupational Health 249
National Safai Karamcharis Finance and Development Corporation 217–18
National Sample Survey Organization (NSSO) 75, 89, 90, 111
Nayar, V. 201
neuroendocrine pathways 50
non-communicable diseases (NCDs) 134–5, 241
  data on 129–30
  and hospitalisation 124, *126*–7
  and mortality 140, *141*
  and occupational classes 133, 142–8, 241
  prevalence of 113, *115–16*, 121–3
  rise in 107, 108–9, 110, 134
  socioeconomic differences in 109, 129–30, 241
NSSO see National Sample Survey Organization
nutrition 2, 178, 184–5, 224


## O


observed morbidity 111
  *see also* diagnosis
occupational classes
  characteristics of 140–2

and chronic NCDs 13–14, 133, 142–8, 241
health inequalities methodology 139–40, 147, 148
typology 136–7, 139–40
occupational health services 248–9
occupational injuries 223
occupational status 70
*see also* economic activity status; employment status
Omran, A. 134
Oraon population 179
organisational justice 32, 37
organisational policy
recommendations 247–9
on work-life balance 192–3, 201–5, 248
organisational strategy 202–3
organisations, role in work-life balance 201–3, 207
Oriflame 192
overcommitment 31

## P

packed cell volume 183
Pagnossin-Aligisakis, E. 88
part-time employment 73–4
passive work 30
Patel, V. 138
Pati, S. 109
patriarchy 193, 194
perception of stress 159
Perez, H.R. 222
physical activity 178
police force, structure and organisation 155–6
police personnel
emotional intelligence of 158–60, 164, 168–9
hierarchy of 156, 158
and stress 15, 153–4, 239–40, 247–8
data analysis 161–4
impacts of stress 154–5
research methodology 160–1
work stressors 157–8, 160, 162–9
suicide rates 156
policy see government policy; organisational policy
political interference 165–7, 169
population growth 11
poverty 1, 238
PricewaterhouseCoopers 192
primary production activities 91, 94–5, 96
private life
stressors in 33
*see also* work-life balance
procedural justice 32, 37
productivity 68
protective equipment 224–5
psychological demands 29–30, 31
psychosocial work environment
measurement of 34–5
policy on 249
relationship with health 3–5, 15, 25–6, 35–7, 239–40
in developing countries 51–60
early research 26, 49–51
in low and middle income countries 51–3
models of 29–34
*see also* police personnel; scavenger community
psychosocial work environment approach 51

## Q

questionnaires 35

## R

Rajadhyaksha, U. 193
Rameshbabu, A. 53
regional differences 237–8
in hospitalisation 124, *125*, *126*–7
in morbidity 109, 111, 112–13, *114–16*, 128–9
*see also* rural/urban locations
religious conversion 216
residence see rural/urban locations
respiratory problems 225–6
rewards see effort-reward imbalance model
routine work 54, 56, 59
Roy, S.K. 16, 53, 177, 240
rural/urban locations
of labour force 69–70, 76–83
and time use 10, *93*, 94–5, 96–9, *100*

## S

Sahoo, H. 11, 107, 241, 243
Salovey, P. 169
sample size 148, 186, 232, 244
scavenger community 17, 240, 243
caste and occupation of 214–19
discrimination and abuse of 214–15, 217, 219, 229–32
government initiatives 217–19, 226
hazardous working conditions of 223–6
health of 219, 221–6
impact of occupation on children 227
nature of 213–14, 232
research methodology 219–20, 232
romanticising of 217
stress and substance use by 219, 228–9

scheduled castes 215, 227, 229
  *see also* scavenger community
secondary production activities 91, 94–5, 96
self-employed 70, 78
self-perceived morbidity 111
self-reports 34, 111, 129–30, 245
Selokar, D. 158
Selye, H. 2
Sen, A. 237–8, 242, 243, 249
service sector 8, 202, 203
Siegrist, J. 30, 35
Sigsgaard, T. 222
Singh, S. 158
skill discretion 29
skilled workers 73
sleep problems 222
small and medium-sized enterprises 8
SNA (System of National Accounts) 88
social class 8, 242–3
  *see also* economic activity status; occupational classes; socioeconomic status
social exclusion 214–17
  *see also* discrimination
social reciprocity 31
social support 30, 36, 197–202, 205–6
society
  Hindu 214
  impact of police stress on 155
socioeconomic inequality 1, 242–3, 249
socioeconomic status
  differences between developing countries 240–1
  and health differences 109, 136–9
  and morbidity 109, 129–30, 241
  *see also* economic activity status; occupational classes
South Korea 75
Srinivas, P.S. 245–6
Srinivasan, S. 158
standard of living 68, 193
state
  role of 74
  *see also* government policy; legislation
status
  of scavengers 213, 214–19, 232
  and stress 50, 51, 158
  *see also* socioeconomic status
stress
  definitions and nature of 2–3, 26–7
  measurement of 160
  models 29–34
  *see also* work-related stress
stress responses 27, 50–1
stressors 50, 159
  impact on health 27
  in police work 157–8, 160, 162–9
  in private life 33
structured interviews 34
Subburaj, A. 159
subsidiary workers 78–9
substance use 178, 219, 228–9
suicide rates 156
supervisors 200–1, 205–6
support see social support
Suresh, R.S. 158
surveys 245
Sustainable Development Goals 6, 45, 60
Swachh Bharat Abhiyan (Clean India Campaign) 218–19
sweepers 215–16, 218, 225–6
sympathy-adrenal pathway 50
System of National Accounts (SNA) 88

## T

tea garden labourers 16, 177, 181, 240
  facilities for 177, 185
  health practices of 181–2
  health traits of 179–80, 182–3
  lifestyle factors in health of 181–2, 183–7
  researching 179–80, 186–7
teamwork 199–200
Theorell, T. 6, 45
Thomas, J. 80
time use data 92–100
time use surveys 88, 89–90
tobacco use 219, 228–9
Toch, H. 166
toilet construction 218
training, for work-life balance 206

## U

undernutrition 182, 184–5, 224
unemployment 28–9, 71, 72
unfairness 167–8
unionisation 54
United Nations (UN) 6, 45, 60
unpaid household work 10–11
  age comparisons 10, 96–100
  data analysis 92
  defining 90–1
  economic value of 87, 88–9, 100–1, 102–3
  gender comparisons 10–11, 87–8, *94*, 95, 99, *100*, 101, 194, 242
  research methods 89–90
  residence comparisons 10, *93*, *94*, 95, 96–9, *100*
  and work-life balance 194, 198

unpaid work, by scavengers 230–1
untouchability 214–15, 229, 230
urban/rural locations
 of labour force 69–70, 76–83
 and time use 10, *93*, 94–5, 96–9, *100*
urbanisation 69–70, 75

## V

Vellakkal, S. 129–30
vulnerable employment 47–9
 *see also* job insecurity

## W

wage employees 70, 78
water, scavenger access to 230
weather conditions 224
Weicko, F. 157
weight, of tea garden labourers 182, 184–5
Westerlund, H. 25
women
 caring activities by *94*, 95, 96, 99, *100*, 102, 195
 economic contribution of 87, 88, 100, 102–3
 and unpaid household work 10–11, 87–8, 95–6, 99, *100*, 101–2, 194, 242
 in workforce 9–10, 70, 76–9, 193, 194–6, 242
 *see also* gender comparisons
work
 relationship with health 28–9, 35–6, 249–51
 vulnerable and insecure 37, 46–9, 226
 *see also* employment sectors; labour force; unpaid household work
work environment
 relationship with health 6, 15, 239–40, 249–51
  occupational examples *see* police personnel; scavenger community; tea garden labourers
 *see also* psychosocial work environment
work schedules 33, 168
work-family conflict 168
work-life balance (WLB) 16–17, 33, 240, 247–8
 benefits of 192, 202–3
 challenges in India 191–2
 countering negativity 205
 employee training 206
 and gender 193, 194–6, 242
 in Indian context 193–7
 organisation responsibility for 207
 policies 192–3, 201–5, 248
 research on 196–7
 role of social support 197–202, 205–6
work-related stress 2–5, 15, 153
 intervention studies 245–6
 models 29–34
 police personnel 15, 153–4, 239–40, 247–8
  data analysis 161–4
  impacts of stress 154–5
  research methodology 160–1
  stressors 157–8, 160, 162–9
 role of emotional intelligence 158–60, 164, 168–9
 scavengers 17, 215, 218–19, 221, 228–9
workforce see labour force
working hours 33, 37, 47, 68, 74, 168, 169, 196
workload 167
World Health Organization (WHO) 6, 178
World Values Survey 53–4
worm infestation 185

## Y

Yerkes-Dodson law 167